BIOCHEMISTRY RESEARCH TRENDS

SAPONINS

PROPERTIES, APPLICATIONS AND HEALTH BENEFITS

BIOCHEMISTRY RESEARCH TRENDS

Additional books in this series can be found on Nova's website under the Series tab.

Additional e-books in this series can be found on Nova's website under the e-book tab.

BOTANICAL RESEARCH AND PRACTICES

Additional books in this series can be found on Nova's website under the Series tab.

Additional e-books in this series can be found on Nova's website under the e-book tab.

BIOCHEMISTRY RESEARCH TRENDS

SAPONINS

PROPERTIES, APPLICATIONS AND HEALTH BENEFITS

RANI KOH
AND
ISAAC TAY
EDITORS

Nova Science Publishers, Inc.
New York

For permission to use material from this book please contact us:
Telephone 631-231-7269; Fax 631-231-8175
Web Site: http://www.novapublishers.com

Library of Congress Cataloging-in-Publication Data

Saponins : properties, applications, and health benefits / editors, Rani Koh and Isaac Tay.
p. ; cm.
Includes bibliographical references and index.
ISBN 978-1-62100-942-9 (hardcover)
I. Koh, Rani. II. Tay, Isaac.
[DNLM: 1. Saponins--chemistry. 2. Saponins--therapeutic use. QU 75]
572.579--dc23
2011040349

Published by Nova Science Publishers, Inc. † New York

CONTENTS

Preface		**vii**
Chapter 1	Saponins: Structural Diversity, Properties and Applications *Ben A. Chindo, Bulus Adzu and Karniyus S. Gamaniel*	**1**
Chapter 2	Saponins from *Panax* Species: Chemistry, Isolation and Analysis *Jian-Bo Wan, Ying Chen, Ping Li,* *Wei-Hua Huang and Qing-Wen Zhang*	**51**
Chapter 3	Triterpenoid Saponins from Genus *Gypsophila L. (Caryophyllaceae)* *M. Yotova, I. Krasteva and S. Nikolov*	**99**
Chapter 4	Potential of Triterpenoids from Ginseng (*Panax quinquefolius and Panax ginseng* C.A. Meyer) to Regulate Cultured Adipocytes *Chia-Rou Yeo and David G. Popovich*	**123**
Chapter 5	Saponin Use as Antimicrobial in Fibrous and Consumer Products *Vivechana Dixit and S. Kay Obendorf*	**135**
Chapter 6	Evidence of Bioactivity from *Ganoderma Lucidum* Triterpenoids in Cultured Cell Models *Weimei Ruan and David G. Popovich*	**145**
Chapter 7	Recent Developments of Soyasaponins from Soy (*Glycine Max* (L.)) Bioactivity in Cell Models *Wei Zhang and David G. Popovich*	**157**
Chapter 8	Occurrence and Properties of Saponins within the Family Chenopodiaceae *Tiwatt Kuljanabhagavad and Michael Wink*	**163**
Index		**207**

PREFACE

Saponins are a diverse group of glycosidic compounds widely distributed in the plant kingdom, which are characterized by structures containing triterpene or steroidal aglycones and one or more sugar chains. Despite their fairly large structural diversity, saponins share some unique biological properties including the ability to foam and lyse erythrocytes. This book presents current research in the study of the properties, applications and health benefits of saponins. Topics discussed include an analysis on the chemical structures and isolation of saponins from Panax species; triterpenoid saponins from genus Gypsophila L. (Caryophyllaceae); the potential of triterpenoids from ginseng to regulate cultured adipocytes and saponin use as antimicrobial in fibrous and consumer products.

Chapter 1 - Saponins are a diverse group of glycosidic compounds widely distributed in the plant kingdom, which are characterized by structures containing triterpene or steroidal aglycones and one or more sugar chains. Despite their fairly large structural diversity, saponins share some unique biological properties including the ability to foam and lyse erythrocytes. The surface activities responsible for the biological properties of this group of compounds are attributed to their characteristic structural features and amphiphilic nature, which is due to the presence of a hydrophilic sugar moiety and a hydrophobic sapogenin. Structurally, saponins possess the aglycones and glycones. The later, mostly consisting of D-glucose, L-rhamnose, D-galactose, D-glucuronic acid, L-arabinose, D-xylose and D-fructose. The aglycones may have a steroidal or triterpenoid structure; and it is on this basis that saponins are classified. Steroidal sapogenins (27C) can have a 6-ring spirostane or a 5-ring furostane skeleton, while triterpenoid sapogenins (30C) are much more structurally diverse and their basic ring system is most often made up of five or more units, seldom of four units. Pentacyclic triterpenoid saponins belong to oleanane-type; other skeleton types include ursane, lupane, hopane, germanicane, dammarane. The presence of different substituent such hydroxyls, hydroxymethyls, carboxyls and acyl groups; and differences in the composition, linkage and number of sugar chains in the polycyclic sapogenin account for significant structural diversity and various bioactivities of saponins. Saponins exhibit a wide range of pharmacological activities including expectorant, anti-inflammatory, vasoprotective, hypocholesterolemic, immunomodulatory, hypoglycaemic, molluscicidal, antifungal, antiparasitic, anticonvulsant and other central nervous activities. Plants rich in saponins have been used for medicinal purposes and have continued to play significant roles in the food and cosmetic industries as sweeteners and emulsifiers. Saponins have also been used as adjuvant in the production of vaccines. Steroidal sapogenins are economically important raw materials for the pharmaceutical industry in the production of steroidal hormones. This chapter examines saponins, discussing their structural diversity, properties and applications.

Chapter 2 - Saponins are very important natural products that show a wide range of pharmacological activities. Ginseng saponins isolated from *Panax* species have attracted worldwide interests owing to their bioactive effects on the immune system, central nervous system, cardiovascular system, cancer and diabetes. These triterpene saponins have been generally considered to be the main bioactive components in *Panax* plants. In this review, the chemistry, isolation and analysis of saponins from *Panax* plants, mainly *P. ginseng* C.A. Mey., *P. quinquefolius* L., *P. notoginseng* (Burk) F.H. Chen were reviewed.

Chapter 3 - Saponins are widespread in medicinal plants and very often are responsible for their pharmacological effects. The genus *Gypsophila,* family *Caryophyllaceae*, is well known to contain triterpenoid saponins with medicinal, industrial and decorative applications. Some species are broadly used as a drug with extensive medical importance, such as an expectorant and diuretic, and are used in treatments of hepatitis, gastritis and bronchitis. *Gypsophila* saponins have anticarcinogenic properties, including direct cytotoxicity, immunomodulating effects, normalization of carcinogen induced cell proliferation, and a cytoprotective effect over hepatocytes, etc. Various triterpene saponins have been reported in *Gypsophila* species including gypsogenin as the major aglycone and other aglycones as quillaic, echinocystic, hederagenin and oleanolic acids. Recently, sulfated triterpene saponins have been reported to occur in the genus. This review deals with the chemistry, methods of purification, structure elucidation and biological activity of triterpene saponins from genus *Gypsophila*.

Chapter 4 - The active component of ginseng (*Panax quinquefolius* and *Panax ginseng* C.A. Meyer), is believed to be dammarane type triterpenoids also known as ginsenosides. They can be generally classified into two main groups based on the attached sugar moieties on either position C3 or C6 of the ring structure. There are differences in biological activities attributed to these minor differences in chemical structure. The objective of this review is to focus on the burgeoning interest in the effect of ginseng and ginsenosides on the reduction of risk or risk factors associated to the risk in metabolic abnormalities such as insulin resistance and the metabolic syndrome. For example ginsenosides have been reported to interact with adipocytes and influencing lipid acquisition and increase adiponectin release that can modulate and improve overall metabolic risks.

Chapter 5 - Natural antimicrobials recently have been used to replace synthesized compounds in materials and consumer products offering the opportunity to reduce hazardous effects on health and environment. Research results show that saponin, a natural biodegradable and non-toxic biopolysaccharide derived from plants, has potential to be used as a natural antimicrobial compound. Saponin has exhibited high antimicrobial activity against a wide variety of pathogenic and microorganisms, including fungi and bacteria. The antimicrobial action is influenced by intrinsic factors such as the type of saponin, the degree of saponin polymerization and extrinsic factors such as the microbial organism, the environmental conditions and presence of the other components. In this article we described properties, a number of applications and health related benefits of saponin when used as biodegradable antimicrobials in fibrous materials and consumer products. Chemical and biochemical antimicrobial saponins derived from natural sources and activities against a range of microorganisms are also outlined.

Chapter 6 - Triterpenoids are a structurally diverse class of potential bioactive molecules found in a variety of plants. This review will focus on a medicinal mushroom *Ganoderma lucidum* which is also known as either lingzhi or reishi mushroom. This mushroom has a long history of use in traditional Chinese medicine. Triterpenoids either isolated or present in extracts of *Ganoderma lucidum* have multiple reported bioactive effects which include chemoprevention by inducing multiple types of programmed cell death. *Ganoderma lucidum* can also influence other metabolic states such as reducing inflammatory markers and possess anti-diabetic properties among others and these may have an influence on improving metabolic control. *Ganoderma lucidum* is a medicinal mushroom (also known as Ling zhi in Chinese and Reshi in Japanese), is a well-known Chinese traditional medicine that has been used to promote longevity and treat weakness for centuries. Research has centered on *Ganoderma lucidum* recently due to its multiple pharmacological activities, including anti-inflammatory, anti-tumorigenic, anti-herpetic, anti-virus, anti-ulcerogenic, anti-allergic, anti-angiogenic, anti-diabetic, hypoglycimic activity, and osteoclastogenesis-regulated effects. Triterpenoids are one of the major classes of potential bioactive compounds in *Ganoderma lucidum*. Hundreds of triterpenoids from *Ganoderma lucidum* have been isolated and identified and these triterpenoids are exclusively found in genus Ganoderma.

Chapter 7 - Soy bean (*Glycine max* (L.)) contains a class of phytochemicals known as soyasaponins which are oleanane triterpenoids. These molecules are diverse, structurally complex and can be classified into two main categories based on their respective soyasapogenols or aglycones. The two main groups of soyasaponins are group A and group B. In terms of biological activity far more in known about group B soyasaponins compared to group A. At the center of the biological activity of these molecules is cytotoxicity leading to apoptosis induction in cultured cancer cell models and it is this ability that has highlighted soy bean possible chemo-preventative properties. In this review the recent literature will be reviewed focusing on both group A and group B soyasaponins on reducing the cultured cancer cell growth and inducing apoptosis in various cancer cell lines. A probably structure function relationship between soyasaponins and cytotoxicity is emerging with the aglycones of both groups being the most cytotoxic than their related glycosides. Recently, soy bean (*Glycine max* (L.)) extracts are under intensive study because of their potential beneficial health effects. Soyasaponins are oleanane triterpenoids and are one of main biological active components in soy bean. Studies indicate that soyasaponins can alter enzyme activities, lower cholesterol, interact with bile acids, and are chemo-preventative. The biological activity of soyasaponins largely depends on their respective chemical structures as well as their polarity, acidity and hydrophobicity. Soyasaponins are classified in two groups, A and B, based on their respective soyasapogenols or aglycones. Both bidesmosidic soyasaponin group A and monodesmosidic soyasaponin group B have varied biological activities. However, the exact mechanism of action and proof of a structure-function relationship of soyasaponins is still ongoing. In this review the reported biological activities of soyasaponins based on their structures classification and plausible mechanism of action will be reviewed.

Chapter 8 - Saponins are a group of glycosides which is widely distributed in the plant kingdom; however, certain lower marine animals such as sea cucumbers and starfish also contain these compounds. They represent a diverse group of chemical compounds which are characterized by a steroid or triterpenoid nucleus to whichone or more carbohydrate chains are attached. The structural diversity of Saponins is reflected in their physicochemical and biological properties which areexploited in several traditions and industrial applications. The plant extracts containing saponins have been widely used in food and industrial applications mainly as surface active and foaming agents. The saponins in foods have traditionally been considered as antinutritional factors which as in quinoa (*Chenopodium quinoa* Willd.) have limited their use due to their bitter taste.

In: Saponins: Properties, Applications and Health Benefits ISBN: 978-1-62100-942-9
Editors: Rani Koh and Isaac Tay

Chapter 1

SAPONINS: STRUCTURAL DIVERSITY, PROPERTIES AND APPLICATIONS

Ben A. Chindo*[*], *Bulus Adzu and Karniyus S. Gamaniel
Department of Pharmacology and Toxicology,
National Institute for Pharmaceutical Research and Development,
Abuja, Nigeria

ABSTRACT

Saponins are a diverse group of glycosidic compounds widely distributed in the plant kingdom, which are characterized by structures containing triterpene or steroidal aglycones and one or more sugar chains. Despite their fairly large structural diversity, saponins share some unique biological properties including the ability to foam and lyse erythrocytes. The surface activities responsible for the biological properties of this group of compounds are attributed to their characteristic structural features and amphiphilic nature, which is due to the presence of a hydrophilic sugar moiety and a hydrophobic sapogenin. Structurally, saponins possess the aglycones and glycones. The later, mostly consisting of D-glucose, L-rhamnose, D-galactose, D-glucuronic acid, L-arabinose, D-xylose and D-fructose. The aglycones may have a steroidal or triterpenoid structure; and it is on this basis that saponins are classified. Steroidal sapogenins (27C) can have a 6-ring spirostane or a 5-ring furostane skeleton, while triterpenoid sapogenins (30C) are much more structurally diverse and their basic ring system is most often made up of five or more units, seldom of four units. Pentacyclic triterpenoid saponins belong to oleanane-type; other skeleton types include ursane, lupane, hopane, germanicane, dammarane. The presence of different substituent such hydroxyls, hydroxymethyls, carboxyls and acyl groups; and differences in the composition, linkage and number of sugar chains in the polycyclic sapogenin account for significant structural diversity and various bioactivities of saponins. Saponins exhibit a wide range of pharmacological activities including expectorant, anti-inflammatory, vasoprotective, hypocholesterolemic, immunomodulatory, hypoglycaemic, molluscicidal, antifungal, antiparasitic, anticonvulsant and other central nervous activities. Plants rich in saponins have been used for medicinal purposes and have continued to play significant roles in the food and

[*] Corresponding author: Email: bachindo@yahoo.com.

cosmetic industries as sweeteners and emulsifiers. Saponins have also been used as adjuvant in the production of vaccines. Steroidal sapogenins are economically important raw materials for the pharmaceutical industry in the production of steroidal hormones. This chapter examines saponins, discussing their structural diversity, properties and applications.

Keywords: Saponins, glycones, sapogenins, haemolysis, emulsifiers, health benefits

INTRODUCTION

The term 'saponin' defines a group of compounds that consist of an isoprenoidal-derived aglycone, designated genin or sapogenin, covalently linked to one or more sugar moieties. The aglycone may have steroidal or triterpenoid structures according to which saponins are usually classified. The name 'saponin' is deduced from the Latin word 'sapo' (meaning soap) reflecting their wide spread ability to form stable soap-like foams in aqueous solutions. Saponins are naturally occurring surface-active secondary metabolites of glycosidic nature that are widely distributed in higher plants, lower marine animals and some bacteria (Riguera, 1997; Yoshiki *et al.,* 1998; Podolak *et al.,* 2010). Despite their fairly large structural diversity, these compounds share some unique biological properties like the ability to lyse erythrocytes and to foam (Bruneton 1995; Rao and Gurfinkel 2000; Francis *et al.,* 2002). Surface activities responsible for foaming properties, as well as some other biological functions including haemolytic activity, are attributed to characteristic structural features of saponins and their amphiphilic nature which results from the presence of a hydrophilic sugar moiety and a hydrophobic sapogenin (Podolak *et al.,* 2010). Haemolysis of red blood cells seems to result from saponins' ability to form complexes with cell membrane cholesterol leading in consequence to pore formation and cell permeabilization, and also to cause alterations in the negatively charged carbohydrate portions on the cell surface (Abe *et al.,* 1978a; Melzig *et al.,* 2001; Gauthier *et al.,* 2009a).

Most known saponins are plant-derived secondary metabolites, though several saponins are also found in marine animals such as sea cucumbers (Holothuroidea) (Van Dyck *et al.,* 2010) and starfish (Asteroidea) (Liu *et al.,* 2008). The presence of saponins has been reported in more than 100 families of plants, and in a few marine sources (Hostettmann and Marston, 1995). The ability to synthesize saponins is rather widespread among plants belonging to the division of Magnoliophyta, covering both dicotyledons and monocotyledons (Vincken *et al.,* 2007). The steroidal saponins are mainly found in monocotyledons (such as *Agavaceae, Dioscoreaceae* and *Liliaceae*), and triterpinoid saponins are predominantly present in dicotyledons (*Leguminosae, Araliaceae, Caryophyllaceae*) (Sparg *et al.,* 2004). In rare cases both types of saponins may accumulate in a plant, like for example in *Avena sp.* (*Monocotyledonous poaceae*) (Osbourn 2003) or *Lysimachia paridiformis* (*Dicotyledonous myrsinaceae*) (Xu *et al.,* 2007). While the main dietary sources of saponins are legumes (soybeans, chickpeas, mungbeans, peanuts, broad beans, kidney beans, lentils), they are also present in oats, allium species (leek, garlic), asparagus, tea, spinach, sugarbeet, and yam (Price *et al.,* 1987). Soap bark tree (*Quillaja saponaria*), fenugreek *(Trigonella foenum-graceum)*, alfalfa (*Medicago sativa*), horse chestnut (*Aesculus hippocastanum*), liquorice (*Glycyrrhiza* species such as *Glycyrrhiza glabra*), soapwort (*Saponaria officinalis)*, Mojave yucca (*Yucca schidigera*), gypsophila genus (such as *Gypsophila paniculata*), sarsaparilla (*Smilax regelii* and other closely related species of Smilax genus) and ginseng (Panax genus) are the main non-food sources of saponins used in health and industrial applications (Hostettmann and Marston, 1995; Balandrin 1996). The saponin content of plant materials is affected by the plant species, genetic origin, and the part of the plant being examined, the environmental and agronomic factors associated with growth of the plant, and post-harvest treatments such as storage and processing (Fenwick *et al.,* 1991).

The unique chemical nature of saponins demands tedious and sophisticated techniques for their isolation from plant material, structure elucidation and analysis. The task is further complicated by the occurrence of many closely related substances in plant tissues, and by the fact that most of the saponins lack a chromophore. Thus, for many years, the complete characterisation of saponins from even well-known saponin-containing plants was not achieved. There are several strategies available for the isolation of saponins (Marston *et al.,* 2000; Muir *et al.,* 2000; Schopke, 2000). As a general rule, they begin with the extraction of the plant material with aqueous methanol or ethanol. Further processing of the extract is carried out after evaporation under reduced pressure, dissolution in a small amount of water and phase separation with n-butanol. It is currently recognized that this step is sometimes undesirable, since only those saponins with short oligosaccharide side chains will eventually be extracted into the butanolic phase. A further purification is then carried out, which involves liquid chromatography over a silica gel column, or a gradient elution from a polymeric support or liquid–liquid partition chromatography, or, as most commonly employed, HPLC separation. In most cases, some of the above steps have to be repeated with a change of support or eluent to achieve high purity. Once the saponin has been purified, it may be subjected to analytical methods including MS, proton and carbon NMR, and infrared spectroscopy. Other classical methods are used to ascertain the presence of saponins in a crude plant extract, and to elucidate their composition throughout purification steps. TLC and staining with dehydrating reagents containing aromatic aldehydes (such as anisyl aldehyde in sulfuric acid) are commonly used. The pure saponin may also be hydrolysed to verify the nature of its glycosidic moieties.

The biological role of saponins in plants is not completely understood. They are generally considered to be part of defense systems due to anti-microbial, fungicidal, allelopathic, insecticidal and molluscicidal, etc. activities (Francis *et al.,* 2002; Sparg *et al.,* 2004). They exhibit a wide range of pharmacological activities including expectorant, anti-inflammatory, vasoprotective, hypocholesterolemic, immunomodulatory, hypoglycaemic, molluscicidal, antifungal, antiparasitic, anticonvulsants and many other central nervous system (CNS) activities (Sparg *et al.,* 2004; Sahu *et al.,* 2008; Chindo *et al.,* 2009). Plants rich in saponins, like *Panax ginseng* or *Glycyrrhiza glabra*, have been used for medicinal purposes since ancient times (Fiore *et al.,* 2005) and to date continue to play significant roles not only in medicine but also in food and cosmetic industry, where they are utilized as emulsifiers or sweeteners (GüclüŪstündağ and Mazza, 2007). Another important application of saponins is their use as adjuvants in the production of vaccines (Sun *et al.,* 2009). Steroidal sapogenins have also been used for many years as economically important raw materials for the pharmaceutical industry in the production of steroidal hormones (Blunden *et al.,* 1975; GüclüŪstündağ and Mazza, 2007). This chapter provides an overview of the structural diversities, properties and applications of saponins. It is hoped that the information collated here will provide the reader with information regarding the various potential applications of saponins, and stimulate further research into these compounds.

STRUCTURES

Saponins are glycosides containing one or more sugar chains on an aglycone backbone also called a sapogenin. The aglycones, which may contain one or more unsaturated C–C bonds, may consist of a triterpenoid (Fig. 1A) or steroid (Fig. 1B) structure and it is on this basis that saponins are classified. Steroidal sapogenins (27C) can have a 6-ring spirostane or a 5-ring furostane skeleton, while triterpenoid sapogenins (30C) are much more structurally diverse and their basic ring system is most often made up of five or more units, seldom of four units. The most common monosaccharides include: D-glucose, L-rhamnose, D-galactose, D-galacturonic acid D-glucuronic acid, L-arabinose, D-xylose and D-fructose. Saponins are also categorized as mono, di-, or tridesmosidic according to the number of sugar chains in their structure. Monodesmosidic saponins have a single sugar chain, normally attached at C-3. Bidesmosidic saponins have two sugar chains, often with one attached through an ether linkage at C-3 and one attached through an ester linkage at C-28 (triterpene saponins) or an ether linkage at C-26 (furastanol saponins). The oligosaccharide chain is normally attached at the C-3 position (monodesmosidic), but many saponins have an additional sugar moiety at the C-26 or C-28 position (bidesmosidic). The great complexity of saponin structure arises from the variability of the aglycone structure, the nature of the side chains and the position of attachment of these moieties on the aglycone.

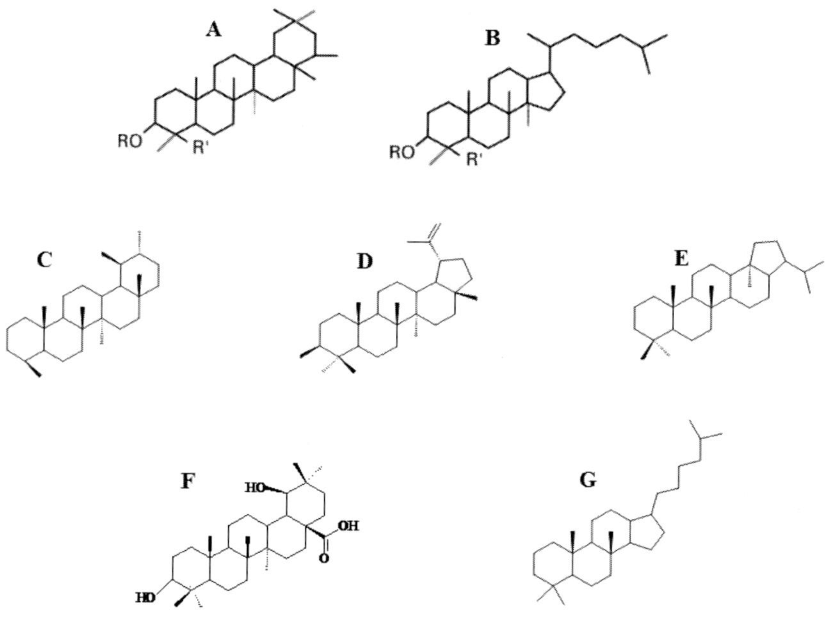

Figure 1. Basic structures of sapogenins: a triterpenoid (A), a steroid (B) and other skeleton types: ursane (C), lupane (D), hopane (E), germanicane (F) and dammarane (G).

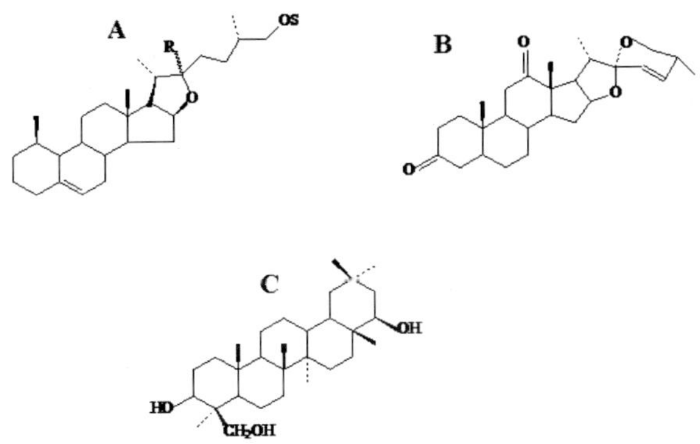

Figure 2. Steroidal sapogenins (27C): 5- ring furostane (A) or 6-ring Spirostane (B) and Triterpenoids saponins (30C) (C).

The main pathway leading to both types of sapogenins is similar and involves the head-to-tail coupling of acetate units. However, a branch occurs, after the formation of the triterpenoid hydrocarbon, squalene, that leads to steroids in one direction and to cyclic triterpenoids in the other.

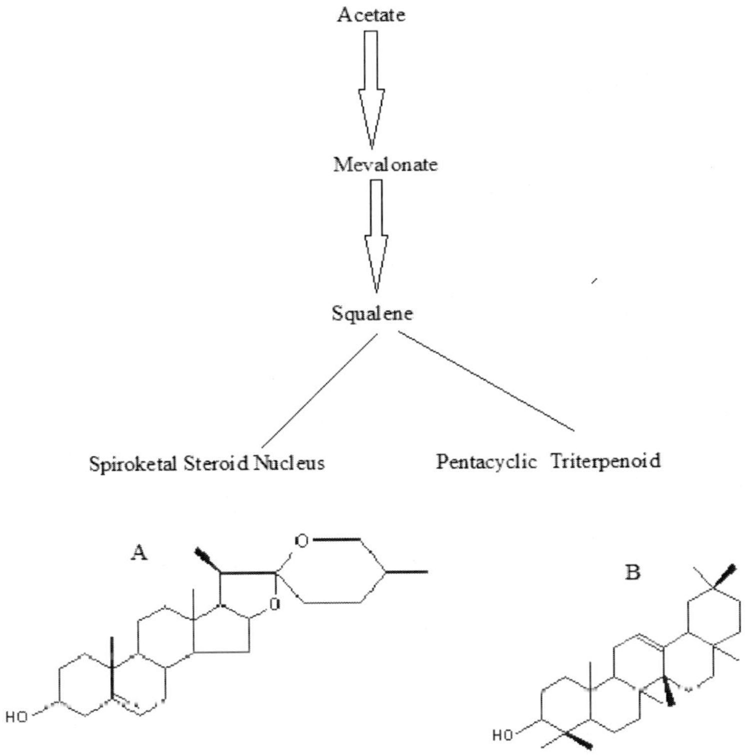

Figure 3. Conversion of acetate to spiroketal steroid nucleus (A) and pentacyclic triterpenoid (B).

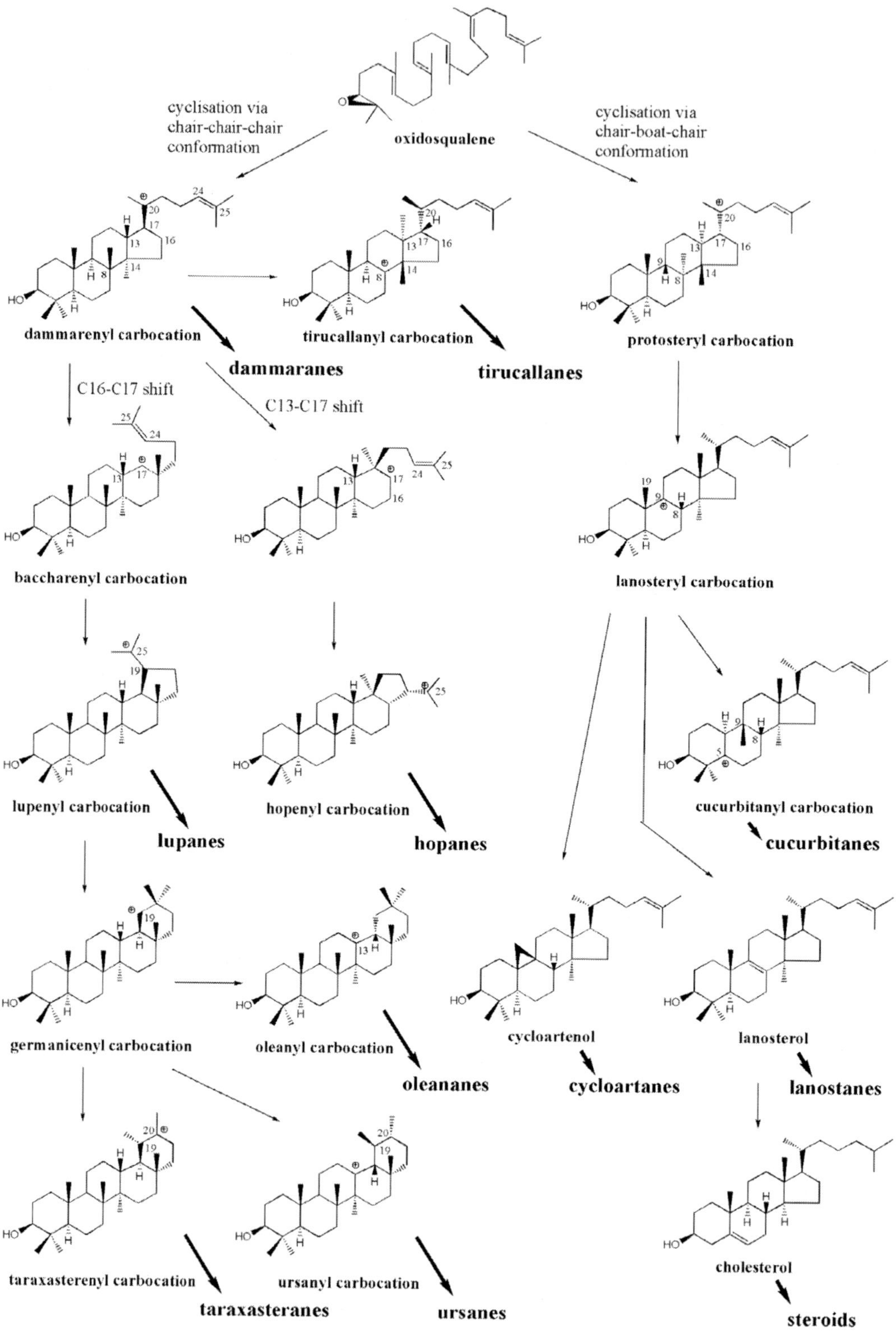

Figure 4. The cyclization of oxidosqualene to the various saponin skeletons (Vincken *et al.,* 2007).

The 11 carbon skeletons shown in Fig. 4, dammaranes, tirucallanes, lupanes, hopanes, oleananes, taraxasteranes, ursanes, cucurbitanes, cycloartanes, lanostanes, and steroids, represent the end products of cyclization, rearrangement and degradation reactions, which cover the main saponin skeletons that have been found in our literature search. There are, however, several other biosynthetic pathways known for triterpenoids, leading to different types of triterpenoid skeletons. Several other triterpene skeletons may occur in nature as glycosides, but have not been characterized as saponins. Although we may have overlooked some of these glycosylated triterpenoids and steroids, this does not interfere with the main principle of classification of saponins based on the biosynthesis of the carbon skeleton of their aglycones. New skeletons can be introduced easily in this system, following the biosynthesis of their carbon skeleton, as soon as sufficient examples of such new skeletons have been found in nature.

Of the 11 main saponin skeletons mentioned in this chapter, several have been found to undergo ring cleavage (leading to seco-skeletons), homologation (leading to homo or bis-homo skeletons), degradation to nor or bis-nor compounds, or minor rearrangement to related skeletons. All these secondary modifications lead to skeletons, which are indicated as separate subclasses as shown in Fig. 5. The skeletons in Fig. 5 are numbered according to the IUPAC rules; in the seco, homo, and nor compounds the numbering of the main skeleton is maintained.

The dammarane skeleton (1) can undergo further processing to give the 3,4-seco-skeleton (1a) (Kennelly *et al.,* 1995), and the 15,16-seco-skeleton (1b) (Oulad-Ali *et al.,* 1994). The lupane skeleton (3) can be cleaved to give the 3,4-seco-skeleton (3a) (Shirasuna *et al.,* 1997). The side chain at the five membered ring in the hopane skeleton can be rearranged to the rearranged hopanes (4a) (Sahu *et al.,* 2001) or be degraded to the bis-nor hopanes (4b) (Sahu *et al.,* 2001). The oleanane skeleton (5) can be fragmented to the 17,22-seco skeleton (5a) (Lavaud *et al.,* 1992), or rearranged to a ring A nor-ring B homo skeleton (5b) (Kanchanapoom *et al*., 2005). Degradation of the oleanane skeleton leads to the 23-nor (5c) (Jia *et al.,* 1998), the 27-nor (5d) (He *et al.,* 2006; Cheng *et al.,* 2002), the 28-nor (5e) (Ueckert *et al.,* 1998), or the 30-nor skeletons (5f) (Ikuta and Itokawa, 1989; Ikuta *et al.,* 1991; Miyase *et al.,* 1995; Junkuszew *et al.,* 1998; Konishi *et al.,* 1998; Pöllmann *et al.,* 1998; Park *et al.,* 2002). The ursane skeleton can be rearranged to the 20- epi skeleton (7a) (Ouyang *et al.,* 1997; Taketa *et al.,* 2000), or cleaved to the 18,19-seco skeleton (7b) (Li *et al.,* 2005). The steroid skeleton (11) can be homologated to the 24-bis-homo skeleton (11a) (Pires *et al.,* 2002). Furthermore, the steroid skeleton can be degraded in the sidechain to the nor-skeleton (11b) (Saijo *et al.,* 1983; Achenbach *et al.*, 1996; Mimaki *et al.,* 1997b; Ahmad *et al.,* 1998; Dong *et al.*, 2001), which belongs to the pregnane type steroids, and to the skeleton (11c) (Mimaki *et al.,* 1997a; Zheng and Yang, 2003), which has been indicated as a 22-homo pregnane skeleton.

Besides the carbon skeleton, the aglycones differ in their number and/or type of substituents attached (e.g —OH, −O, —CH_3, CH_2OH, —CHO, —COOH, and/or glycosyl residues), the number and position of double bonds, lactones, and spirocompounds.The nature of the aglycone and the functional groups such hydroxyls, hydroxymethyls, carboxyls and acyl on the aglycone backbone and number and nature of the sugar chains in the polycyclic sapogenin account for significant structural diversity and various bioactivities of saponins (Price *et al.,* 1987; Hostettmann and Marston, 1995).

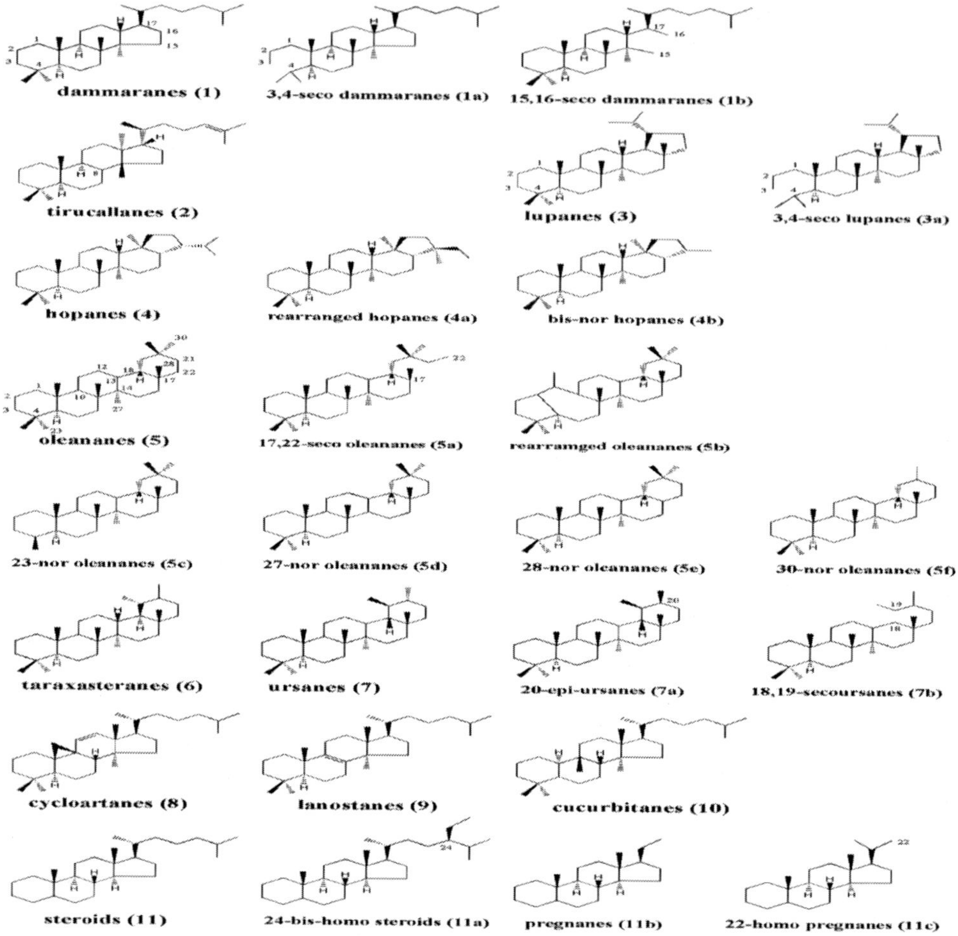

Figure 5. Structures of the 11 main classes of carbon skeletons of saponins after cyclization, and their various derivatives (Vincken *et al.*, 2007).

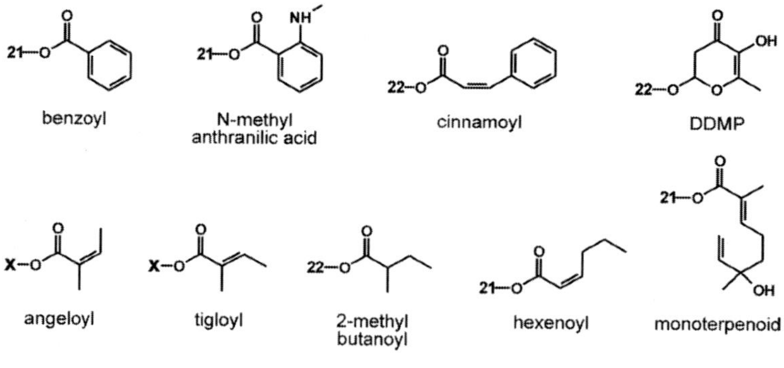

Figure 6. Structures of substituents at the hydroxyl group of the C-21 and C-22 atoms of the oleanane skeleton (5). 21 and 22 indicate the position of the oleanane skeleton at which the substituent is attached. X represents both positions 21 and 22 of the oleanane skeleton. The groups include benzoyl (Trojanowska *et al.*, 2000), N-methyl anthranilic acid (Germonprez *et al.*, 2004; Trojanowska *et al.*, 2000), cinnamoyl (Germonprez *et al.*, 2004), DDMP (Kudou *et al.*, 1993), angeloyl (Germonprez *et al.*, 2004; Lu *et al.*, 2000), tigloyl (Yoshikawa *et al.*, 2000), 2-methyl butanoyl (Lu *et al.*, 2000), hexenoyl (Yoshikawa *et al.*, 2000), and monoterpenoid (Zou *et al.*, 2005) substituents.

PROPERTIES

The structural complexity of saponins results in a number of physical, chemical, and biological properties, only a few of which are common to all members of this diverse group of compounds. Due to the presence of a lipid-soluble aglycone and water soluble sugar chain(s) in their structure (amphiphilic nature), saponins are surface active compounds with detergent, wetting, emulsifying, and foaming properties (Mitra and Dungan, 1997; Ibanoglu and Ibanoglu, 2000; Wang *et al.*, 2005). Saponins, including soybean saponins, saponins from *Saponaria officinalis,* and *Quillaja saponaria*, form micelles in aqueous solutions, the size and structure of which are dependent on type of saponin (Oakenfull, 1986). The micelle forming properties are affected by temperature, salt concentration, and pH of the aqueous phase (Mitra and Dungan, 1997). The incorporation of cholesterol into the saponin micelles increased their critical micellar concentration, size, viscosity, and the aggregation number (Mitra and Dungan, 1997) resulting in the solubility enhancement of cholesterol as much as a factor of 10^3 at room temperature (Mitra and Dungan, 1997).

A significant decrease in the solubilizing effect on saikosaponin-a was observed upon methylation or reduction of the glucuronide carboxyl group of ginsenoside-Ro indicating the role of the glucuronide moiety in the observed effect (Tanaka, 1987). Solubility enhancement may have important implications for the bioactivity and processing of saponins. Monodesmosides, while poorly soluble in water in purified form, can be extracted readily due to the solubilizing effect of co-occuring compounds (Kimata *et al.,* 1983). Micellar solubilization by saponins can be exploited for the development of micellar extraction processes or to affect the solubilization of ingredients in cosmetic, pharmaceutical or food formulations (Shirakawa *et al.,* 1986). Solubility of saponins is also affected by the properties of the solvent (as affected by temperature, composition, and pH). While water, alcohols (methanol, ethanol) and aqueous alcohols are the most common extraction solvents for saponins, solubility of some saponins in ether, chloroform, benzene, ethyl acetate, or glacial acetic acid has also been reported (Hostettmann and Marston, 1995).

Bitterness has been observed to be the most common sensory attribute associated with saponins (Price *et al.,* 1987), but the occurrence of sweet saponins is also well known (Kennelly *et al.,* 1996). For example, the sweetness of licorice is attributed to its main saponin, glycyrrhizic acid, which is 50 times sweeter than sugar (Muller and Morris, 1966). The complex structure of saponins may undergo chemical transformations during storage or processing which in turn may modify their properties/activity. The glycosidic bond (between the sugar chain and the aglycone), and the interglycosidic bonds between the sugar residues can undergo hydrolysis in the presence of acids/alkali, due to hydrothermolysis (heating in presence of water) or enzymatic/microbial activity resulting in the formation of aglycones, prosapogenins, sugar residues or monosaccharides depending on the hydrolytic method and conditions (Hostettmann and Marston, 1995).

Complete acid hydrolysis yields the constituent aglycone and monosaccharides, whereas under basic hydrolysis conditions, cleavage of O-acylglycosidic sugar chains results in the formation of prosapogenins (Hostettmann and Marston, 1995). DDMP (2,3-dihydro-2,5-dihydroxy-6-methyl-4*H*-pyran-4-one) conjugated saponins, which were determined to be the genuine saponins in intact soybeans, are hydrolyzed into saponins upon heating, in alkaline solutions, and in the presence of iron (Kudou *et al.,* 1993; Okubo and Yoshiki, 1995). The conversion of saponins to their aglycones may also result in the loss of activity. For example the hydrolysis of saponins by ruminal bacteria results in the loss of antiprotozoal activity, which requires the intact saponin structure (Cheeke, 1999). The aglycones, which might be naturally present in the plants or formed by hydrolysis of saponins *in vivo* or during storage and/or processing of the plant material, may have biological activity which is absent or present in a lower degree in their corresponding saponins. The solubility behavior of the parent aglycone can be markedly different than the saponin due to its lipophilic nature.

The interaction of sterols (Walter *et al.*, 1954; Shany *et al.*, 1970; Gestetner *et al.*, 1971, 1972), minerals (West *et al.*, 1978), and proteins (Potter *et al.*, 1993; Tanaka *et al.*, 1995) with saponins may result in the modification of the physicochemical properties and biological activities of these compounds. Steroid saponins such as digitonin (Gestetner *et al.*, 1972), alfalfa saponins (Walter *et al.*, 1954), and triterpenoid saponins such as Lucerne (Shany *et al.*, 1970; Gestetner *et al.*, 1971, 1972) form water insoluble addition products with cholesterol and phytosterols such as sitosterol and stigmasterol. Interaction of sterols and lucerne saponins has been shown to be dependent on the structure of the saponin and sterols (Gestetner *et al.*, 1971, 1972). While cholesterol and β-sitosterol formed complexes with lucerne saponins containing medicagenic acid, which possess carboxyl groups at C-23 and C-28 positions, saponins with soyasapogenol aglycones did not precipitate (Gestetner *et al.*, 1971). Insoluble complexes were also formed between ammoniated glycyrrhizic acid and alfalfa root saponins and the minerals zinc and iron (West *et al.*, 1978).

The nature and effect of the saponin-protein interaction has been shown to depend on the type of protein (Potter *et al.*, 1993) and the type of the saponin mixture (Tanaka *et al.*, 1995). Upon heating at 78°C (upto 26 min) quillaja saponin interacts with casein to form high molecular weight complexes, whereas soybean proteins form insoluble aggregates independent of saponin addition (Potter *et al.*, 1993). Similarly, while heating salt soluble proteins from walleye pollack meat at 40–100°C for up to 10 min in the presence of quillaja saponins increased protein aggregation, tea seed saponins inhibited the aggregation of the protein (Tanaka *et al.*, 1995). Complex formation between beet saponin and protein (as evidenced by turbidity and interfacial tension measurements) and destabilization of a model dispersion of sucrose, oil, saponin, and protein in acidic conditions point to the role of beet saponin and protein in the formation of the acid beverage floc in sucrose-sweetened carbonated soft drinks and acidified syrups (Morton and Murray, 2001). The interaction of saponins and proteins also results in modifications of protein properties such as heat and enzyme stability (Ikedo *et al.*, 1996; Shimoyamada *et al.*, 1998), and surface properties (Chauhan *et al.*, 1999). Heat stability of bovine serum albumin (BSA) (Ikedo *et al.*, 1996) and resistance of BSA (Ikedo *et al.*, 1996) and soybean protein (Shimoyamada *et al.*, 1998) to chymotryptic hydrolyses improved upon addition of soybean saponins. The stability of whey proteins to chymotryptic hydrolyses however decreases upon addition of soybean saponins (Shimoyamada *et al.*, 2000). Similarly, unlike soybean protein whose sensitivity to tryptic hydrolysis improved, whey proteins show higher sensitivity in the presence of soya saponins (Shimoyamada *et al.*, 2000). The influence of soybean saponin on the trypsin hydrolysis of bovine milk α-lactalbumin was attributed to the modification of the protein's tertiary structure (Shimoyamada *et al.*, 2005). Desaponization of quinoa protein increases water hydration capacity and lowers the fat binding and buffer capacity, and total nitrogen solubility (Chauhan *et al.*, 1999). Removal of saponins reduces the emulsion and foaming capacity of the proteins but increases the stability of the foams and emulsions (Chauhan *et al.*, 1999).

Biological Activity

Saponins have been reported to possess a wide range of biological activities (Hostettmann and Marston, 1995; Milgate and Roberts, 1995; Lacaille-Dubois and Wagner, 1996; Francis *et al.,* 2002) with the ability to swell and rupture erythrocytes causing a release of haemoglobin (the *in vitro* haemolytic activity) being the most investigated property of these compounds (Oda *et al.,* 2000). However, even for this activity, which has been related to the saponin structure (type of aglycone and the presence of sugar side chains), there is no apparent consistency among members of this diverse group of compounds (Oda *et al.,* 2000). While crude isolates, extracts, and saponin containing plants have been utilized in the investigation of biological activity, especially in the earlier studies, developments in the isolation/purification and characterization techniques have enabled the investigation of the bioactivity of well characterized saponins and led to the emergence of structural-bioactivity relationships (Oda *et al.,* 2000; Gurfinkel and Rao, 2003). The toxicity of saponins to insects, parasitic worms, molluscs, and fish and their antifungal, antiviral, and antibacterial activity are well documented (Milgate and Roberts, 1995; Lacaille-Dubois and Wagner, 1996; Francis *et al.,* 2002). Saponins have a diverse range of properties, which include sweetness and bitterness (Grenby, 1991; Kitagawa, 2002; Heng *et al.,* 2006), foaming and emulsifying properties (Price *et al.,* 1987), pharmacological and medicinal properties (Attele *et al.,* 1999) and haemolytic properties (Oda *et al.,* 2000; Sparg *et al.,* 2004). Numerous reports also emphasize on the allelopathic (Waller *et al.,* 1993), antimicrobial (Avato *et al.,* 2006; Sung and Lee, 2008b), insecticidal (Sandermann and Funke, 1970; Shinoda *et al.,* 2002; Kuzina *et al.,* 2009; Nielsen *et al.,* 2010a), fungicidal (Lee *et al.,* 2001; Morrissey and Osbourn, 1999; Saha *et al.,* 2010; Sung and Lee, 2008a) and molluscicidal activities (Gopalsamy *et al.,* 1990; Huang *et al.,* 2003; Sparg *et al.,* 2004; Aladesanmi, 2007) activity of various saponins. However, the molecular mechanisms behind these deterrent and toxic effects are not completely elucidated.

Effects on Cell Membranes

A large number of the biological effects of saponins have been ascribed to their action on membranes, which is the most intensively studied effect of several saponins and many steroidal glycoalkaloids. Although interference with the integrity of biological membranes is probably the most abundant effect of saponins, their activities are not limited to this type of action, and not all saponins show significant hemolytic activity (Chwalek *et al.,* 2006; Gauthier *et al.,* 2009a,b; Nakamura *et al.,* 1979). Several structure–activity relation studies further emphasized that the ability to cause hemolysis often does not correlate with other known activities of saponins such as their anti-fungal and cytotoxic properties or their applicability as adjuvants (Adams *et al.,* 2010; Chwalek *et al.,* 2006; Gauthier *et al.,* 2009a,b; Oda *et al.,* 2000; Santos *et al.,* 1997).

The action of saponins on cell membranes, which is often referred to as their 'hemolytic activity', is thought to be the molecular basis for the observed ability of saponins to cause lysis of mammalian erythrocytes (Baumann *et al.,* 2000; Chwalek *et al.,* 2006). This effect towards membranes was first described by Dourmashkin *et al.* (1962) in their study on saponin-inactivated *Rous sarcoma* virus particles by electron microscopy. The observed formation of pores (or pits) in the viral membrane coat as a consequence of the saponin treatment inspired Bangham and Horne (1962) and Glauert *et al.* (1962) to pursue additional experiments in this direction. Both groups concurrently reported the occurrence of cholesterol in the target membrane to be essential for saponin induced pore formation. Since then, several research groups further elucidated the molecular basis behind the membrane penetration activity by studying various sets of saponins or steroidal glycoalkaloids on natural occurring or artificial membrane systems. The results of these studies confirmed the influence of membrane composition, especially in regards to concentration levels as well as the structure of incorporated membrane sterols, on the ability of saponins and steroidal glycoalkaloids to cause membrane perturbation (Armah *et al.,* 1999; Keukens *et al.,* 1992, 1995; Nishikawa *et al.,* 1984; Rosenqvist *et al.,* 1980; Steel and Drysdale, 1988; Stine *et al.,* 2006; Walker *et al.,* 2008; Yu and Jo, 1984). In addition, it became obvious that the overall hemolytic potential of saponins and steroidal glycoalkaloids is affected by virtually all characteristics of their chemical composition, including structure of the aglycone (Gauthier *et al.,* 2009a,b; Oda *et al.,* 2000; Takechi *et al.,* 2003; Ullah *et al.,* 2000; Voutquenne *et al.,* 2002; Yu and Jo, 1984), number of saccharide side chains (Hase *et al.,* 1981; Hu *et al.*, 1996; Voutquenne *et al.,* 2002; Woldemichael and Wink, 2001), length of these side chains (Armah *et al.,* 1999; Chwalek *et al.,* 2006; Keukens *et al.,* 1995; Nishikawa *et al.,* 1984; Oda *et al.,* 2000; Plé *et al.,* 2004; Seebacher *et al.,* 1999b; Voutquenne *et al.,* 2002) as well as the types and linkage variants of the incorporated sugar units (Chwalek *et al.,* 2006; Hu *et al.,* 1996; Seebacher *et al.,* 1999a,b, 2000; Takechi *et al.,* 2003). The sides chains present on the aglycone acyl residues (Matsuda *et al.,* 1997) or the epoxy-framework system (Abe *et al.,* 1978b) also contribute to the effects on membranes. These effects however were not uniform; some saponins with acyl residue for instance, did not show haemolytic activity (Oda *et al.,* 2000), while acylated triterpenoid saponins in low concentrations were able to alter membrane activity (Melzig *et al.,* 2001). It was suggested that only acetylated saponins might integrate transiently into membranes, thus inducing pore-like structures. It has been suggested that the haemolytic activity of saponins increases with increasing numbers of polar groups in the aglycone moiety (Namba *et al.,* 1973).

The precise mechanisms of the interactions between saponins and membranes are not well understood. The interactions are complex and may involve different mechanisms including the formation of the saponin–cholesterol complex, alterations in the organization of sarcolemmal membrane phospholipids, and the formation of phospholipid breakdown products such as phosphatidic acid (Yamasaki *et al.,* 1987) in addition to saponin structure and three-dimentional orientation are all involved in the actions of saponins on membranes. The haemolytic action of saponins is believed to be the result of the affinity of the aglycone moiety for membrane sterols, particularly cholesterol, with which they form insoluble complexes with the amount of glycosides required for permeabilisation much lower for cholesterol-rich lipid layers than cholesterol-free membranes (Gŏgelein and Hŭby, 1984).

Glauert *et al.* (1962) proposed the first model of saponin action towards membranes. According to this model, spontaneous formation of complexes between saponins and cholesterol in membranes is followed by association of these complexes into 'two-dimensional micellar-type structures' within the membrane. The hydrophilic sugar chains of the saponins, which are thought to be centrally orientated in the micellar- like complex, lead to formation of an aqueous pore. Such pores would cause an increase in membrane permeability enabling ions and macromolecules up to proteins to pass the membrane bilayer. More recent models of the molecular mechanism behind the membrane permeabilizing activity of saponins and steroidal glycoalkaloids (Armah *et al.,* 1999; Keukens *et al.,* 1995;

Nishikawa *et al.,* 1984) expand this initial hypothesis. The first step in these modes of action is the incorporation of saponins or steroidal glycoalkaloids into the facing membrane monolayer. This step occurs spontaneously, driven by the lipophilic character of the aglycone as it is expected to favor the hydrophobic conditions of membrane layers over aqueous surroundings. Within the membranes, saponins and steroidal glycoalkaloids then assemble into 1:1-complexes with membrane sterols as, e.g., cholesterol in mammalian cell membranes. Subsequently, the saponin–sterol or glycoalkaloid– sterol complexes accumulate into matrices or plaques by processes whose driving force is not currently understood. Armah *et al.* (1999) and Keukens *et al.* (1995) proposed interactions between the sugar moieties of the incorporated saponins/glycoalkaloids to cause these phase-separation phenomena. Finally, as a consequence of such accumulation, the sterical properties of saponins and steroidal glycoalkaloids may cause membrane curvature as a final step in the membrane perturbation mechanism. This curvature could result in the formation of either pores (Armah *et al.,* 1999) within these saponin/sterol plaques, or hemitubular protuberances that may eventually lead to sterol extraction via vesiculation (Keukens *et al.,* 1995). The observation of pore-like structures and holes in electron microscopy images of membranes and cells treated with saponins (Bangham and Horne, 1962; Baumann *et al.,* 2000; Dourmashkin *et al.,* 1962; Glauert *et al.*, 1962; Mazzucchelli *et al.*, 2008; Seeman *et al.*, 1973) supports the concept of pore formation. In addition, formation of pores may provide the simplest explanation for the observed changes in ion conductivity (e.g. Armah *et al.,* 1999; Gŏgelein and Hŭby, 1984) and protein mobility through the membrane (e.g. Krawczyk *et al.,* 2010; Mazzucchelli *et al.,* 2008). However, microscopy studies based on membranes treated with steroidal glycoalkaloids did not reveal similar pores (Keukens *et al.,* 1992, 1995; Stine *et al.,* 2006; Walker *et al.,* 2008).

An alternative model of saponin activity towards membranes originates from coarse-grained molecular dynamics simulations (Lin and Wang, 2010). In this model, saponins migrate in the membrane to sphingomyelin and cholesterol enriched membrane domains, the so-called lipid rafts (Brown and London, 2000; Fantini *et al.,* 2002), and form a complex with the cholesterols therein. Such saponin interaction with specific membrane domains is supported by recent studies on saponin-induced lipid raft disruption (Xu *et al.,* 2009; Yi *et al.,* 2009; Zhuang *et al.,* 2002) and microdomain alteration (Naruse *et al.,* 2010). Consequently, the earlier indicated plaque formation may originate from complex formation following preexisting phase separation rather than resulting from membrane reorganization processes triggered by saponin–sterol complex accumulation.

Cholesterol enrichment is shown to have an inhibitory effect on many membrane ATPases. It is probable that cholesterol may directly interact with the boundary lipids of ATPase and alter the intermolecular hydrogen bonds of the protein. Ginsenosides (from *Panax quinquefolius* and *P. japonicus*) share the steroid backbone and amphipathic nature with cholesterol. The desacyl-jego-saponin (from *Styrax japonica*) and gensenoside-Rd, which had little or no effect on membrane permeability, were capable of stimulating Na^+ - Ca^{2+} exchange activity in canine cardiac sarcolemmal vesicles (Yamasaki *et al.*, 1987; Choi *et al.,* 2001). Ginsenosides have variable Na^+ - K^+ ATPase and Ca^{2+} - Mg^{2+} ATPase activities in neurones (Choi *et al.,* 2001). It is possible that some ginsenosides interact with membrane cholesterol and displace it from the immediate environment of ATPases. Removal of cholesterol will lead to an increase in membrane fluidity; conformational changes that ATPases undergo during their transport cycle may be facilitated. Membrane fluidity controls the enzyme activity of biological membranes and has an important role in ion transport (Ma and Xiao, 1998) and the ability of saponins to affect this parameter may explain their effects on cellular function. The inotropic action of saponins may be caused by their effect on membrane Ca^{2+} channels, which may have no correlation with membrane permeability effect (Enomoto *et al.*, 1986).

Membrane proteins are thought to be localized selectively in cholesterol-rich domains (acetylcholine receptor) or in cholesterol-poor domains (the sarcoplasmic Ca^{2+} ATPase). Therefore, the biophysical properties of the different domains, rather than the bulk lipid, may selectively influence transmembrane protein function and mimic specificity at the effector level. Saponins may interact with the polar heads of membrane phospholipids and the -OH group of cholesterol through OH groups at C-3 or C-28, which will result in their later ability to form micelle-like aggregates. Moreover, their hydrophobic aglycone backbone could intercalate into the hydrophobic interior of the bilayer. Both of these effects may contribute to the alteration of the lipid environment around membrane proteins. It has become increasingly evident that the lipid environment of membrane proteins, including ion channels, transporters, and receptors, plays an important role in their function. The changed-function proteins or glycoproteins in the plasma membranes have been suggested to be the cause of secondary biochemical responses induced by saponins (Abe *et al.*, 1978b; Rao and Sung, 1995).

Hypoglycaemic Activity

Saponins isolated from plants such as fenugreek (Petit *et al.*, 1993), *Phellodendron cortex* and *Aralia cortex* (Kim *et al.*, 1998c), *Pueraria thunbergiana* (Lee *et al.*, 2000a), and *Calendula officinalis* (Yoshikawa *et al.*, 2001) have been shown to have hypoglycaemic effects. Petit *et al.* (1993) found chronically higher plasma insulin levels, probably caused by stimulation of the β-cells in male Wistar rats given fenugreek extract mixed with food, while Matsuda *et al.* (1999b) did not find insulin-like or insulin-releasing activity in rats given oleanolic acid glycosides orally. The hypoglycaemic action here was due to suppression of the transfer of glucose from the stomach to the small intestine and the inhibition of glucose transport across the brush border of the small intestine. The saponin momordin Ic was also found to significantly and dose-dependently inhibit gastric emptying (Matsuda *et al.*, 1999a), which dependent on the level of serum glucose and mediated at least in part by the capsaicin-sensitive sensory nerves and the central nervous system. Yoshikawa *et al.* (2001) showed that the oleanolic acid 3-monodesmosides with hypoglycaemic activity also inhibited gastric emptying showing a correlation between the two effects, while other saponins showing no hypoglycaemic activity in the mixture also did not affect gastric emptying. Studies have also shown that both Asian ginseng and American ginseng roots (Xie *et al.*, 2005), *Terminalia arjuna* (Biswas *et al.*, 2011), possess significant hypoglycemic abilities in animal models of diabetic.

Effects on Cholesterol Metabolism

A number of studies have shown that saponins from different sources lower serum cholesterol levels in a variety of animals including human subjects (Southon *et al.*, 1988; Harwood *et al.*, 1993; Potter *et al.*, 1993; Matsuura, 2001; Al-Habori and Raman, 1998). Saponins also reduced the more harmful LDL-cholesterol selectively in the serum of rats, gerbils and human subjects (Potter *et al.*, 1993; Harris *et al.*, 1997; Matsuura, 2001). It has also been noted that a saponin-induced reduction of serum cholesterol occurred only when a hypercholesterolaemic diet had been fed (Jenkins and Atwal, 1994). The synthetic saponins tiqueside and pamaqueside are much more potent than naturally occurring saponins (such as those from Lucerne) in preventing hypercholesterolaemia (Morehouse *et al.,* 1999).

Cholesterol-lowering activity of saponins has been attributed to inhibition of the absorption of cholesterol from the small intestine, or the reabsorption of bile acids (Oakenfull and Sidhu, 1990; Kim *et al.,* 2003b). This mechanism of action of saponins was luminal and did not involve stoichiometric complexation with cholesterol (Morehouse *et al.,* 1999) without interference with the entero-hepatic bile acid recirculation (Harwood *et al.,* 1993). Since cholesterol binding takes place in the intestinal lumen, factors such as quantity of saponins and cholesterol, and the presence of other ligands of both these compounds may play a role and these may have caused the observed discrepancies among the various results. Knowledge of the nature of the interaction between the particular saponin and cholesterol, and the nature of the cholesterol moieties and other ligands in the diet are essential to arrive at an effective dietary dose of that particular saponin that could have a significant hypocholesterolaemic effect.

Large mixed micelles formed by the interaction of saponins with bile acids account for their increased excretion when saponin-rich foods such as soyabean, lucerne and chickpea are consumed (Oakenfull, 1986; Oakenfull and Sidhu, 1990). There is also evidence of increased cholesterol synthesis to compensate for saponin-induced excretion (Jenkins and Atwal, 1994). The resulting accelerated metabolism of cholesterol in the liver causes its serum levels to go down. Other suggested mechanisms of action of saponins include delaying the intestinal absorption of dietary fat by inhibiting pancreatic lipase activity (Han *et al.,* 2000).

Effects on Animal Reproduction

The negative effects of saponins on animal reproduction, which have been ascribed to their abortifacient, antizygotic and anti-implantation properties, are well documented (Tewary *et al.,* 1973; Stolzenberg and Parkhurst, 1976). Saponins from broom weed (Gutierrezia sp.) and lechuguilla (*Agave lecheguilla*) or commercial pharmaceutical grade saponins caused abortion or death or both in rabbits, goats and cows (Dollahite *et al.,* 1962). Saponins isolated from the crude extract of *Gleditischia horrida, Costus speciosus* and *Phytolacca dodecandra* caused sterility in mice (Chou *et al.,* 1971; Tewary *et al.,* 1973; Stolzenberg and Parkhurst, 1976). Quin and Xu (1998) found that the butanol extract of *Mussaenda pubescens* was capable of terminating pregnancy in rats. Extracts of this plant are used as a contraceptive in the Fujian traditional medicine. Saponins were found to be extremely strong stimulators of luteinising hormone release from cultured hypophysial cells (El Izzi *et al.,* 1989; Benie *et al.,* 1990) but their action was neutralised in the presence of serum suggesting a passive membrane-permeabilising effect (El Izzi *et al.*, 1992) in this case. However, saponin-rich extracts from *Combretodendron africanum* injected into female rats stimulated uterine growth, lowered luteinizing hormone release, and blocked the oestrous cycle (Benie *et al.,* 1990). The steroid saponin was found to directly inhibit the genes responsible for steroidogenesis, and also suppress the proliferation of follicle-stimulating hormone-modulated granulosa cells in the ovarian follicle. The mechanism of suppression of cell proliferation here might be through a similar mechanism as saponin-induced proliferation of tumour cells. Saponins have been shown to have both positive and negative effects on the viability of human sperm cells *in vitro* with some ginseng saponins increasing motility as well as progression of sperm (Chen *et al.,* 1998) while *Sesbania sesban* saponins are shown to possess spermicidal activity at 1·0–1·3 mg/ml (Dorsaz *et al.*, 1988). Saponin-rich extracts of *Turnera diffusa and Pfaffia paniculata* improves the copulatory performance of sexually sluggish or impotent rats while being ineffective in sexually potent rats (Arletti *et al.,* 1999), which may be ascribed to increased central noradrenergic and dopaminergic tone, and possibly oxytocinergic transmission. The inhibitory effects of dietary Quillaja saponins on egg production in Nile tilapia have also been reported (Francis *et al.,* 2001b). Saponins also reportedly affect functioning of the male reproductive system. The gonado-somatic index of 6-month-old male tilapia fed a diet containing Quillaja saponins during the initial part of the life-cycle was significantly higher than that of the control, whereas male tilapia receiving a continuous supply of dietary saponins tended to have lower gonado-somatic index (unpublished data). The mechanism of action in these instances remains to be clarified. The *in vivo* effects of saponins on the reproductive functioning seem to suggest more than a simple permeabilising effect on secretary cell membranes and could possibly be linked to interactions between saponins and steroid receptors given the similarities between the basic chemical structures of saponins and steroid hormones. Ginseng saponins were found to compete strongly with oestradiol and R5020 (a synthetic progestin) for oestrogen- and progesterone-binding sites in the human myometrial cytosol (Punnonen and Lukola, 1980). *C. africanum* extract was shown to compete with oestradiol and with progesterone on uterine receptors (Benie *et al.,* 1990). The spirostanol-steroid saponin, digitonin, stimulates binding of progesterone to bovine luteal membrane and this action is mediated by its ability to specifically complex with membrane sterols rather than by a non-specific detergent effect (Menzies *et al.,* 1999). The saponin receptor complexes may then translocate into the nucleus and affect transcription patterns. Ginsenoside Rg3 (20(s) protopanaxadiol type) exhibited a dose-dependent inhibitory activity on the expression of marker genes coding for androgen receptors and 5α-reductases that converts testosterone into the more potent dihydrotestosterone, which in turn binds to androgen receptors for eliciting its actions (Liu *et al.,* 2000).

Effects on the Immune System

Saponins modulate the immune system through their adjuvant activity, their ability to improve effectiveness of orally administered vaccines by facilitating the absorption of large molecules, and their immunostimulatory effects (Cheeke, 1999). The ability of saponins to act as immunological adjuvants by enhancing the immune response to antigens has been recognized since 1940s (Bomford *et al.,* 1992; Francis *et al.,* 2002). In addition to quillaja saponins, which have been almost exclusively used in the production of saponin adjuvants (Bomford *et al.*, 1992), adjuvant activity of soyasaponins, lablabosides, jujubosides, quinoa, gypsophila, and saponaria saponins has also been reported (Bomford *et al.*, 1992; Oda *et al.*, 2000; Estrada *et al.*, 1998).

Saponin-based adjuvants have the unique ability to stimulate the cell-mediated immune system, as well as to enhance antibody production, and only a low dose is needed for adjuvant activity (Oda *et al.,* 2000). Saponins are known to have immunostimulatory activity (Kensil, 1996; Barr *et al.,* 1998; Sjolander *et al.,* 1998). Studies thus far have focused on Quillaja saponins and derivatives such as immune-stimulating complex vaccines (immunestimulating complexes formed by the combination of cholesterol, saponin, phospholipid and amphiphatic proteins). Quillaja and other saponins either as crude mixtures or as purified compounds have been reported to increase immune-cell proliferation *in vitro* (Chavali *et al.* 1987; Plohmann *et al*., 1997; Lacaille-Dubois *et al.,* 1999). Purified Quillaja saponins boosted antibody production without producing any reaginic antibodies (So *et al,*. 1997). The varied action of saponins might suggest that their immunostimulatory effects are the result of specific targeting of physiological intermediaries rather than the result of a non-specific effect on cell membrane permeability.

Immune-stimulating complexes formulated with Quillaja saponin preparations induced specific cytotoxic T-lymphocyte responses (Coulter *et al.,* 1998) and have been reported to induce antibody responses and/or protective immunity in guinea-pig, turkey, cat, rabbit, dog, seal, sheep, pig, cow, horse and monkeys (Mowat *et al.,* 1999).

The mechanisms of immune-stimulating action of saponins have not been clearly understood, but many explanations have been put forward. For instance, saponins reportedly induced production of cytokines such as interleukins and interferons that might mediate their immunostimulant effects (Jie *et al.,* 1984; Kensil, 1996; Chindo *et al.,* 2010). It is likely that they interact with antigen-presenting cells to induce many of these responses (Barr *et al.,* 1998). The incorporation of the saponins into cell or endosomal membranes might expose the incorporated antigen to cytosolic proteases. There is evidence that saponins may increase the immune response by increasing the uptake of antigens from the gut and other membranes. Oral administration of *Panax ginseng* C. A. Meyer saponins (Jie *et al.,* 1984), *Quillaja* saponins (Maharaj *et al.,* 1986), and the butanol extract of *Lonicera japonica* (Lee *et al.,* 1998), and de-acylated saponin-1 administered on the nasal mucosa (Recchia *et al.,* 1995), all stimulated the immune responses *in vivo*. Purified *Quillaja* saponin-21 was able to act as a mucosal adjuvant in DNA vaccination against HIV-1 (Sasaki *et al.,* 1998).

The adjuvant activity of saponins is believed to be related to branched sugar chains or aldehyde groups (Bomford *et al.,* 1992) or to an acyl residue bearing the aglycone (Kensil, 1996). Soyasaponins and lablabosides were later found to show strong adjuvant activity despite lacking acyl residues and possessing only unbranched sugar chains (Oda *et al.,* 2000). Also most of the escins that have acyl residues and branched sugar chains did not show adjuvant activity. Adjuvant activity and toxicity, but not the cholesterol-binding capacity of QH-B, a Quillaja fraction, declined on peroxidate oxidation due to alterations in the structure of the sugars, galactose and xylose. Modification of the apiose moiety may influence adjuvant activity but not toxicity *in vivo* (Ronnberg *et al.,* 1997).

As against the stimulatory effects on specific immunity components, saponins have also been shown to be able to prevent some non-specific immune reactions such as inflammation (de Oliveira *et al.,* 2001; Haridas *et al.,* 2001a) and monocyte proliferation (Delmas *et al.,* 2000; Yui *et al.,* 2001). Triterpenoid saponins from *Acacia victoriae* having a, b ester groups at C-28 and the outer monoterpene chains could have reacted with cysteine residues in the nuclear transcription factor-kB (NF-kB) molecule and this might have modified this molecule and prevented it from performing its normal function of stimulating genes involved in immune and inflammatory pathways in response to stress signals. One downstream effector substance whose activity has shown to be lowered by saponin is phospholipase A2 (de Oliveira *et al.,* 2001) that cause a decrease in hydrolysis in membrane phospholipids and thereby decreased membrane fluidity.

Anticancer Activity

Anticancer activity has been reported for a number of triterpene and steroid saponins including but not limited to soyasaponins (Rao and Sung, 1995; Kerwin, 2004; Berhow *et al.,*

2000; Plewa *et al.*, 1998), ginsenosides (Huang and Jia, 2005; Liu *et al.*, 2000), saikosaponin-d (Hsu *et al.*, 2004), diosgenin (Raju *et al.*, 2004), and glycyrrhizic acid (Hsiang *et al.*, 2002). The pursuit of natural substances capable of controlling malignancies has stimulated considerable research on this property of saponins. Methyl protoneogracillin (Hu and Yao, 2003), methyl protogracillin (Hu and Yao, 2001), steroidal saponins isolated from the rhizomes of *Dioscorea collettii*, protoneodioscin (Hu and Yao, 2002a), and protodioscin (Hu and Yao, 2002b), furastanol saponins isolated from the rhizomes *of Dioscorea collettii,* have been identified as potential anticancer agents by the National Cancer Institute's (NCI) anticancer drug screen program. Anticancer activities of saponin containing plants such as ginseng and licorice have also being documented (Wang and Nixon, 2001; Yun and Choi, 1998; Shin *et al.*, 2000). The cancer preventive effects of ginseng have been demonstrated in experimental models and in epidemiological studies. Saponins isolated from different plants and animals have been shown to specifically inhibit the growth of cancer cells *in vitro* (Kuznetzova *et al.*, 1982; Rao and Sung, 1995; Konoshima *et al.* 1998; Marino *et al.*, 1998; Mimaki *et al.* 1998a; Podolak *et al.*, 1998). Other aglycones with anticancer activity include dammarane sapogenins from ginseng (Huang and Qi, 2005), betulinic acid (Yogeeswari and Sriram, 2005; Wick *et al.*, 1999), and oleanolic acid (Liu, 1995; Hsu *et al.*, 1997).

The depressive effect of saponins against cancer cells may take place through diverse and complex mechanisms unrelated to the destructive activity of saponins against cells such as erythrocytes (Mimaki *et al.*, 1998b). Triterpenoid saponins (avicins from *Acacia victoriae*) selectively inhibited growth of tumour cell lines by cell cycle arrest in human breast cancer cell line and apoptosis in leukaemia cell line (Mujoo *et al.*, 2001) and reduced both tumour incidence and multiplicity in a murine skin carcinogenesis model (Hanausek *et al.*, 2001). Ginsenoside Rg3 was found to exert multiple anti-proliferative activities towards human prostate carcinoma cells including cell cycle arrest at G1 phase and stimulation of apoptosis. Saponin (triterpenoid or steroid)-induced apoptosis is primarily caused by stimulating the cytochrome c–caspase 9–caspase 3 pathway in the human cancer and other cell lines (Liu *et al.*, 2000; Haridas *et al.*, 2001b; Yui *et al.*, 2001; Cai *et al.*, 2002), a property that is shared by a ginseng saponin derivative (20-O- (b-D-glucopyranosyl)-20(S)-protopanaxadiol) produced in the intestine by bacteria and absorbed into blood (Lee *et al.*, 2000c). Yui *et al.* (2001) detected specific toxic activity against macrophage colony-stimulating factor-induced growth of macrophages by terpenoids (securiosides) having specific structural features such as presence of dimethoxycinnamoyl group. Apoptosis seemed to be induced by mechanisms similar to those reported for Jurkat cells (Haridas *et al.* 2001b) by stimulating the cytochrome c–caspase pathway. Interestingly the securiosides seemed to have no or considerably weaker effects against other cells including thymocytes, bone marrow cells and tumour cell lines or even macrophages stimulated by growth factors other than macrophage colony-stimulating factor, revealing a high degree of structure- related specificity. Saponin-initiated cytotoxicity thus begins non-specifically with cell aggregation caused by detergent action (Mimaki *et al.*, 2001), followed by specific toxicity determined by receptors on the cell surface and saponin structure leading to what seems to be a mechanism of apoptosis that is independent of saponin structure. The tumour-specificity of the cytotoxic action seems to be influenced by the structure of the sugar portion of the saponins (Kuroda *et al.*, 2001) after the hydrophobic aglycone core allowed saponins to traverse the mitochondrial membrane.

The mechanism of the cytochrome c release is not caused by the anticipated passive permeabilisation of the mitochondrial membrane by saponin. A cell cycle arrest mediated by inhibition of the phosphatidylinositol- 3-kinase–protein kinase signalling pathway (Mujoo *et al.,* 2001) or direct suppression of protein kinase complex genes (Liu *et al.,* 2000) is stimulated by saponins either along with the apoptotic pathway (Mujoo *et al.,* 2001) or independently (Oh and Sung, 2001), based on the structure of saponin. The complexity of effects and interactions involved could be seen from the fact that the ginsenosides Rb1 and Rg1 are able to inhibit apoptosis in a human neuroblastoma cell line induced by toxins (Rudakewich *et al.,* 2001) and the abolishment by orally administered ginseng total saponins of morphine-induced apoptosis of thymocytes (Kim *et al.*, 1999). The inhibition of the phosphatidylinositol-3-kinase–protein kinase pathway is considered important in apoptosis, given the role of protein kinases in inactivating the caspases (apoptotic enzymes). Avicins also decreased the release of reactive oxygen species from mitochondria, which along with the inhibition of reactive nitric oxide synthetase (Haridas *et al.*, 2001b) might be the reason for the prevention of chromosomal damage reported in (Hanausek *et al.*, 2001). These activities may be considered as antioxidative in nature. But the above saponins lack an H atom-donating group and thus their effect must be at the physiological levels of specific induction. Saponins have been observed to decrease microsomal enzyme activity (Sindambiwe *et al.*, 1998; Nguyen *et al.*, 2000). Triterpenoid saponins from *Acacia victoriae* decreased expression of NF-kB regulated proteins such as inducible nitric oxide synthase and cyclo-oxygenase in human leukaemia cells *in vitro*, changes that may help prevent development of malignancies by reducing oxidative and nitrosative stress (Haridas *et al.*, 2001a). Saponins also reduce occurrence of reactive oxygen species such as H_2O_2 (Haridas *et al.*, 2001a; Pawar *et al.*, 2001), probably by enhancing its breakdown by activation of peroxiredoxins and catalase, and/or glutathione peroxidase (Deng and Zhang, 1991) as well as by suppressing its production by inhibiting the phosphatidylinositol- 3-kinase signalling pathway (Haridas *et al.*, 2001a). Direct effects on genetic material have also been reported. Ginseng saponins have been found to be specific inducers of the superoxide dismutase gene that codes for one of the major antioxidant enzymes, through transcription factor AP2 binding site and its induction (Kim *et al.*, 1996).

Saponins might also exert an anti-cancer effect at the intestinal level. Bile acids are metabolized by intestinal microbes to form secondary bile acids that are implicated as causative agents of colon cancer. The binding of saponins to bile acids in the intestine could reduce the availability of bile acids to the microbial population, thus reducing the formation of carcinogenic substances in the colon (Cheeke, 1996). Saponin metabolites, for example the ginseoside metabolite M1 produced in the intestine by the action of microbes on ingested ginseng saponins, may also have anti-cancer effects (Wakabayashi *et al.,* 1998). Hederagenin glycosides from *Kalopanax pinctus* could effectively prevent the metabolic activation of aflatoxin B-1 or scavenge the electrophilic intermediate capable of inducing mutation (Lee *et al.,* 2000b). Theasaponin E-1 from seeds of the tea plant *Camellia sinensis* L. var. Assamica Pierre exhibit considerable gastroprotective activity and the whole saponin fraction from tea seed protect gastric mucosal lesions induced by ethanol in rats (Murakami *et al.,* 1999).

Anti-inflammatory Activity

There are a number of reports of saponins with anti-inflammatory properties. The significant ameliorative activity of the saponins may be due to inhibition of the mediators of inflammation such as histamine, serotonin and prostaglandin along with its antioxidant property which inhibits the formation of ROS which also plays a major role in inflammation

(Sayyah *et al.,* 2004; Tatiya *et al.,* 2007). Many saponins isolated from plant sources produce an inhibition of inflammation in the mouse albumin- an carrageenan-induced oedema assay. In a study by Just *et al.* (1998), Fruticesaponin B, a bidesmosidic saponin with an unbranched saccharide moiety isolated from *Bupleurum fruticescens* L. (Apiaceae), was shown to have the highest anti-inflammatory activity of the all the saponins tested in the mouse oedema assays. Just *et al.* (1998) suggested that the anti-inflammatory activity of saponins isolated from *Bupleurum fruticescens* is related to the chemical structure of the saponins. *In vivo* studies on saponins isolated from *Bupleurum rotundifolium* L. (Apiaceae) were reported to have anti-inflammatory activity against both 12-O-tetradecanoylphorbol-13-acetate (TPA) induced ear oedema and chronic skin inflammation (Navarro *et al.*, 2001). Of the seven saponins tested, five were fairly active in reducing the TPA-induced ear oedema. The saponins produced a dose-dependent oedema reduction. Only two saponins were active in reducing the chronic skin inflammation, and also caused a parallel decrease in neutrophile infiltration.

Aescin, a mixture of triterpenoid saponins that forms the major active principle of *Aesculus hippocastanum* L. (Hippocastanaceae), has been shown to have anti-inflammatory, anti-oedematous and venotonic properties (Sirtori, 2001). Li *et al.* (2002) isolated two triterpenoid saponins from the stem bark of *Kalopanax pictus* Nakai (Araliaceae). We also reported the anti-inflammatory of saponin-rich fraction of *Ficus platyphylla* (Moraceae) stam bark in rats (Chindo *et al.,* 2010).

A novel steroidal saponin isolated from the leaves of *Agave attenuata* Salm-Dyck (Agavaceae) was evaluated for anti-inflammatory activity using the capillary permeability assay (da Silva *et al.,* 2002). The steroidal saponin inhibited the increase in vascular permeability caused by acetic acid which is a typical model for the first stage inflammatory reaction. However, the activity was not accompanied by an undesirable haemolytic effect and warrants further investigation as an anti-inflammatory drug.

The triterpenoid saponin loniceroside C isolated from the aerial parts of *Lonicera japonica* Thunb. (Caprifoliaceae), a medicinal plant known as an anti-inflammatory agent for centuries, showed anti-inflammatory activity when tested *in vivo* in the mouse ear oedema provoked by croton oil (Kwak *et al.,* 2003).

Kim *et al.* (1998a) investigated the anticomplementary activity of ginseng (*Panax ginseng* C.A. Mey., Araliaceae) saponins. Ginsenoside Ro and oleanolic acid showed the highest anticomplementary activity of the tested saponins. Kim *et al.* (1998a) suggested that the anti-inflammatory activity of these saponins is related to anticomplementary action through the classical inflammation pathway.

Molluscicidal Activity

The molluscicidal properties of saponins were first observed by Lemma (1965) who noticed the toxic effects of extracts of unripe berries of *Phytolacca dodecandra* on river snails in Ethiopia. Efforts were then mounted to utilize this property of saponins to control diseases such as schistosomiasis, which are transmitted by molluscs. Saponins have been investigated as molluscicides in the control of schistosomiasis (Sindambiwe *et al.,* 1998; Abdel-Gawad *et al.,* 1999). *Bulinus* and *Biomphalaria* species in particular, act as intermediate hosts in the life cycle of schistosomes, which cause urinary bilharzia. Many trials have been run in African countries where schistosomiasis has a high prevalence. In a study by Sindambiwe *et al.* (1998) a six-oleanane-type triterpenoid saponin mixture (maesasaponin mixture, isolated from

Maesa lanceolata) was tested for molluscicidal activity against *Biomphalaria glabrata*. *Phytolacca dodecandra* L• fHer. (Phytolaccaceae) and *Phytolacca icosandra* L. berries contain saponins with highly potent molluscicidal activity (Treyvaud *et al.*, 2000). Aqueous extracts of *Phytolacca icosandra* had a very high molluscicidal activity against *Biomphalaria glabrata* snails. According to Treyvaud *et al.*, (2000), the activity can be attributed to the presence of monodesmosidic saponins of serjanic and spergulagenic acids. Molgaard *et al.*, (2000) investigated the biodegradability of molluscicidal water-extracted saponins from the berries of *Phytolacca dodecandra*. Results showed that the saponins in an aqueous extract of *Phytolacca dodecandra* readily biodegraded. The saponins were completely consumed within 10 days which indicates their abilities to degrade in aquatic environments under aerobic conditions. As a result, the use of *Phytolacca dodecandra* berries for snail control in schistosomiasis-infested water bodies is environmentally acceptable. Apers *et al.* (2001) tested 10 saponins isolated from the leaves of *Maesa lanceolata* for molluscicidal activity against *Biomphalaria glabrata* snails.

The molluscicidal activity of the saponins may be due to their characteristic detergent effect on the soft body membranes of the molluscs. Saponins extracted from many other sources were also seen to have similar molluscicidal properties, for example purified *Sesbania sesban* saponins (Dorsaz *et al.*, 1988) and purified saponin mixtures from *Maesa lanceolata* at above 5 parts per million (Sindambiwe *et al.*, 1998) have been found to be active against *Biomphalaria glabrata*. Monodesmodic triglycosides from the pericarp of the fruits of Sapindus rarak (Hamburger *et al.*, 1992), a spirostanol glycoside from the inflorescence of *Y. aloifolia* (Kishor and Sati, 1990), and some 21,22 diacylated maesasaponins (Apers *et al.*, 2000) are also found to be molluscicides.

Antimicrobial Activity

Saponins have also been reported to have antimicrobial activity (Killeen *et al.*, 1998). They show the antimicrobial activity by inhibiting the growth of Gram +ve or Gram -ve microorganism. Some saponins are not effective against Gram -ve microorganisms because of the reason that they are not able to penetrate into the cell membranes of the microorganisms (Jain *et al.*, 2007; Soetan *et al.*, 2006)

Three butanol-extractable 5β-spirostan-3β-ol saponins were shown to have antimicrobial activity on both prokaryotic and eukaryotic organisms, but only at low cell densities. The saponins did not inhibit microbial growth of dense populations.

Three new triterpenoid saponins, Nudicaucins A, B, and C and a known saponin guaiacin D were isolated from *Hedyotis nudicaulis* Wight and Arn. (Rubiaceae) were tested against *Bacillus subtilis* (Konishi *et al.*, 1998). All four of the isolated saponins showed weak antibacterial activity. Results indicated that the tetraglycoside saponins have stronger activity than the triglycoside saponins.

A new jujubogenin saponin isolated from *Colubrina retusa* L. (Rhamnaceae), jujubogenin 3-*O*—α-L-arabinofuranosyl-(1 → 2)-[3-*O*-(*trans*)-*p*-coumaroyl-β-d-glucopyranosyl-(1→3)]-α-L-arabinopyranoside, had antimycobacterial activity when tested against *Mycobacterium intracellulare* (ElSohly *et al.*, 1999).

Iorizzi *et al.* (2002) isolated three new furostanol saponins along with seven known saponins from the seeds of *Capsicum annuum* L. var. *acuminatum* Fingerh. (Solanaceae). The saponins showed weak or no growth inhibition against both Gram-positive and Gram-negative bacteria.

Antifungal Activity

Saponins have high toxicity against fungi (Delmas *et al.*, 2000; Wang *et al.*, 2000a) and fungicidal activity against *Trichoderma viride* was previously used as an identification method for saponins. Kalopanaxsaponins A and I isolated from *Kalopanax pinctus* exhibited strong and specific antifungal activity against *Candida albicans* and *Cryptococcus neoformans* (Kim *et al.*, 1998b). Asparagus saponin-1, from the lower leaves of *Asparagus officinalis*, has antifungal properties depending on the type of fungus (Shimoyamada *et al.*, 1990). The monodesmosidic spirostanol saponins from *Y. schidigera* destroy certain food-deteriorating yeasts, film-forming yeasts, and dermatophytic yeasts and fungi (Miyakoshi *et al.*, 2000).

The antifungal activity of the steroidal saponins is associated with their aglycone moieties and the number and structure of monosaccharide units in their sugar chains (Chong-Ren *et al.*, 2006). The major mechanism suggested for the antifungal activity of saponins is their interaction with membrane sterols. Synthetic steroid saponins prepared by Takechi *et al.* (1999) were both antifungal and haemolytic but in many cases haemolytic triterpenoid saponins show little antifungal activity. It was observed that those saponins having a branched-chain trisaccharide moiety without any oxygen-containing groups at C-2 and C-12 exhibited the anti-yeast activity, while saponins with 2b-hydroxyl or 12 keto groups showed very weak or no activity (Miyakoshi *et al.*, 2000). A saponin with a disaccharide moiety exhibited relatively low activity and the aglycones or bidesmodic furostanol saponins showed no activity. Some reports describe the anti-yeast activity of saponins as having an anti-food deteriorating effect (Miyakoshi *et al.*, 2000).

Antiviral Activity

Some saponins and sapogenins have been shown to be capable of deactivating viruses; for example, purified saponin mixture from *Maesa lanceolata* (Sindambiwe *et al.*, 1998). Maesasaponins with 21,22 diacylation have antiviral activity (Apers *et al.*, 2000). The triterpenoid sapogenin oleanolic acid inhibits HIV-1 virus replication probably by inhibiting HIV-1 protease activity (Mengoni *et al.*, 2002). Anti-viral (anti-HIV) activity has been demonstrated for betulinic acid and its derivatives (Yogeeswari and Sriram, 2005).

Antiprotozoal Activity

Saponins from different sources have been found to be detrimental to protozoa and have been identified as possible defaunating agents in the rumen (Wallace *et al.*, 1994; Newbold *et al.*, 1997). This property could be exploited in treatment of protozoal infections in other animals. Triterpenoid and steroid saponins have been found to be detrimental to several infectious protozoans such as *Plasmodium falciparum* (Traore *et al.*, 2000), Giardia trophozoites (McAllister *et al.* 2001) and Leishmania species (Delmas *et al.*, 2000; Plock *et al.*, 2001). The toxicity of saponins to protozoans seems to be widespread, nonspecific and obviously the result of their detergent effect on the cell membranes. The antiprotozoal property of saponins may be lost upon deglycosylation (Wang *et al.*, 2000a).

Antioxidant Effects

The term 'antioxidants' that is to describe chain-breaking inhibitors of lipid peroxidation as free radicals generated *in vivo* damage many targets other than lipids, including proteins,

DNA and small molecules, is important in foods both as preservatives and supplying essential antioxidants *in vivo*. These oxidation reactions might lead to an array of adverse biological effects. Zilversmit (1979) hypothesised that atherogenesis might result from phenomena that occur immediately after eating, and that it might be affected by chylomicron remnants. Several investigators (Staprans *et al.*, 1994; Wolff and Nourooz-Zadeh, 1996; Ursini *et al.*, 1998) expanded Zilversmit's hypothesis and suggested that dietary lipid hydroperoxides, which may be partly generated during digestion in the alkaline pH of the intestine, are the source of chylomicron remnants of lipid hydroperoxides, which are elevated in the postprandial state. These findings emphasize the importance of natural antioxidants in food, and throughout the digestive tract. Usually, polyphenols and carotenoid pigments, being the major nutritional antioxidants in food, attract most of the attention in this area. Some saponins have also been found to have antioxidative or reductive activity.

A group of saponins produced in legumes, namely, group B soyasaponins, contain an antioxidant moiety attached at C-23 (Yoshiki *et al.*, 1998). This unique sugar residue, 2, 3-dihydro-2, 5-dihydroxy-6-methyl-4H-pyran-4-one (DDMP), allows saponins to scavenge superoxides by forming hydroperoxide intermediates, thus preventing bio-molecular damage by free radicals (Yoshiki and Okubo, 1995; Hu *et al.*, 2002). Previously it was suggested that the DDMP residue is lost during soyabean processing. However, it has been shown that soya ingredients (soyabean flour, toasted soya hypocotyls, soya protein isolates, textured vegetable protein, soya protein concentrates, and Novasoy) and soya foods (commercial soya milk, tofu, and tempeh) contain the group B soyasaponins from (Hu *et al.*, 2002). The DDMP moiety is widely distributed among legumes such as kidney beans, peanuts, chickpeas, clover, and Japanese bushclover (Yoshiki *et al.*, 1998).

Central Nervous System Activity

Ginseng extract has been shown to have neurotrophic and neuroprotective effects (Rudakewich *et al.*, 2001). It significantly improves learning ability and cognitive functions in brain-damaged rats in a dose-dependent manner, and enhances the strategic performance of normal rats. These effects are thought to be due to membrane-stabilising effects such as the inhibition of Na^+ and Ca^{2+} channels (Zhao and McDaniel, 1998). Ginseng total saponins injected intracerebroventricularly inhibit stress-induced hypothalamo– pituitary–adrenal responses by inducing NO production in the brain (Kim *et al.*, 1998a). This may be beneficial in preventing the harmful effects of excessive increases in plasma corticosterone on the target organs under stressful circumstances. *Panax notoginseng* saponins administered intraperitoneally significantly inhibited abnormal increases in platelet aggregation and platelet adhesiveness in rats subjected to permanent occlusion of the middle cerebral artery. Similar effects were observed with *in vitro* preparations. The anticerebral ischemic effect of *Panax notoginseng* saponins is probably due to changes in the rank and structure of functional membrane proteins induced by fluidity of membranes that lead to changes in protein activities (Ma and Xiao, 1998). Platelet membrane glycoproteins play a key role in the adhesion of platelets to the walls of blood vessels, in the accretion of platelets and in the formation of thromboses.

Zhang *et al.* (2001) studied inhibition of gap junction mediated intercellular communication (GJIC) by ginsenosides. Gap junctions are believed to be involved in the pathogenesis of many inherited and acquired human diseases. Some ginsenosides reduced GJIC by activating tyrosine kinase, while others produced the same effect by activating protein kinase C. Tyrosine kinase and protein kinase C are the two primary kinases that phosphorylate connexins, leading to GJIC down regulation. Still other ginsenosides inhibited GJIC by directly modulating the gap junction channels. They were, for example, found to inhibit striatal dopamine release stimulated by psychostimulants (Shim *et al.,* 2000) probably due to their effects on receptor-operated Na^+ channels in dopaminergic nerve terminals or on presynaptic nicotinic acetylcholine receptors. Even among the chemically related ginsenosides prominent structure–activity relationships were difficult to find, even among chemically-related ginsenosides.

Glucocorticoid-like Activity

Another intriguing mode of action for some saponins is the ability to bind to glucocorticoid receptors. Glucocorticoids represent a class of steroidal hormones known to be involved in regulation of a manifold of physiological processes. In mammals, they play an important role in regulation of development, metabolism, neurobiology and apoptosis, etc. (Yudt and Cidlowski, 2002). Due to the structural resemblance of saponin aglycones and steroids, it is therefore not surprising that several pharmacological activities of saponins such as anti-inflammatory (Giner *et al.,* 2000) and neuroprotective (Zhang *et al.,* 2008) effects as well as induction of adipogenesis (Niu *et al.,* 2009) or apoptosis (Jia *et al.,* 2004), are linked to interaction with receptors of glucocorticoid hormones.

Lee *et al.* (1997) reported that the ginsenoside Rg1 suppressed growth in rat hepatoma cells through transactivation induced by its binding to the glucocorticoid receptor (GR). By using the antiglucocorticoid RU486 it was found that Rg1 induced gene expression through a GRmediated mechanism. This GR-mediated gene induction by Rg1 was coupled with other signalling pathways, as in the case of glucocorticoids, evidenced by synergistic induction in the presence of increasing doses of a cyclic adenosine monophosphate analogue (Chung *et al.,* 1998). Again, Rg1 also caused a down regulation of GR in a manner similar to glucocorticoids. In contrast, chronic infusion of Rg1 restored binding capacity of type 1 corticosterone- preferring receptors in the hippocampal region of aged rats (de Kloet *et al.,* 1987). Orally administered ginseng total saponins were shown to restore morphineinduced elevation of plasma corticosterone to the control level (Kim *et al.,* 1999), probably through negative feedback exerted by ginseng saponin or metabolite–GR complexes. Other reports point out that saponin ingredients act by mechanisms other than binding to steroid receptors. Glycyrrhetinic acid, the active aglycone of a liquorice saponin, for example, was found to be a highly efficient inhibitor of corticosteroid 11b-dehydrogenase (Monder *et al.,* 1989) and showed mineralocorticoid-like activity. This enzyme catalyses the oxidation of the biologically active steroid cortisol to its inactive metabolite cortisone. [Glycyrrhizic acid and glycyrrhetinic acid glucuronide given orally to rats were reported to inhibit renal 11bdehydrogenase in the Monder *et al.* (1989) study, providing further evidence of absorption of active saponin derivatives from the intestine]. Oral administration of saponins from *Hernaria glabra*, on the other hand, resulted in a significant decrease in blood pressure in hypertensive rats and increased salt and water transport in the renal tubules (Rhiouani *et al.,* 1999). The glucocorticoid-like action of saponins could possibly explain the diverse effects of saponins in biological systems. Glucocorticoids, acting through GR, are involved in the regulation of numerous physiological processes (Gagliardo *et al.,* 2001). Upon ligand binding GR inhibits or stimulates gene transcription. On nuclear translocation GR transactivate DNA elements compatible with glucocorticoid response elements. Activated GR also antagonize transcription factors, particularly NF-kB, directly and indirectly through gene transcription and protein synthesis of the NF-kB inhibitor (Almawi and Melemedjian, 2002). NF-kB regulates a number of genes involved in immune and inflammatory pathways such as various pro-inflammatory cytokines, adhesion molecules, and apoptosis and has been shown to be affected by saponins (see Haridas *et al.,* 2001a,b). Higher glucocorticoid activity has been described to have negative effects on female reproductive function (Andersen, 2002). Contradictory results are, however, common when the action of glucocorticoids is described, as several local mechanisms modulate its potency and availability at the tissue level. The end effects of glucocorticoid-like activity of saponins could hence be unpredictable and different from that of glucocorticoids itself as it is not known whether the modulatory machinery works in the same manner for saponins. The action of saponins that evolved in plants as important defence adaptation against highly conserved key pathways such as the NF-kB pathway in potential rivals may also have evolutionary significance (Haridas *et al.,* 2001a).

Applications

Structural diversity of saponins is reflected in their physicochemical and biological properties, which are exploited in a number of traditional (as soaps, fish poison, and molluscicides) and industrial applications (Price *et al*., 1987; Oakenfull, 1981; Fenwick *et al.,* 1991; Hostettmann and Marston, 1995; Oakenfull and Sidhu, 1989). While plant extracts containing saponins have been widely used in food and other industrial applications mainly as surface active and foaming agents (San Martin and Briones, 1999); saponins in foods have traditionally been considered as "antinutritional factors" (Thompson, 1993) and in some cases their use have limited to their bitter taste (Ridout *et al*., 1991). Therefore, most of the earlier research on processing of saponins targeted their removal to facilitate human consumption (Khokhar and Chauhan, 1986; Ridout *et al.,* 1991). However, food and non-food sources of saponins have come into renewed focus in recent years due to increasing evidence of their health benefits such as cholesterol lowering and established anticancer properties of saponins (Gurfinkel and Rao, 2003; Kim *et al.,* 2003b). They have also being established as the active components in many herbal medicines (Liu and Henkel, 2002; Alice *et al.,* 1991) and the contributions to the health benefits of foods such as soybeans (Kerwin, 2004; Oakenfull, 2001) and garlic (Matsuura, 2001) are highlighted. The commercial potential of saponins has resulted in the development of new processes/processing strategies and reevaluation of existing technologies (Muir *et al.,* 2002) for their extraction and concentration (Rickert *et al.,* 2004b). Saponins have found wide applications in beverages and confectionery, as well as in cosmetics (Price *et al.,* 1987; Petit *et al.,* 1995; Uematsu *et al.,* 2000) and pharmaceutical products (Sparg *et al.,* 2004).

Health Applications

Steroidal saponin-containing plant materials gained commercial significance in 1950s as raw materials for the production of steroid hormones and drugs. The synthesis of progesterone from the sapogenin diosgenin obtained from Mexican yam by Marker *et al.*

(1947) was the beginning of a remarkable era in steroid research culminating in the synthesis of the first oral contraceptive in 1951. Diosgenin isolated from *Dioscorea* species and to a lesser extent structurally similar sapogenins such as hecogenin from *Agave* species have been widely used as raw materials by the steroid industry (Blunden *et al.,* 1975). Saponins have been used as immunological adjuvants in veterinary vaccine formulations due to their immune enhancing properties since 1950s (Dalsgaard, 1974). Their use in human vaccines, however, has been limited by their complexity and toxicity.

Purification of the quillaja extract to yield fractions with differing chemical and biological properties enabled the characterization and thus reproducible production of the fractions for optimal adjuvant activity and minimal haemolytic activity and toxicity (Cox *et al.,* 2002; Kensil and Marciani, 1991). Consequently, there have been significant advances in the development of saponins as human vaccine adjuvants in the last decade leading to the development of a new generation of vaccines against cancer and infectious diseases which are at various phases of clinical trials (Kensil *et al.,* 2004). The use of quillaja extracts (even at concentrations commonly used in foods) as oral adjuvants in human clinical tests requires supporting toxicology and general safety data due to their non-GRAS status (Dirk and Webb, 2005).

The wealth of information on the biological activity of saponins and aglycones from a variety of sources is providing leads for the development of drugs. The chemopreventive and chemotherapeutic activities of ginseng dammarane sapogenins have prompted the development of anticancer drugs which are at various stages of development (Panagin Pharmaceuticals Inc., 2005). A new class of HIV drugs called Maturation Inhibitors (PA-457, in Phase 2 clinical trials) is being developed using betulinic acid derivatives (Panacos, 2005).

Pharmaceutical compositions or plant extracts containing saponins have been patented for the prevention and/or treatment of a variety of conditions such as inflammation (Forse and Chavali, 1997; Bombardelli *et al.,* 2001), infection (Forse and Chavali, 1997), alcoholism (Bombardelli and Gabetta, 2001), pre- and post-menopausal symptoms (Bombardelli and Gabetta, 2001), cardiovascular and cerebrovascular diseases such as coronary heart disease and hypertension (Yao *et al.,* 2005; Hidvegi, 1994), dementia (Ma *et al.*, 2003), cataract, and carcinoma cutaneum (Satoshi *et al.,* 2004), gastritis, gastric ulcer, and duodenal ulcer (Kim *et al.,* 2003a). The use of saponins in pharmaceutical preparations as adjuvants to enhance absorption of pharmacologically active substances or drugs has also been patented (Kensil *et al.,* 1996; Tanaka and Yata, 1985).

Saponin-containing plants such as ginseng, yucca, horse chestnut, sarsaparilla, and liquorice have been used in traditional medicine by various cultures for centuries for the prevention/treatment of various ailments (Liu and Henkel, 2002; Hostettmann and Marston, 1995). Characterization of the medicinal plants and their extracts points to the role of saponins in conjuction with other bioactive components such as polyphenols in the observed health effects (Liu and Henkel, 2002; Alice *et al.,* 1991). Over 85% of the herbs most commonly used in Traditional Chinese Medicine were observed to contain saponins (in addition to polyphenols) in significant detectable amounts, while the herbal products in the eight best known and most commonly used formulae were explicitly rich in these components (Liu and Henkel, 2002). It should be noted that while some of the health benefits associated with these plants have been supported by clinical data or described in pharmacopeias and in traditional systems of medicine, a variety of uses attributed to these medicinal plants have not been substantiated.

Food Applications

Yucca (Mohave yucca, *Yucca schidigera* Roezl Fla) and quillaja (quillaia, soap bark, *Quillaja saponaria* Mol Fla) are classified as food additives in the US under section (US Food and Drug Administration, 2003). The food additives from natural origins containing saponins used in Japan include enzymatically modified soybean saponin, *Pfaffia paniculata* extract; quillaja extract, tea seed saponins, and yucca foam extract (Japanese Ministry of Health and Welfare, 2005). Quillaja extract is classified by the European Union as a foaming agent for use in water-based, flavored non-alcoholic drinks (Office for Official Publications of the European Communities, 1996). Although quillaja and yucca are not considered Generally Recognized as Safe (GRAS) by the US Food and Drug Administration (FDA), they have been given GRAS designation by Flavor and Extract Manufacturers' Association (Ash and Ash, 2002).

Quillaja extract (type 1) is used in foods and beverages mainly for its foaming properties at concentrations of 100 ppm (dry basis, undiluted extract) in soft drinks, and at concentrations up to 250 ppm in frozen carbonated beverages (Joint FAO/WHO Expert Committee on Food Additives, 2004). Quillaja extract, (type 2) is used in Japan as an emulsifier for preparations containing lipophilic colors or flavors that are added to soft drinks and fermented vegetables (Joint FAO/WHO Expert Committee on Food Additives, 2004). Liquorice and liquorice derivatives, which are considered as GRAS by FDA, are used in foods such as baked foods, beverages, chewing gum, candy, herbs and seasonings, plant protein products, and vitamin and mineral dietary supplements as a flavoring agent only with specific limitations (U.S. Food and Drug Administration, 2005b). Saponins have also been proposed for use in foods as antimicrobial (Sogabe *et al.*, 2003) and anti-yeast agents (Ashida and Matsuda, 1999). Other commercial saponin products for food applications include soybean concentrates marketed as functional food ingredients and nutraceuticals (OrganicTechnologies, 2005), and a Korean ginseng extract called saponia (Godwithus Co Ltd., 2005). The presumed health benefits of oleanolic acid led to the development of methods to fortify food products (such as olive oil) with oleanolic acid (van Putte, 2002). Proposed applications for oleanolic acid include as a flavoring agent to modify the aftertaste/taste of the artificial sweetener (Kang *et al.*, 1999) and in fat blends as crystal modifier (Bhaggan *et al.*, 2001).

The physicohemical properties of saponins can also be utilized in food processing applications. Thus, while complex formation of saponins with cholesterol has been used for the removal of cholesterol from dairy products such as butter oil (Micich *et al.*, 1992; Richardson and Jimenez-Flores, 1994), the interaction of saponins with cell membranes has been considered for the selective precipitation of fat globule membranes from cheese whey (Hwang and Damodaran, 1994). In this last application, saponins are used to increase the hydrophobicity of the fat membrane to facilitate flocculation and precipitation of the formed complexes (Hwang and Damodaran, 1994).

Due to their surface active properties, saponins are being utilized as natural surfactants in cleansing products in the personal care sector such as shower gels, shampoos, foam baths, hair conditioners and lotions, bath/shower detergents, liquid soaps, baby care products, mouth washes, and toothpastes (Indena, 2005; Olmstead, 2002; Brand and Brand, 2004). Natural surfactants containing saponins available commercially include Juazarine from the bark of *Zizyphus joazeiro* tree (Anonymous, 2004), horse chestnut saponins (Indena, 2005) and mixture of plant saponins (Bio-Saponins, Bio-Botanica, Inc., 2005). Saponins and sapogenins are also marketed as bioactive ingredients in cosmetic formulations with claims to delay the aging process of the skin (Yoo *et al.*, 2003; Bonte *et al.*, 1998), and prevent acne (Bombardelli *et al.*, 2001).

Commercial Applications

The diverse physicochemical and biological properties of saponins have been successfully exploited in a number of commercial applications in food, cosmetics, agricultural and pharmaceutical industries. Market trends towards the use of natural ingredients and increasing evidence of their biological activity have increased the demand for saponins (Brown, 1998; Malcolm, 1995). As natural non-ionic surfactants, they find widespread use as emulsifying and foaming agents, and detergents (San Martin and Briones, 1999; Balandrin, 1996). Other investigated/proposed applications of saponins and saponin containing plants include as feed additives (Cheeke, 1999; Zhan, 1999; Aoun *et al.*, 2003; Jensen and Elgaard, 2001), antibacterial (Henderson, 2001) and vegetable growth regulators (Yamauchi *et al.*, 2000), and for soil remediation (Roy *et al.*, 1997). While the two major commercial sources of saponins are *Quillaja saponaria* and *Yucca schidigera* extracts (San Martin and Briones, 1999; Balandrin, 1996), a number of other plant materials such as horse chestnut (Indena, 2005), tea seed (Zhan, 1999), and soybeans (Organic Technologies, 2005) are being utilized/evaluated for use as commercial sources of saponins. Pharmaceutical applications of saponins include as raw materials for production of hormones (Blunden *et al.,* 1975), immunological adjuvants (Kensil *et al.,* 2004), and as drugs (Panagin Pharmaceuticals Inc., 2005; Panacos, 2005). Saponins have also been reported to be the active ingredients in various natural health products, such as herbal extracts (Balandrin, 1996).

Conclusion

Saponins are a diverse family of secondary metabolites. Many plants used in traditional medicines worldwide contain saponins, which can often account for their biological and therapeutic action. It is believed that the natural role of these compounds in plants is to protect against attack by potential pathogens, which would account for their antimicrobial activity. Saponins can be utilized for their insecticidal, antibiotic, fungicidal, and other pharmacological properties. The membrane-permeabilising activity seems to be possessed by a large number of saponins, whether steroidal or triterpenoid. The adjuvant effect of specific saponins and their derivatives on the specific immune system function have been proved in animal models. Saponins also show wide-ranging cytostatic effects against cancer cells. The ability of saponins to lower the serum cholesterol level of animals has also been reported. These favourable effects point to the potentials of saponins, including those present in the diet, as a remedy against two of the major health hazards in many countries; obesity and cancer. Similarly, the sterol-mediated antiprotozoal and antifungal effects, and molluscicidal and antiviral effects, also offer considerable potentials in managing various diseases. Other properties ascribed to saponins such as the beneficial effects that some of them are reported to have on the efficiency of feed utilisation and growth in ruminants, single-stomached animals and fish need further experimental proof to be conclusively established, and studies need to be directed towards understanding the factors, dietary- or animal- or saponin-related, for presence or absence of these beneficial effects. Another important area that calls for further investigation relates to the effects of saponins or their derivatives on animal and human reproductive cycles and hormonal balance. It is difficult to establish clear functionality and structure–activity relationships regarding the effects of saponins in biological systems. This is largely due to the occurrence of a vast number of saponins with similar chemical structures, and to the complexity of cellular physiological reactions, which are often differently influenced by small and subtle differences in stereo-structures of effector ligands. Other factors that could have substantial influence on saponin actions could be their interactions with other dietary constituents. This chapter has provided an overview of the structural diversity, properties and applications of saponins, thus providing the reader with information regarding the various potential applications of saponins, and should stimulate further research into these compounds.

REFERENCES

Abe H, Odashima S. and Arichi S. (1978a). The effects of saikosaponins on biological membranes. 2. Changes in electron spin resonance spectra from spin labelled erythrocyte and erythrocyte ghost membranes. *Planta Medica* 34, 287–290.

Abe, H., Sakaguchi, M., Konishi, H., Tani, T. and Arichi, S. (1978b). The effects of saikosaponins on biological membranes. 1. The relationship between the structures of saikosaponins and haemolytic activity. *Planta Medica* 34, 160–166.

Achenbach, H., Hŭbner, H. and Reiter, M. (1996). Cholestane- and pregnanetype glycosides from the roots of *Tribulus cistoides*. *Phytochem.* 41, 907–917.

Adams, M.-M., Damani, P., Perl, N.R., Won, A., Hong, F., Livingston, P.O., Ragupathi, G. and Gin, D.Y. (2010). Design and synthesis of potent Quillaja saponin vaccine adjuvants. *J. Am. Chem. Soc.* 132, 1939–1945.

Ahmad, V.U., Khaliq-uz-Zaman, S.M., Shameel, S., Perveen, S. and Ali, Z. (1998). Steroidal saponins from *Asparagus dumosus*. *Phytochem.* 50, 481–484.

Aladesanmi, A.J. (2007). Tetrapleura tetraptera: molluscicidal activity and chemical constituents. *Afr. J. Tradit. Compl. Altern. Med.* 4, 23–36.

Al-Habori, M. and Raman, A. (1998). Antidiabetic and hypocholesterolaemic effects of *fenugreek* (Review). *Phytother. Res.* 12, 233–242.

Alice, C.B., Vargas, V.M.F., Silva, G.A.A.B., de Siqueira, N.C.S., Schapoval, E.E.S., Gleye, J., Henriques, J.A.P. and Henriques, A.T. (1991). Screening of plants used in south Brazilian folk medicine. *J. Ethnopharmacol.* 35,165–171.

Almawi, W.Y. and Melemedjian, O.K. (2002). Negative regulation of nuclear factor-kappa B activation and function by glucocorticoids. *J. Mol. Endocrinol.* 28, 69–78.

Andersen, C.Y. (2002). Possible new mechanism of cortisol action in female reproductive organs: physiological implications of the free hormone hypothesis. *J. Endocrinol.* 173, 211–217.

Anonymous. (2004). The fine line. *Soap, Perfumery and Cosmetics*, July:57.

Aoun, M., Amiand, G., Garres, P. and Boide, P. (2003). Food supplement used in feed formulations in ruminants. *WO Patent* 03/056935 A1.

Apers, S., Baronikova, S., Sindambiwe, J.B., Witvrouw, M., De Clercq, E., Vanden Berghe, D., Van Marck, E., Vlietinck, A. and Pieters, L. (2000). Antiviral, haemolytic and molluscicidal activities of triterpenoid saponins from *Maesa lanceolata*: establishment of structure-activity relationships. *Planta Medica* 67, 528–532.

Arletti, R., Benelli, A., Cavazzuti, E., Scarpetta, G. and Bertolini, A. (1999). Stimulating property of *Turnera diffusa* and *Pfaffia paniculata* extracts on the sexual behavior of male rats. *Psychopharmacol.* 143, 15–19.

Armah, C.N., Mackie, A.R., Roy, C., Price, K., Osbourn, A.E., Bowyer, P. and Ladha, S. (1999). The membrane-permeabilising effect of avenacin A-1 involves the reorganization of bilayer cholesterol. *Biophysical J.* 76, 281–290.

Ash, M., and Ash, I. (2002). *Handbook of Food Additives.* Synapse Information Resources, Inc., NY.

Ashida, T. and Matsuda, S. (1999). Food additive and its production. *JP Patent11*, 225,724.

Attele, A.S., Wu, J.A. and Yuan, C.S. (1999). Ginseng pharmacology. Multiple constituents and multiple actions. *Biochem. Pharmacol.* 58, 1685–1693.

Avato, P., Bucci, R., Tava, A., Vitali, C., Rosato, A., Bialy, Z. and Jurzysta, M. (2006). Antimicrobial activity of saponins from Medicago sp.: structure–activity relationship. *Phytother. Res.* 20, 454–457.

Balandrin, M.F. (1996). Commercial utilization of plant-derived saponins: An overview of medicinal, pharmaceutical, and industrial applications. In: G. R. Waller, and K. Yamasaki, Eds., *Saponins Used in Traditional Medicine,* pp. 1–14. Plenum Press, New York.

Bangham, A.D. and Horne, R.W. (1962). Action of saponins on biological cell membranes. *Nature* 196, 952–953.

Barr, I.G., Sjolander, A. and Cox, J.C. (1998). ISCOMs and other saponin based adjuvants (Review). *Adv. Drug Del. Rev.* 32, 247–271.

Baumann, E., Stoya, G., Volkner, A., Richter, W., Lemke, C. and Linss, W. (2000). Hemolysis of human erythrocytes with saponin affects the membrane structure. *Acta Histochem.* 102, 21–35.

Benie, T., El-Izzi, A., Tahiri, C., Duval, J. and Thieulant, M.L.T.I. (1990). Combretodendron africanum bark extract as an antifertility agent. I: Estrogenic effects *in vivo* and LH release by cultured gonadotrope cells. *J Ethnopharmacol.* 29, 13–23.

Berhow, M.A.,Wagner, E.D., Vaughn, S.F., and Plewa, M.J. (2000). Characterization and antimutagenic activity of soybean saponins. *Mut. Res.*, 448, 11–22.

Bhaggan, K., Cain, F.W., Pierce, J.H., Rogers, J.S. and Schmid, U. (2001). Fat blends with crystal modifiers. *EP Patent 1*,123,659 A1.

Bio-Saponin, Bio-Botanica Inc. (2005). Bio-saponins™ The natural surface active agent. *http://www.bio botanica.com/articles/articles.asp#,* accessed 11/10/2005.

Biswas, M., Kar, B., Bhattacharya, S., Kumar, R.B.S., Ghosh, A.K. and Haldar, P.K. (2011). Antihyperglycemic activity and antioxidant role of *Terminalia arjuna* leaf in streptozotocin induced diabetic rats. *Pharm. Biol.* 49(4): 335–340

Blunden, G., Culling, M.C. and Jewers, K. (1975). Steroidal sapogenins: a review of actual and potential plant sources. *Trop. Sci.* 17:139–154

Bombardelli, E. and Gabetta, B. (2001). Soya extract, process for its preparation and pharmaceutical composition. *US Patent* 6,280,777.

Bombardelli, E., Morazzoni, P., Cristoni, A. and Seghizzi, R. (2001). Pharmaceutical and cosmetic formulations with antimicrobial activity. *US Patent Application* 2001/0046525 A1.

Bomford, R., Stapleton, M., Winsor, S., Beesly, J.E., Jessup, E.A., Price, K.R. and Fenwick, G.R. (1992). Adjuvancity and ISCOM formation by structurally diverse saponins. *Vaccine*, 10, 572–577.

Bonte, F.,Meybeck, A. and Massiot, G. (1998). Method of treatment for combating the effects of aging on the condition of skin and hair.*US Patent* 5,770,223.

Brain, K., Hadgraft, J. and Al-Shatalebi M. (1990). Membrane modification in activity of plant molluscicides. *Planta Medica* 56, 663.

Brand, H. and Brand, E. (2004). A weighty issue. *Soap, Perfumery and Cosmetics Asia*, March: 27–31.

Brown, D.A. and London, E. (2000). Structure and function of sphingolipid- and cholesterol-rich membrane rafts. *J. Biol. Chem.* 275, 17221–17224.

Brown, R. (1998). The natural way in cosmetics and skin care. *Chemical Market Reporter*, 254(2), FR8–9.

Bruneton, J. (1995). *Pharmacognosie, Phytochimie, Plantes Médicinales; Ěditions Technique and Documentation*, Paris, p 1120

Cai, J., Liu, M., Wang, Z. and Ju, Y. (2002). Apoptosis induced by dioscin in Hela cells. *Biol. Pharm. Bull.* 25, 193–196.

Chauhan, G.S., Cui, W. and Eskin, N.A.M. (1999). Effect of saponin on the surface properties of quinoa proteins. *Int. J. Food Prop.* 2, 13–22.

Chavali, S.R., Francis, T. and Campbell, J.B. (1987). An *in vitro* study of immunodilatory effects of some saponins. *Int. J. Immunopharmacol.* 9, 675–683.

Cheeke, P.R. (1996). Biological effects of feed and forage saponins and their impact on animal production. In: GR Waller and Y Yamasaki, eds. *Saponins Used in Food and Agriculture,* pp. 377–386. New York: Plenum Press.

Cheeke, P.R. 1999. Actual and potential applications of *Yucca schidigera* and *Quillaja saponaria* saponins in human and animal nutrition. *Proceedings of the American Society of Animal Science, 1999.*

Chen, J.C., Xu, M.X., Chen, L.D., Chen, Y.N. and Chiu, T.H. (1998). Effect of *Panax notoginseng* saponins on sperm motility and progression *in vitro*. *Phytomed.* 5, 289–292.

Chen, R.J.Y., Chung, T.-Y., Li, F.-Y., Lin, N.-H. and Tzen, J.T.C. (2009). Effect of sugar positions in ginsenosides and their inhibitory potency on Na+/K+-ATPase activity. *Acta Pharmacol. Sin.* 30, 61–69.

Cheng, Z., Yu, B. and Yang, X. (2002). 27-Nor-triterpenoid glycosides from *Mitragyna inermis*. *Phytochem.* 61, 379–382.

Chindo, B.A., Anuka, J.A., Isaac, E., Ahmadu, A.A., Tarfa, F.D. and Gamaniel, K.S. (2010). Saponins are involved in the analgesic and anti-inflammatory properties of *Ficus platyphylla* stem bark. *Int. J. Biol. Chem. Sc.* 4, 415 – 423

Chindo, B.A., Anuka, J.A., McNeil, L., Yaro, A.H., Adamu, S.S., Amos, S., Connelly, W.K., Lees, G. and Gamaniel, K.S. (2009). Anticonvulsant properties of saponins from *Ficus platyphylla* stem bark. *Br. Res. Bull.* 78, 276 – 282

Choi, S., Jung, S.Y., Kim, C.H., Kim, H.S., Rhim, H., Kim, S.C. and Nah, S.Y. (2001). Effect of Ginsenosides on voltage-dependent Ca^{2+} channel subtypes in bovine chromaffin cells. *J. Ethnopharmacol.* 74, 75–81.

Chong-Ren Yang., Ying Zhang., Melissa R. Jacob., Shabana I. Khan., Ying-Jun Zhang and Xing-Cong Li. (2006). Antifungal Activity of C-27 Steroidal Saponins. *Antimicrob. Agents and Chem.* 50, 1710-1714

Chou, S.C., Ramanathan, S., Matsui, A., Rojers, J. and Cutting, W.C. (1971). Isolation of saponins with antifertility activity from *Gleditschia horrida. Indian J. Exp. Biol.* 9, 503–504.

Chung, E., Lee, K.Y., Lee, Y.J., Lee, Y.H. and Lee, S.K. (1998). Ginsenoside Rg1 down-regulates glucocorticoid receptor and displays synergistic effects with cAMP. *Steroids* 63, 421–424.

Chwalek, M., Lalun, N., Bobichon, H *et al.* (2006). Structure activity relationships of some hederagenin diglycosides: haemolysis, cytotoxicity and apoptosis induction. *Biochim Biophys Acta* 1760, 1418–1427

Coulter, A., Wong, T.Y., Drane, D., Bates, J., Macfarlan, R. and Cox, J. (1998). Studies on experimental adjuvanted influenza vaccines: comparison of immune stimulating complexes (Iscoms (TM)) and oil-in-water vaccines. *Vaccine* 16, 1243–1253.

Cox, J.C., Coulter, A.R., Morein, B., Lovgren-Bengtsson, K. and Sundquist, B. (2002). Saponin preparations and use thereof in ISCOMS. *US Patent* 6,352,697.

Dalsgaard, K. (1974). Saponin adjuvants III. Isolation of a substance from *Quillaja saponaria* Molina with adjuvant activity in foot-and-mouth disease vaccines. *Archiv fur die gesamte Virusforschung*, 44:243–254.

de Kloet, E.R., Reul, J.M., van den Bosch, F.R., Tonnaer, J.A. and Saito H (1987). Ginsenoside RG1 and corticosteroid receptors in rat brain. *Endocrinol. Japan* 34, 213–220.

de Oliveira, C.A.C., Perez, A.C., Merino, G., Prieto, J.G. and Alvarez, A.I. (2001). Protective effects of Panax ginseng on muscle injury and inflammation after eccentric exercise. *Comp. Biochem. Physiol.* 130, 369–377.

Delmas, F., D., Giorgio, C., Elias, R., Gasquet, M., Azas, N., Mshvildadze, V., Dekanosidze, G., Kemertelidze, E. and Timon-David, P. (2000). Antileishmanial activity of three saponins isolated from ivy, alpha-hederin, beta-hederin and hederacolchiside A(1), as compared with their action on mammalian cells cultured *in vitro. Planta Medica* 66, 343–347.

Deng, H.L. and Zhang, J.T. (1991). Anti-lipid peroxilative effect of ginsenoside Rb1 and Rg1. *Chinese Med. J.* 104, 395–398.

Dirk, D.D. and Webb, S.R. (2005). The next 15 years: Taking plant vaccines beyond proof of concept. *Immunol. Cell Biol.*, 83:248–256.

Dollahite, J.W., Shaver, T. and Camp, B.J. (1962). Injected saponins as abortifacients. *Amer. J. Vet. Res.* 23, 1261–1263.

Dong, M., Feng, X., Wang, B., Wu, L. And Ikejima, T. (2001). Two novel furostanol saponins from the rhizomes of *Dioscorea panthaica* Prain et Burkill and their cytotoxic activity. *Tetrahedron* 57, 501–506.

Dorsaz, A-C., Hostettmann, M. and Hostettmann, K. (1988). Molluscicidal saponins from *Sesbania sesban. Planta Medica* 54, 225–227.

Dourmashkin, R.R., Dougherty, R.M. and Harris, R.J.C. (1962). Electron microscopic observations on *Rous sarcoma* virus and cell membranes. *Nature* 194, 1116–1119.

El Izzi, A., Benie, T., Thieulant M-L., Le Men-Oliver, L. and Duval, J. (1992) Stimulation of LH release from cultured pituitary cells by saponins of *Petersianthus macrocarpus*: a permeabilising effect. *Planta Medica* 58, 229–233.

El Izzi, A., Duval, J. and Delaude, C. (1989). Effet d'une serie de saponines extrites de vegetaux de L'Afrique tropicale sur la liberation d'hormone luteinisante par les cellules hypophysaires en culture (Effect of a series of saponin extracts from African plants on the release of luteinizing hormone by hypophysial cells in culture). *Bulletin de la Societe´ Royale des Sciences de Liege* 58, 53–56.

ElSohly, H.N., Danner, S., Li, X.-C., Nimrod, A.C. and Clark, A.M. (1999). New antimycobacterial saponin from *Colubrina retusa*. *J. Nat. Prod.* 62, 1341–1342.

Enomoto, Y., Ito, K., Kawagoe, Y., Morio, Y. and Yamasaki, Y. (1986). Positive inotropic action of saponins on isolated atrial and papillary muscles from the guinea pig. *Br. J Pharmacol.* 88, 259–267.

Estrada, A., Li, B. and Laarveld, B. 1998. Adjuvant action of *Chenopodium quinoa* saponins on the induction of antibody responses to intragastric and intranasal administered antigens in mice. *Comp. Immunol. Microb.* 21, 225–236.

Fantini, J., Garmy, N., Mahfoud, R. and Yahi, N. (2002). Lipid rafts: structure, function and role in HIV, Alzheimer's and prion diseases. *Expert Rev. Mol. Med.* 4, 1–22.

Fenwick, G. R., Price, K. R., Tsukamoto, C. and Okubo, K. 1991. Saponins. In: J.P.F. D'Mello, C.M. Duffus, and J.H. Duffus, Eds. *Toxic Substances in Crop Plants*. pp. 285–327. *The Royal Society of Chemistry,* Cambridge.

Fiore. C., Eisenhut, M., Ragazzi E *et al.* (2005). A history of the therapeutic use of liquorice in Europe. *J. Ethnopharmacol.* 99, 317–324

Forse, R. A. and Chavali, S. (1997). Enternal formulations for treatment of inflammation and infection. *US Patent* 5,674,853.

Francis, G., Makkar, H.P.S. and Becker, K. (2001a). Antinutritional factors present in plant-derived alternate fish feed ingredients and their effects in fish. *Aquaculture* 199, 197–227.

Francis, G., Makkar, H.P.S. and Becker, K. (2001b). Effects of Quillaja saponins on growth, metabolism, egg production, and muscle cholesterol in individually reared Nile tilapia (*Oreochromis niloticus*). *Comp. Biochem. Physiol.* 129, 105–114.

Francis, G., Kerem, Z., Makkar, H.P.S. and Becker, K. (2002). The biological action of saponins in animal systems: A review. *Brit. J. Nutr.* 88, 587–605.

Gagliardo, R., Vignola, A.M. and Mathieu, M. (2001). Is there a role for glucocorticoid receptor beta in asthma? *Resp. Res.* 2, 1–4.

Gauthier, C., Legault, J., Girard-Lalancette K *et al.* (2009a). Haemolytic activity, cytotoxicity and membrane cell permeabilization of semi-synthetic and natural lupane- and oleanane-type saponins. *Bioorg. Med. Chem.* 17, 2002–2008

Gauthier, C., Legault, J. and Pichette, A. (2009b). Recent progress in the synthesis of naturally occurring triterpenoid saponins. *Mini-Rev. Org. Chem.* 6, 321–344

Gee, J.M., Price, K.R., Johnson, I.T. and Rhodes, M.J. (1998). The relationship between saponin structure and bioactivity – a preliminary study. In: Bardocz, S. and Pusztai, P., eds. Cost 98, *Effects of Antinutrients on the Nutritional Value of Legume Diets* no. 4, pp. 8–14. Luxemburg: European Commission.

Germonprez, N., van Puyvelde, L., Maes, L., van Tri, M., and de Kimpe, N. (2004). New pentacyclic triterpene saponins with strong anti-leishmanial activity from the leaves of *Maesa balansae*. *Tetrahedron* 60, 219–228.

Gestetner, B., Assa, Y., Henis, Y., Tencer, Y., Rotman, M., Birk, Y., and Bondi, A. (1972). Interaction of lucerne saponins with sterols. *Biochim. Biophys. Acta*, 270:181–187.

Gestetner, B., Assa,Y., Henis,Y., Birk,Y. and Bondi, A. (1971). Lucerne saponins IV. Relationship between their chemical constitution, and haemolytic and antifungal activities. *J. Sci. Food Agric.*, 22:168–172.

Giner, R.-M., Villalba, M.-L., Recio, M.-C., Manez, S., Cerda-Nicolas, M. and Rios, J.-L. (2000). Anti-inflammatory glycoterpenoids from *Scrophularia auriculata*. *Eur. J. Pharmacol.* 389, 243–252.

Glauert, A.M., Dingle, J.T. and Lucy, J.A. (1962). Action of saponin on biological cell membranes. *Nature* 196, 953–955.

Grenby, T.H. (1991). Intense sweeteners for the food industry: an overview. *Trends Food Sci. Technol.* 2, 2–6.

Godwithus Co., Ltd. (2005). Saponia [Korean Ginseng Oil]. *http://godwithus.en.ec21.com/GC00513155/Saponia [Korean Ginseng oil].html,* accessed on 11/10/2005.

Gogelein, H. and Huby, A. (1984). Interaction of saponin and digitonin with black lipid membranes and lipid monolayers. *Biochim. Biophys. Acta* 773, 32–38.

Gopalsamy, N., Gueho, J., Julien, H.R., Owadally, A.W. and Hostettmann, K. (1990). Molluscicidal saponins of *Polyscias dichroostachya*. *Phytochem.* 29, 793–795.

GüclüŪstündağ, O. and Mazza, G. (2007). Saponins: properties, applications and processing. *Crit. Rev. Food Sci. Nutr.* 47, 231–258.

Gurfinkel, D.M. and Rao, A.V. (2003). Soyasaponins: The relationship between chemical structure and colon anticarcinogenic activity. *Nutr. Cancer*, 47, 24–33.

Hamburger, M., Slacanin, I., Hostettmann, K., Dyatmiko, W. and Sutarjadi (1992). Acetylated saponins with molluscicidal activity from *Sapindus rarak*: unambiguous structure determination by proton nuclear magnetic resonance and quantitative analysis. *Phytochem. Anal.* 3, 231–237.

Han, L.K., Xu, B.J., Kimura, Y., Zheng, Y.N. and Okuda, H. (2000). *Platycodi radix* affects lipid metabolism in mice with high fat diet induced obesity. *J. Nutr.* 130, 2760–2764.

Hanausek, M., Ganesh, P., Walaszek, Z., Arntzen, C.J., Slaga, T.J. and Gutterman, J.U. (2001). Avicins, a family of triterpenoid saponins from *Acacia victoriae* (Bentham), suppress H-ras mutations and aneuploidy in a murine skin carcinogenesis model. *Pr. Nat. Acad. Sc. USA* 98, 11551–11556.

Haridas, V., Arntzen, C.J. and Gutterman, J.U. (2001a). Avicins, a family of triterpenoid saponins from *Acacia victoriae* (Bentham), inhibit activation of nuclear factor-kappa B by inhibiting both its nuclear localization and ability to bind DNA. *Pr. Nat. Acad. Sc. USA* 98, 11557–11562.

Haridas, V., Higuchi, M., Jayatilake, G.S., Bailey, D., Mujoo, K., Blake, M.E., Arntzen, C.J. and Gutterman JU (2001b) Avicins: triterpenoid saponins from *Acacia victoriae* (Bentham) induce apoptosis by mitochondrial perturbation. *Pr. Nat. Acad. Sc. USA* 98, 5821–5826.

Harris, W.S., Dujovne, C.A., Windsor, S.L., Gerrond, L.L.C., Newton, F.A. and Gelfand, R.A. (1997) Inhibiting cholesterol absorption with CP-88,818 (beta-tigogenin cellobioside; tiqueside): Studies in normal and hyperlipidemic subjects. *J. Cardiovas. Pharmacol.* 30, 55–60.

Harwood, H.J. Jr, Chandler, C.E., Pellarin, L.D., Bangerter, F.W., Wilkins, R.W., Long, C.A., Cosgrove, P.G., Malinow, M.R., Marcetta, C.A., Pettini, J.L., Savoy, Y.E. and Mayne, J.T. (1993). Pharmacologic consequences of cholesterol absorption inhibition: alteration in cholesterol metabolism and reduction in plasma cholesterol concentration induced by the synthetic saponin b-tigogenin cellobioside (CP-88818; tiqueside). *J. Lipid Res.* 34, 377–395.

Hase, J., Kobashi, K., Mitsui, K., Namba, T., Yoshizaki, M. and Tomimori, T. (1981). The structure–hemolysis relationship of oleanolic acid derivatives and inhibition of the saponin-induced hemolysis with sapogenins. *J. Pharmacobiodyn.* 4, 833–837.

He, X., Qiao, A., Wang X *et al.* (2006). Structural identification of methyl protodioscin metabolites in rats' urine and their antiproliferative activities against human tumor cell lines. *Steroids* 71:828–833

Henderson, G. M. (2001). Bio-enhancer. *US Patent* 6,228,265 B1.

Heng, L., Vincken, J.-P., van Koningsveld, G.A., Legger, L., Gruppen, H., van Boekel, M.A.J.S., Roozen, J.P. and Voragen, A.G.J. (2006). Bitterness of saponins and their content in dry peas. *J. Sci. Food Agric.* 86, 1225–1231.

Hidvegi, M. (1994). *Process for the preparation of a pharmaceutical composition selectively lowering the blood-lipid level.* US 5,277,910.

Hostettmann, K. and Marston, A. (1995). *Saponins.* Cambridge University Press, Cambridge, New York.

Hsiang, C.-Y., Lai, I.-L., Chao, D.-C., and Ho, T.-Y. (2002). Differential regulation of activator protein 1 activity by glycyrrhizin. *Life Sci.*, 70:1643–1656.

Hsu, H.-Y., Yang, J.-J. and Lin, C.-C. (1997). Effects of oleanolic acid and ursolic acid on inhibiting tumor growth and enhancing the recovery of hematopoietic system postirradiation in mice. *Cancer Lett.*, 111:7–13.

Hsu, Y.-L., Kuo, P.-L. and Lin, C.-C. (2004). The proliferative inhibition and apoptotic mechanism of Saikosaponin D in human non-small cell lung cancer A549 cells. *Life Sci.*, 75:1231–1242.

Hu, J., Lee, S.O., Hendrich, S. and Murphy, P.A. (2002). Quantification of the group B soyasaponins by high-performance liquid chromatography. *J. Agri. Food Chem.* 50, 2587–2594.

Hu, M., Konoki, K. and Tachibana, K. (1996). Cholesterol-independent membrane disruption caused by triterpenoid saponins. *Biochimica et Biophysica Acta – Lipid Metabolism* 1299, 252–258.

Hu, K. and Yao, X. (2001). Methyl protogracillin (NSC-698792): the spectrum of cytotoxicity against 60 human cancer cell lines in the National Cancer Institute's anticancer drug screen panel. *Anti-Cancer Drug* 12:541–547.

Hu, K. and Yao, X. (2002a). The cytotoxicity of protoneodioscin (NSC-698789), a furostanol saponin from the rhizomes of *Dioscorea collettii* var. *hypoglauca*, against human cancer cells *in vitro*. *Phytomed.* 9:560–565.

Hu, K. and Yao, X. (2002b). Protodioscin (NSC-698 796): its spectrum of cytotoxicity against sixty human cancer cell lines in an anticancer drug screen panel. *Planta Medica* 68:297–301.

Hu, K. and Yao, X. (2003). The cytotoxicity of methyl protoneogracillin (NSC-698793) and gracillin (NSC-698787), two steroidal saponins from the rhizomes of *Dioscorea collettii* var. hypoglauca, against human cancer cells *in vitro*. *Phytother. Res.*, 17:620–626.

Huang, H.-C., Liao, S.-C., Chang, F.-R., Kuo, Y.-H. and Wu, Y.-C. (2003). Molluscicidal saponins from *Sapindus mukorossi,* inhibitory agents of golden apple snails, *Pomacea canaliculata. J. Agric. Food Chem.* 51, 4916–4919.

Huang, D. and Qi, D. F. (2005). Dammarane sapogenins, their use as anti-cancer agents, and a process producing same. *US Patent* 6,888,014 B2.

Huang,W. and Jia,W. (2005). Use of ginsenosides Rh2 and Rg3, and aglycon ginsenosides for the prevention of cancer. *WO Patent Application* 2005/034963 A1.

Hwang, D.-C. and Damodaran, S. (1994). Selective precipitation of fat globule membranes of cheese whey by saponin and bile salt. *J. Agric. Food Chem.*, 42, 1872–1878.

Ibanoglu, E. and Ibanoglu, S. (2000). Foaming behavior of liquorice (*Glycyrrhiza glabra*) extract. *Food Chem.*70, 333–336.

Ikedo, S., Shimoyamada, M. and Watanabe, K. (1996). Interaction between bovine serum albumin and saponin as studied by heat stability and protease digestion. *J. Agric. Food Chem.* 44, 792–795.

Ikuta, A. and Itokawa, H. (1989). 30-Noroleanane saponins from callus tissues of *Akebia quinata. Phytochem.* 28, 2663–2665

Ikuta, A., Morikawa, A. and Kubota, K. (1991). A saponin from callus tissue of *Stauntonia hexaphylla. Phytochem.* 30, 2425–2427

Indena. (2005). Horse chestnut saponins. *http://www.indena.com/pdf/cosmleaf. pdf,* accessed 24/8/2005.

Iorizzi, M., Lanzotti, V., Ranalli, G., De Marino, S. and Zollo, F. (2002). Antimicrobial furostanol saponins from the seeds of *Capsicum annuum* L. var. *acuminatum. J. Agric. Food Chem.* 50, 4310–4316.

Jain, A.S., Surana, S.J., Gokhale, S.B., Tatiya, A.U. and Bothara, R.C. (2007). Antimicrobial properties of *Eranthemum roseum* (Vahl) R. *Br. Iranian J. Pharm. Res.* 6, 131-133

Jenkins, K.J. and Atwal, A.S. (1994) Effects of dietary saponins on fecal bile acids and neutral sterols, and availability of vitamins A and E in the chick. *J. Nut. Biochem.* 5, 134–138.

Jensen, J. M. and Elgaard, T. (2001). Natural feed additive, a method of preparing said feed additive, a feed mixture containing the feed additive as well as a method of breeding farm animals. *EP Patent* 1,129,627 A1.

Jia, W.W.-G., Bu, X., Philips, D., Yan, H., Liu, G., Chen, X., Bush, J.A. and Li, G. (2004). Rh2, a compound extracted from ginseng, hypersensitizes multidrug-resistant tumor cells to chemotherapy. *Can. J. Physiol. Pharmacol.* 82, 431–437.

Jia, Z., Koike, K., Kudo, M., Li, H. and Nikaido, T. (1998). Triterpenoid saponins and sapogenins from *Vaccaria segetalis. Phytochem.* 48, 529–536.

Junkuszew, M., Oleszek, W., Jurzysta, M., Piancente, S. and Pizza, C. (1998). Triterpenoid saponins from the seeds of *Amaranthus cruentus. Phytochem.* 49, 195–198.

Just, M.J., Recio, M.C., Giner, R.M., Cuéllar, M.J., Mañez, S., Bilia, A.R. and R′ıos, J.-L. (1998). Anti-inflammatory activity of unusual lupine saponins from *Bupleurum fruticescens. Planta Medica* 64, 404–407.

Kanchanapoom, T., Noiarsa, P., Kasai, R., Otsuka, H. and Ruchirawat, S. (2005). Justiciosides E–G, triterpenoidal glycosides with an unusual skeleton from *Justicia betonica*. *Tetrahedron* 61, 2583–2587.

Kensil, C.R. (1996) Saponins as vaccine adjuvants. *Cr. Rev. Ther. Drug Carrier Sys.* 13, 1–55

Kang, R. K. L., Zyzak, L. L. and Nakatsu, T. (1999). Flavored product additive and method for using same. *US Patent* 5, 948,460.

Kennelly, E.J., Cai, L., Long, L., Shamon, L., Zaw, K., Zhou, B.-N., Pezzuto, J.M., Kinghorn, A.D., 1995. Novel highly sweet secodammarane glycosides from *Pterocarya paliurus*. *J. Agric. Food Chem.* 43, 2602–2607.

Kensil, C. A. and Marciani, D. J. (1991). Saponin adjuvant. *US Patent* 5,057,540.

Kensil, C. R., Mo, A. X. and Truneh, A. (2004). Current vaccine adjuvants: an overview of a diverse class. *Frontiers in Bioscience* 9, 2972–2988.

Kerwin, S. M. (2004). Soy saponins and the anticancer effects of soybeans and soy-based foods. *Curr. Med. Chem. - Anti-Cancer Agents*, 4, 263–272.

Keukens, E.A.J., de Vrije, T., Fabrie, C.H.J.P., Demel, R.A., Jongen, W.M.F. and de Kruijff, B., (1992). Dual specificity of sterol-mediated glycoalkaloid induced membrane disruption. *Biochim. Biophys. Acta* 1110, 127–136.

Keukens, E.A.J., de Vrije, T., van den Boom, C., de Waard, P., Plasman, H.H., Thiel, F., Chupin, V., Jongen, W.M.F. and de Kruijff, B., (1995). Molecular basis of glycoalkaloid induced membrane disruption. *Biochim. Biophys. Acta* 1240, 216–228.

Khokhar, S. and Chauhan, B. M. (1986). Antinutritional factors in moth bean (*Vigna aconitifolia*): Varietal differences and effects of methods of domestic processing and cooking. *J. Food Sci.* 51, 591–594

Killeen, G.F., Madigan, C.A., Connolly, C.R., Walsh, G.A., Clark, C., Hynes, M.J., Timmins B.F., James P., Headon, D.R. and Power, R.F. (1998) Antimicrobial saponins of *Yucca Schidigera* and the implications of their *in vitro* properties for their *in vivo* impact. *J. Agric. Food Chem.* 46, 3178–3186.

Kim, D.H., Jung, J.S., Suh, H.W., Huh, S.O., Min, S.K., Son, B.K., Park, J.H., Kim, N.D., Kim, Y.H. and Song, D.K., (1998a). Inhibition of stressinduced plasma corticosterone levels by Ginsenosides in mice: involvement of nitric oxide. *Neuroreport* 9, 2261–2264.

Kim, D.W., Bang, K.H., Rhee, Y.H., Lee, K.T. and Park, H.J. (1998b). Growth inhibitory activities of kalopanaxsaponins A and I against human pathogenic fungi. *Arch. Pharm. Res.* 21, 688–691.

Kim, S.J., Kim, Y.Y., Ko, K.H., Hong, E.K., Han, Y.B., Kang, B.H. and Kim, H. (1998c). Butanol extract of 1 : 1 mixture of Phellodendron cortex and Aralia cortex stimulates PI3-kinase and ERK2 with increase of glycogen levels in HepG2 cells. *Phytother. Res.* 12, 255–260.

Kim, Y.H., Park, K.H. and Rho, H.M. (1996). Transcriptional activation of the Cu, Zn-superoxide dismutase gene through the AP2 site by ginsenoside Rb2 extracted from a medicinal plant, *Panax ginseng*. *J. Biol. Chem.* 271, 24539–24543.

Kim, Y.R., Lee, S.Y., Shin, B.A. and Kim, K.M. (1999) *Panax ginseng* blocks morphine-induced thymic apoptosis by lowering plasma corticosterone level. *Gen. Pharmacol.* 32, 647–652.

Kim, D.-H., Bae, E.-A., Han, M.-J., Choo, M.-K., Park, E.-K., and Park, J.-H. (2003a). Novel use of the extract of processed panax genus plant and saponin compound isolated therefrom. *US Patent Application* 2003/0190377 A1.

Kim, N. D., Park, M. K., Lee, S. K., Park, J. H., and Kim, J. M. (1998b). Processed ginseng product with enhanced pharmacological effects. *USPatent* 5,776,460.

Kim, S.-W., Park, S.-K., Kang, S.-I., Kang, H.-C., Oh, H.-J., Bae, C.-Y. and Bae, D.-H. (2003b). Hypocholesterolemic property of *Yucca schidigera* and *Quillaja saponaria* extracts in human body. *Arch. Pharm. Res.,* 26:1042–1046.

Kimata, H., Nakashima, T., Kokubun, S., Nakayama, K., Mitoma, Y., Kitahara, T.,Yata, N., andTanaka, O. (1983). Saponins of pericarps of *Sapindus mukurossi* GAERTN. and solubilization of monodesmosides by bidesmosides. *Chem. Pharm. Bull.* 31, 1998–2005.

Kishor, N. and Sati, O.P. (1990) A new molluscicidal spirostanol glycoside of *Yucca alufolia*. *J. Nat. Prod.* 53, 1557–1559.

Kitagawa, I. (2002). Licorice root. A natural sweetener and an important ingredient in Chinese medicine. *Pure Appl. Chem.* 74, 1189–1198.

Konishi, M., Hano, Y., Takayama, M., Nomura, T., Hamzah, A.S., Ahmad, R.B., and Jamani, H. (1998). Triterpenoid saponins from *Hedyotis nudicaulis*. *Phytochem.*48, 525–528.

Konoshima, T., Takasaki, M., Tokuda, H., Nishino, H., Duc, N.M., Kasai, R. and Yamasaki, K. (1998) Anti-tumor-promoting activity of majonoside-R2 from *Vietnamese ginseng, Panax vietnamensis* SHV. (I). *Biol. Pharmac. Bull.* 21, 834–838.

Krawczyk, E., Suprynowicz, F.A., Sudarshan, S.R., Schlegel, R.. (2010). Membrane orientation of the human papillomavirus type 16 E5 oncoprotein. *J. Virol.* 84, 1696–1703.

Kudou, S., Tonomura, M., Tsukamoto, C., Uchida, T., Sakabe, T., Tamura, N., and Okubo, K. (1993). Isolation and structural elucidation of DDMP conjugated soyasaponins as genuine saponins from soybean seeds. *Biosci. Biotech. Biochem.* 57, 546–560.

Kuroda M, Mimaki Y, Hasegawa F, Yokosuka A, Sashida Y and Sakagami H (2001). Steroidal glycosides from the bulbs of *Camassia leichtlinii* and their cytotoxic activities. *Chem. Pharm. Bull.* 49, 726–731.

Kuzina, V., Ekstrom, C.T., Andersen, S.B., Nielsen, J.K., Olsen, C.E., Bak, S. (2009). Identification of defense compounds in *Barbarea vulgaris* against the herbivore *Phyllotreta nemorum* by an ecometabolomic approach. *Plant Physiol.* 151, 1977–1990.

Kuznetzova, T.A., Anisimov, M.M. and Popov, A.M. (1982). A comparative study *in vitro* of physiological activity of triterpene glycosides of marine invertebrates of echinoderm type. *Comp. Biochem. Phy.* 73C, 41–43.

Kwak, W.J., Han, C.K., Chang, H.W., Kim, H.P., Kang, S.S. and Son, K.H. (2003). Loniceroside C, an antiinflammatory saponin from *Lonicera japonica*. *Chem. Pharm. Bull.* 51, 333–335.

Lacaille-Dubois, M.A., Hanquet, B., Cui, Z.H., Lou, Z.C. and Wagner, H. (1999) A new biologically active acylated triterpene saponin from *Silene fortunei*. *J. Nat. Prod.* 62, 133–136.

Lacaille-Dubois, M.A., and Wagner, H. (1996). A review of the biological and pharmacological activities of saponins. *Phytomed.* 2, 363–386.

Lavaud, C., Massiot, G., Le Men-Olivier, L., Viari, A., Vigny, P., Delaude, C. (1992). Saponins from *Steganotaenia araliacea*. *Phytochem.* 31, 3177–3181.

Lee, K.T., Sohn, I.C., Kim, D.H., Choi, J.W. and Kwon, S.H. (2000a) Hypoglycaemic and hypolipidemic effects of tectorigenin and kaikasaponin III in the streptozotocin-induced diabetic rat and their antioxidant activity *in vitro*. *Arch. Pharm. Res.* 23, 461–466.

Lee, K.T., Sohn, I.C., Park, H.J., Kim, D.W. and Jung, G.O. (2000b). Essential moiety for antimutagenic and cytotoxic activity of hederagenin monodesmosides and bisdesmosides isolated from the stem bark of *Kalopanax pictus*. *Planta Medica* 66, 329–332.

Lee, S.J., Ko, W.G., Kim, J.H., Sung, J.H., Lee, S.J., Moon, C.K. and Lee, B.H. (2000c). Induction of apoptosis by a novel intestinal metabolite of ginseng saponin via cytochrome c-mediated activation of caspase-3 protease. *Biochem. Pharmacol.* 60, 677–685

Lee, Y.J., Chung, E., Lee, K.Y., Lee, Y.H., Huh, B. and Lee, S.K. (1997). Ginsenoside-Rg1, one of the major active molecules from *Panax ginseng*, is a functional ligand of glucocorticoid receptor. *Mol. Cell. Endocr.* 133, 135–140.

Lee, M.-W., Kim, S.U. and Hahn, D.-R. (2001). Antifungal activity of modified hederagenin glycosides from the leaves of *Kalopanax pictum* var. chinese. *Biol. Pharm. Bull.* 24, 718–719.

Lemma A (1965) A preliminary report on the molluscicidal property of endod (*Phytolacca dodecandra*). *Ethiop. Med. J.* 3, 187.

Li, W., Asada, Y., Koike, K., Nikaido, T., Furuya, T. and Yoshikawa, T. (2005). Bellisosides A–F, six novel acylated triterpenoid saponins from *Bellis perennis* (compositae). *Tetrahedron* 61, 2921–2929

Lin, F. and Wang, R. (2010). Hemolytic mechanism of dioscin proposed by molecular dynamics simulations. *J. Mol. Model* 16, 107–118.

Liu, J. (1995). Pharmacology of oleanolic acid and ursolic acid. *J. Ethnopharmacol.* 49:57–68.

Liu, J. and Henkel, T. (2002). Traditional Chinese Medicine (TCM): Are polyphenols and saponins the key ingredients triggering biological activities? *Curr. Med. Chem.* 9, 1483–1485.

Liu, W. K., Xu, S. X., and Che, C. T. (2000). Anti-proliferative effect of ginseng saponins on human prostate cancer cell line. *Life Sci.* 67, 1297–1306.

Lu, Y., Umeda, T., Yagi, A., Sakata, K., Chaudhuri, T., Ganguly, D.K., Sarma, S., (2000). Triterpenoid saponins from the roots of tea plant (*Camellia sinensis* var. assamica). *Phytochem.* 53, 941–946

Liu, H.-W., Li, J.-K., Zhang, D.-W., Zhang, J.-C., Wang, N.-L., Cai, G.-P., Yao and X.-S. (2008). Two new steroidal compounds from starfish *Asterias amurensis* Lutken. *J. Asian Nat. Prod. Res.* 10, 521–529.

Lucas, E. A., Khalil, D. A., Daggy, B. P., and Arjmandi, B. H. (2001). Ethanolextracted soy protein isolate does not modulate serum cholesterol in golden syrian hamsters: a model of postmenopausal hypercholesterolemia. *J. Nutr.* 131, 211–214.

Ma, L.Y. and Xiao, P.G. (1998). Effects of *Panax notoginseng* saponins on platelet aggregation in rats with middle cerebral artery occlusion or *in vitro* and on lipid fluidity of platelet membrane. *Phytother. Res.* 12, 138–140.

Ma, B., Dong, J. and Wang, B. 2003. Use of steroidal saponins for the propylaxis or treatment of dementia, and novel steroidal saponin compounds. *US Patent* 6,593,301.

Maharaj, K., Froh, K.H. and Campbell, J.B. (1986). Immune responses of mice to inactivated rabies vaccine administered orally: potentiation by Quillaja saponin. *Canadian J. Microbiol.* 32, 414–420.

Malcolm, C. (1995). Teetertottering between synthetic and 'natural'. *DCI*, 156 (5):50.

Marino, S.D., Iorizzi, M., Palagiano, E., Zollo, F. and Roussakis, C. (1998). Starfish saponins. 55. Isolation, structure elucidation, and biological activity of steroid oligoglycosides from an Antarctic starfish of the family Asteriidae. *J. Nat. Prod.* 61, 1319–1327.

Marker, R. E., Wagner, R. B., Ulshafer, P. R., Wittbecker, G. P. J., and Ruof, C. H. (1947). Steroidal sapogenins. *J. Am. Chem. Soc.* 69, 2167–2230.

Marston, A., Wolfender, J.L. and Hostettmann, K. (2000). Analysis and isolation of saponins from plant material. In *Saponins in Food, Feedstuffs and Medicinal Plants, Annual Proceedings of the Phytochemical Society*, pp. 1–12 [W Oleszek and A Marston, editors]. Oxford and London: Clarendon Press.

Matsuda, H., Li, Y., Yamahara, J. and Yoshikawa, M. (1999a). Inhibition of gastric emptying by triterpene saponin, momordin Ic, in mice: Roles of blood glucose, capsaicin-sensitive sensory nerves, and central nervous system. *J. Pharmacol. Exp. Ther.* 289, 729–734.

Matsuda, H., Li, Y.H., Murakami, T., Yamahara, J. and Yoshikawa, M. (1999b). Structure-related inhibitory activity of oleanolic acid glycosides on gastric emptying in mice. *Bioorg. Med. Chem.* 7, 323–327.

Matsuda, H., Murakami, K., Ninomiya, K., Yamahara, J. and Yoshikawa, M. (1997). Effects of escins 1a, 1b, 11a, and 11b from horse chestnut, the seeds of *Aesculus hippocastanum* L, on acute inflammation in animals. *Chem. Pharm. Bull.* 20, 1092–1095.

Matsuura, H. (2001). Saponins in garlic as modifiers of the risk of cardiovascular disease. *J. Nutr.* 131, 1000S–1005S.

Mazzucchelli, G.D., Cellier, N.A., Mshviladzade, V., Elias, R., Shim, Y.-H., Touboul, D., Quinton, L., Brunelle, A., Laprevote, O., de Pauw, E.A. and de Pauw-Gillet, M.-C. (2008). Pores formation on cell membranes by hederacolchiside A1 leads to a rapid release of proteins for cytosolic subproteome analysis. *J. Proteome Res.* 7, 1683–1692.

McAllister, T.A., Annett, C.B., Cockwill, C.L., Olson, M.E., Wang, Y. and Cheeke, P.R. (2001). Studies on the use of *Yucca schidigera* to control giardiosis. *Vet. Parasitol.* 97, 85–99.

Melzig, M.F., Bader, G. and Loose, R. (2001). Investigations of the mechanism of membrane activity of selected triterpenoid saponins. *Planta Medica* 67, 43–48.

Mengoni, F., Lichtner, M., Battinelli, L., Marzi, M., Mastroianni, C.M., Vullo, V. and Mazzanti, G. (2002). *In vitro* anti-HIV activity of oleanolic acid on infected human mononuclear cells. *Planta Medica* 68, 111–114.

Menzies, G.S., Howland, K., Rae, M.T. and Bramley, T.A. (1999). Stimulation of specific binding of [3H]-progesterone to bovine luteal cell-surface membranes: specificity of digitonin. *Mol. Cell. Endocrinol.*153, 57–69.

Micich, T. J., Foglia, T. A., and Holsinger, V. H. (1992). Polymer-supported saponins: An approach to cholesterol removal from butteroil. *J. Agric. Food Chem.* 40, 1321–1325

Milgate, J., and Roberts, D. C. K. (1995). The nutritional and biological significance of saponins. *Nutr. Res.* 15, 1223–1249.

Mimaki, Y., Kuroda, M., Kameyama, A., Yokosuka, A. and Sashida, Y. (1998b). Steroidal saponins from the rhizomes of *Hosta sieboldii* and their cytostatic activity on HL-60 cells. *Phytochem.* 48, 1361–1369.

Mimaki, Y., Kuroda, M., Kameyama, A., Yokosuka, A. and Sashida, Y., Francis *et al.* (1998a). Steroidal saponins from the underground parts of *Ruscus aculeatus* and their cytostatic activity on HL-60 cells. *Phytochem.* 48, 485–493.

Mimaki, Y., Kameyama, A., Kuroda, M., Sashida, Y., Hirano, T., Oka, K., Koike, K. and Nikaido, T. (1997a). Steroidal glycosides from the underground parts of *Hosta plantaginea* Var. japonica and their cytostatic activity on leukaemia HL-60 cells. *Phytochem.* 44, 305–310.

Mimaki, Y., Takaashi, Y., Kuroda, M., Sashida, Y., 1997b. Steroidal glucosides from leaves of *Cordyline stricta*. *Phytochem.* 45, 1229–1234.

Mitra, S., and Dungan, S.R. (1997). Micellar properties of quillaja saponin. 1. Effects of temperature, salt and pH on solution properties. *J. Agric. Food Chem.* 45, 1587–1595.

Miyakoshi, M., Tamura, Y., Masuda, H., Mizutani, K., Tanaka, O., Ikeda, T., Ohtani, K., Kasai, R. and Yamasaki, K. (2000). Antiyeast steroidal saponins from *Yucca schidigera* (Mohave yucca), a new anti-food-deteriorating agent. *J. Nat. Prod.* 63, 332–338.

Miyase, T., Andoh, T. and Ueno, A. (1995). Linderniosides A and B, oleanane saponins from *Lindernia pyxidaria*. *Phytochem.* 40, 1499–1502.

Mølgaard, P., Chihaka, A., Lemmich, E., Furu, P., Windber, C., Ingerslev, F. and Halling-Sørensen, B., 2000. Biodegradability of the molluscicidal saponins of *Phytolacca dodecandra*. *Regul. Tox. Pharmacol.*32, 248–255.

Monder, C., Stewart, P.M., Lakshmi, V., Valentino, R., Burt, D. and Edwards, C.R.W. (1989). Licorice inhibits corticosteroid 11bdehydrogenase of rat kidney and liver: *in vivo* and *in vitro* studies. *Endocrinol.* 125, 1046–1053.

Morehouse, L.A., Bangerter, F.W., DeNinno, M.P., Inskeep, P.B., McCarthy, P.A., Pettini, J.L., Savoy, Y.E., Sugarman, E.D., Wilkins, R.W., Wilson, T.C., Woody, H.A., Zaccaro, L.M. and Chandler, C.E. (1999). Comparison of synthetic saponin cholesterol absorption inhibitors in rabbits: evidence for a non-stoichiometric, intestinal mechanism of action. *J. Lipid Res.* 40, 464–474.

Morrissey, J.P. and Osbourn, A.E. (1999). Fungal resistance to plant antibiotics as a mechanism of phatogenesis. *Mol. Biol. Rev.* 63, 708–724.

Morton, P.A.J. and Murray, B.S. (2001). Acid beverage floc: Protein-saponin interaction and an unstable emulsion model. *Colloid. Surface Biointerfaces* 21, 101–106.

Mowat, A.M., Smith, R.E., Donachie, A.M., Furrie, E., Grdic, D. and Lycke, N. (1999). Oral vaccination with immune stimulating complexes. *Immunol. Lett.* 65, 133–140.

Muir, A.D., Ballantyne, K.D. and Hall, T.W. (2000). LC-MS and LC-MS/MS analysis of saponins and sapogenins – comparison of ionization techniques and their usefulness in compound identification. In Saponins in Food, Feedstuffs and Medicinal Plants, *Annual Proceedings of the Phytochemical Society*, pp. 35–42 [W Oleszek and A Marston, editors]. Oxford and London: Clarendon Press

Muir, A. D., Paton, D., Ballantyne, K., and Aubin, A. A. (2002). Process for recovery and purification of saponins and sapogenins from quinoa (*Chenopodium quinoa*). *US Patent 6,355,249.*

Mujoo, K., Haridas, V., Hoffmann, J.J., Wachter, G.A., Hutter, L.K., Lu, Y., Blake, M.E., Jayatilake, G.S., Bailey, D., Mills, G.B. and Gutterman, J.U. (2001). Triterpenoid saponins from *Acacia victoriae* (Bentham) decrease tumor cell proliferation and induce apoptosis. *Cancer Res.* 61, 5486–5490.

Muller, R.E., and Morris, R.J. Jr. (1966). Sucrose-ammoniated glycyrrhizin sweetening agent. *US Patent* 3,282,706.

Murakami, T., Nakamura, J., Matsuda, H. and Yoshikawa, M. (1999). Bioactive saponins and glycosides. XV. Saponin constituents with gastroprotective effect from the seeds of tea plant, *Camellia sinensis* L var. assamica Pierre, cultivated in Sri Lanka: Structures of assamsaponins A, B, C, D, and E. *Chem. Pharm. Bull.* 47, 1759–1764.

Nakamura, T., Inoue, K., Nojima, S., Sankawa, U., Shoji, J., Kawasaki, T. and Shibata, S. (1979). Interaction of saponins with red blood cells as well as with the phosphatidylcholine liposomal membranes. *J. Pharm. Dyn.* 2, 374–382.

Namba, T., Yoshsaki, M., Tomimori, T., Kobashi, K., Mitsui, K. and Hase, J. (1973). Haemolytic and protective activity of ginseng saponins. *Chem. Pharm. Bull.* 21, 459–461.

Naruse, M., Suetomo, H., Matsubara, T., Sato, T., Yanagawa, H., Hoshi, M. and Matsumoto, M. (2010). Acrosome reaction-related steroidal saponin, Co-ARIS, from the starfish induced structural changes in microdomains. *Dev. Biol.* 347, 147–153.

Navarro, P., Giner, R.M., Recio, M.C., Máñez, S., Cerdá-Nicolàs, M. and Rìos, J.-L., 2001. *In vivo* anti-inflammatory activity of saponins from *Bupleurum rotundifolium*. *Life Scien.* 68, 1199–1206.

Newbold, C.J., El Hassan, S.M., Wang, J., Ortega, M.E. and Wallace, R.J. (1997). Influence of foliage from African multipurpose trees on activity of rumen protozoa and bacteria. *Brit. J. Nutrit.* 78, 237–249.

Nguyen, T.D., Villard, P.H., Barlatier, A., Elsisi, A.E., Jouve, E., Duc, N.M., Sauze, C., Durand, A. and Lacarelle, B. (2000). *Panax vietnamensis* protects mice against carbon tetrachloride-induced hepatotoxicity without any modification of CYP2E1 gene expression. *Planta Medica* 66, 714–719.

Nielsen, J.K., Nagao, T., Okabe, H. and Shinoda, T. (2010). Resistance in the plant, *Barbarea vulgaris,* and counter-adaptions in flea beetles mediated by saponins. *J. Chem. Ecol.* 36, 277–285.

Nishikawa, M., Nojima, S., Akiyama, T., Sankawa, U. and Inoue, K. (1984). Interaction of digitonin and its analogs with membrane cholesterol. *J. Biochem.* 96, 1231–1239.

Niu, C.-S., Yeh, C.-H., Yeh, M.-F. and Cheng, J.-T., 2009. Increase of adipogenesis by ginsenoside (Rh2) in 3T3-L1 cell via an activation of glucocorticoid receptor. *Horm. Metab. Res.* 41, 271–276.

Oakenfull, D. (1981). Saponins in food-a review. *Food Chem.*, 6, 19–40.

Oakenfull, D. (1986). Aggregation of saponins and bile acids in aqueous solution. *Aust. J. Chem.* 39, 1671–1683.

Oakenfull, D. (2001). Soy protein, saponins and plasma cholesterol. *J. Nutr.* 131, 2971.

Oakenfull, D., and Sidhu, G.S. (1989). Saponins. In: Cheeke, P. R., Ed., *Toxicants of Plant Origin, Vol II Glycosides*. CRC Pres, Inc. Boca Raton, Florida, pp. 97–141.

Oakenfull, D., and Sidhu, G.S. 1990. Could saponins be a useful treatment for hypercholesterolaemia? *Eur. J. Clin. Nutr.* 44, 79–88.

Oda, K., Matsuda, H., Murakami, T., Katayama, S., Ohgitani, T. and Yoshikawa, M. (2000). Adjuvant and haemolytic activities of 47 saponins derived from medicinal and food plants. *Biol. Chem.* 381, 67–74.

Oh, Y.J. and Sung, M.K. (2001). Soybean saponins inhibit cell proliferation by suppressing PKC activation and induce differentiation of HT-29 human colon adenocarcinoma cells. *Nutrit. Cancer* 39, 132–138.

Okubo, K. and Yoshiki, Y. (1996). Oxygen-radical-scavenging activity of DDMP-conjugated saponins and physiological role in leguminous plant. In*: Waller, G.R., Yamasaki, K. (Eds.), Saponins Used in Food and Agriculture*. Plenum Press, New York, pp. 141–154.

Olmstead, M. J. (2002). Organic toothpaste containing saponin. *US Patent* 6,485,711 B1.

Organic Technologies. (2005). Organic Technologies Products. http://www.organictech.com/products/index.html, accessed 11/10/2005. Panacos. 2005. A new generation of anti-infective drugs. *http://www. panacos.com/product 2.htm,* accessed 11/10/2005.

Osbourn, A.E. (2003). Saponins in cereals. *Phytochem.* 62, 1–4

Oulad-Ali, A., Guillaume, D., Weniger, B., Jiang, Y. and Anton, R. (1994). Mabiosides C–E: Triterpenoid saponins from the bark of *Colubrina elliptica. Phytochem.* 36, 445–448

Ouyang, M.-A., Wang, H.-Q., Liu, Y.-Q., Yang, C.-R., 1997. Triterpenoid saponins from the leaves of *Ilex latifolia. Phytochem.* 45, 1501–1505.

Panacos. (2005). A new generation of anti-infective drugs. http://www. panacos.com/product 2.htm, accessed 11/10/2005.

Panagin Pharmaceuticals Inc. (2005). *http://www.panagin.com/index.htm,* accessed 23/8/2005.

Park, I. H., Piao, L. Z., Kwon, S. W., Lee, J. Y., Cho, S. Y., Park, M. K., and Park, J. H. (2002). Cytotoxic dammarane glycosides from processed ginseng. *Chem. Pharm. Bull.* 50, 538–540.

Park, S.-Y., Chang, S.-Y., Oh, O.-J., Yook, C.-S. and Nohara, T. (2002). Nor- Oleanene type triterpene glycosides from the leaves of *Acanthopanax japonicus. Phytochem.* 59, 379–384 .

Pawar, R., Gopalakrishnan, C. and Bhutani, K.K. (2001). Dammarane triterpene saponin from *Bacopa monniera* as the superoxide inhibitor in polymorphonuclear cells. *Planta Medica* 67, 752–754.

Petit, P.R., Sauvaire, Y., Ponsin, G., Manteghetti, M., Fave, A. and Ribes, G. (1993). Effects of a fenugreek seed extract on feeding behaviour in the rat: metabolic endocrine correlates. *Pharmaco. Biochem. Behav.* 45, 369–374.

Petit, P.R., Sauvaire, Y.D., Hillairebuys, D.M., Leconte, O.M., Baissac, Y.G., Ponsin, G.R. and Ribes, G.R. (1995). Steroid saponins from fenugreek seeds – extraction, purification, and pharmacological investigation on feeding behavior and plasma cholesterol. *Steroids* 60, 674–680.

Pires, V.S., Taketa, A.T.C., Gosmann, G. and Schenkel, E.P. (2002). Saponins and sapogenins from *Brachiaria decumbens* Stapf. J. *Braz. Chem. Soc.* 13, 135–139.

Plock, A., Sokolowska-Kohler, W. and Presber, W. (2001). Application of flow cytometry and microscopical methods to characterize the effect of herbal drugs on Leishmania spp. *Exp. Parasitol.* 97, 141–153.

Plohmann, B., Bader, G., Hiller, K. and Franz, G. (1997). Immunomodulatory and antitumoral effects of triterpenoid saponins. *Pharmazie* 52, 953–957.

Pöllmann, K., Schaller, K., Schweizer, U., Elgamal, M.H.A., Shaker, K.H. and Seifert, K. (1998). Triterpenoid saponins from *Zygophyllum decumbens. Phytochem.* 48, 875–880.

Podolak, I., Elas, M. and Cieszka, K. (1998). *In vitro* antifungal and cytotoxic activity of triterpene saponosides and quinoid pigments from *Lysimachia vulgaris* L. *Phytother. Res.*12, S70–S73.

Podolak, I., Galanty, A., Sobolewska, D. (2010). Saponins as cytotoxic agents: a review. *Phytochem. Rev.* 9, 425–474

Potter, S. M., Jimenez-Flores, R., Pollack, J., Lone, T. A., and Berber-Jimenez, M. D. (1993). Protein-saponin interaction and its influence on blood lipids. *J. Agric. Food Chem.* 41,1287–1291.

Price, K. R., Johnson, I. T., and Fenwick, G.R. (1987). The chemistry and biological significance of saponins in foods and feeding stuffs. *CRC Crit. Rev. Food Sci.* 26, 27–135.

Punnonen, R. and Lukola, A. (1980). Oestrogen-like effect of ginseng. *Brit. Med. J.* 281, 1110.

Quin, G-W. and Xu, R-S. (1998). Recent advances in bioactive natural products from Chinese medicinal plants. *Med. Res. Rev.* 18, 375–382.

Raju, J., Patlolla, J.M.R.,Swamy,M.V. and Rao, C.V. (2004). Diosgenin, a steroid saponin of *Trigonella foenum* graecum (Fenugreek), inhibits azoxymethaneinduced aberrant crypt foci formation in F344 rats and induces apoptosis in HT-29 human colon cancer cells. *Cancer Epidem. Biomar.*, 13,1392–1398.

Rao, A.V. and Gurfinkel, D.M. (2000). The bioactivity of saponins: triterpenoid and steroid glycosides. *Drug Metab. Drug Interact.* 17, 211–235

Rao, A.V. and Sung, M.-K. (1995). Saponins as anticarcinogens. *J. Nutr.*, 125, 717S–724S.

Recchia, J., Lurantos, M.H.A., Amsden, J.A., Storey, J. and Kensil, C.R .(1995). A semisynthetic Quillaja saponin as a drug delivery agent for aminoglycosaide antibiotics. *Pharm. Res.* 12, 1917–1923.

Rhiouani, H., Settaf, A., Lyoussi, B., Cherrah, Y. and Lacaille-Dubois, A. (1999). Effects of saponins from *Herniaria glabra* on blood pressure and renal function in spontaneously hypertensive rats. *Therapie* 54, 735–739.

Richardson, T. and Jimenez-Flores, R. (1994). *Process to remove cholesterol from dairy products* 5,326,579.

Rickert, D. A.,Meyer, M. A., Hu, J., and Murphy, P. A. (2004). Effect of extraction pH and temperature on isoflavone and saponin partitioning and profile during soy protein isolate production. *J. Food Sci.* 69, C623–C630.

Ridout, C. L., Price, K. R., DuPont, M. S., Parker, M. L., and Fenwick, G. R. (1991). Quinoa saponins-Analysis and preliminary investigations into the effects of reduction by processing. *J. Sci. Food Agric.* 54, 165–176.

Riguera, R. (1997). Isolating bioactive compounds from marine organisms. *J. Marine Biotech.* 5, 187–193.

Ronnberg, B., Fekadu, M., Behboudi, S., Kenne, L. and Morein, B. (1997). Effects of carbohydrate modification of *Quillaja saponaria* Molina QH-B fraction on adjuvant activity, cholesterol binding capacity and toxicity. *Vaccine* 15, 1820–1826.

Rosenqvist, E., Michaelsen, T.E. and Vistnes, A.I. (1980). Effect of streptolysin O and digitonin on egg lecithin/cholesterol vesicles. *Biochim. Biophys. Acta* 600, 91–102.

Roy, D., Kommalapati, R. R., Mandava, S. S., Valsaraj, K. T. and Constant, W. D. (1997). Soil washing potential of a natural surfactant. *Environ. Sci. Technol.* 31, 670–695.

Rudakewich, M., Ba, F. and Benishin, C.G. (2001). Neurotrophic and neuroprotective actions of Ginsenosides Rb(1) and Rg(1). *Planta Medica* 67, 533–537.

Sahu, N.P, Banerjee, S., Mondal, N.B. and Mandal, D. (2008). Steroidal saponins. In: *Fortschritte der Chemie Organischer Naturstoffe/progress in the chemistry of organic natural products, fortschritte der chemie organischer naturstoffe/progress in the chemistry of organic natural products*, vol 89. Springer, Vienna, pp 45–141

Sahu, N.P., Koike, K., Banerjee, S., Achari, B. and Nikaido, T. (2001). Triterpenoid saponins from *Mollugo spergula*. *Phytochem.* 58, 1177–1182

Saijo, R., Fuke, C., Murakami, K., Nohara, T. and Tomimatsu, T. (1983). Two steroidal glycosides, aculeatiside A and B from *Solanum aculeatissimum*. *Phytochem.* 22, 733–736.

San Martin, R. and Briones, R. (1999). Industrial uses and sustainable supply of *Quillaja saponaria* (Rosaceae) saponins. *Econ. Bot.* 53, 302–311.

Santos, W.R., Bernardo, R.R., Pecanha, L.M.T., Palatnic, M., Parente, J.P, and de Sousa, C.B. (1997). Haemolytic activities of plant saponins and adjuvants. Effect of *Periandra mediterranea* saponin on the humoral response to the FML antigen of *Leishmania donovani*. *Vaccine* 15, 1024–1029.

Sasaki S, Sumino K, Hamajima K, Fukushima J, Ishii N, Kawamoto S, Mohri H, Kensil CR and Okuda K (1998) Induction of systemic and mucosal immune responses to human immunodeficiency virus type 1 by a DNA vaccine formulated with QS-21 saponin adjuvant via intramuscular and intranasal routes. *J. Virology* 72, 4931–4939.

Satoshi, M., Erihi, O., and Satariyo, G. (2004). Composition for preventing or ameliorating ultraviolet damage. *JP Patent* 2,004,131,431.

Sayyah, M., Hadidi, N. and Kamalinejad, M. (2004). Analgesic and anti-inflammatory activity of *Lactuca sativa* seed extract in rats. *J. Ethnopharmacol.* 92, 325-329

Seaforth, C.E., Mohammed, S., Maxwell, A., Tinto, W.F. and Reynolds, W.F. (1992). Mabioside A, a new saponin from *Colubrina elliptica*. *Tetrahed. Lett.* 33, 4111–411.

Schopke, T. (2000). Non-NMR methods for structure elucidation of saponins. In *Saponins in Food, Feedstuffs and Medicinal Plants, Annual Proceedings of the Phytochemical Society*, pp. 106–113 [W Oleszek and A Marston, editors]. Oxford and London: Clarendon Press.

Seebacher, W., Haslinger, E., Rauchensteiner, K., Jurenitsch, J., Presser, A. and Weis, R.. (1999a). Synthesis and haemolytic activity of randianin isomers. *Monatsh. Chem.* 130, 887–897.

Seebacher, W., Weis, R., Jurenitsch, J., Rauchensteiner, K. and Haslinger, E. (1999b). Synthesis and haemolytic activity of oleanolic acid trisaccharides. *Monatsh. Chem.* 130, 1383–1391.

Seeman, P. (1974). Ultrastructure of membrane lesions in immune lysis, osmotic lysis and drug-induced lysis. *Fed. Proceedings* 33, 2116–2124.

Segal, R., Shatkovsky, P. and Milo-Goldzweig, I. (1974). On the mechanism of saponin hemolysis -1. Hydrolysis of the glycosidic bond. *Biochem. Pharmacol.* 23, 973–981.

Shany, S., Gestetner, B., Birk, Y., and Bondi, A. (1970). Lucerne saponins III. Effect of lucerne saponins on larval growth and their detoxification by various sterols. *J. Sci. Food Agric.* 21, 508–510.

Shim, I., Javaid, J.I. and Kim, S.E. (2000). Effect of ginseng total saponin on extracellular dopamine release elicited by local infusion of nicotine into the striatum of freely moving rats. *Planta Medica* 66, 705–708.

Shimoyamada, M., Suzuki, M., Sonta, H., Maruyama, M. and Okubo, K. (1990). Antifungal activity of saponin fraction obtained from *Asparagus Officinalis* L. and its active principle. *Agric. Biol. Chem.*54, 2553–2557.

Shimoyamada, M., Ikedo, S., Ootsubo, R., and Watanabe, K. (1998). Effects of soybean saponins on chymotryptic hydrolyses. *J. Agric. Food Chem.* 46, 4793–4797.

Shimoyamada, M., Okada, Y., Watanabe, K., and Yamauchi, R. (2005). Characterization of tryptic hydrolysis of lactalbumin/saponin mixture and structural change of lactalbumin interacting with soybean saponin. *Arch. Biochem. Biophys.* 435, 273–279.

Shimoyamada, M., Ootsubo, R., Naruse, T. and Watanabe, K. (2000). Effects of soybean saponin on protease hydrolyses of ß-lactoglobulin and α-lactalbumin. *Biosci. Biotechnol. Biochem.* 64, 891–893.

Shimoyamada, M., Osugi, Y., Shiraiwa, M., Okubo, K. and Watanabe, K. (1993). Solubilities of soybean saponins and their solubilization with a bidesmoside saponin. *J. Jpn. Soc. Food Sci.* 40, 210–213.

Shin, H.R., Kim, J.Y., Yun, T.K., Morgan, G. and Vainio, H. (2000). The cancerpreventive potential of *Panax ginseng*: A review of human and experimental evidence. *Cancer Causes Control* 11, 565–576.

Shirakawa, Y., Itoh, M.,Koyama, K. and Minowa,Y. (1986). Aqueous preparation containing vitamin E and saponins. *US Patent* 4,568,667.

Shirasuna, K., Miyakoshi, M., Mimoto, S., Isoda, S., Satoh, Y., Hirai, Y., Ida, Y. and Shoji, J. (1997). Lupane triterpenoid glycosyl esters from leaves of *Acanthopanax divaricatus. Phytochem.* 45, 579–584

Sjolander, A., Cox, J.C. and Barr, I.G. (1998). ISCOMs: an adjuvant with multiple functions (Review). *J. Leukocyte Biol.* 64, 713–723.

So, H.S., Yoon, H.S., Kwoon, Y.S., Sung, J.H., Lee, T.G., Park, E.N., Cho, H.S., Lee, B.M., Cho, J.M. and Ryu, W.S. (1997). Effect of a novel saponin adjuvant derived from *Quillaja saponaria* on immune response to recombinant hepatitis B surface antigen. *Mol. Biol. Cells* 7, 176–186.

Soetan, K.O., Oyekunle, M.A., Aiyelaagbe, O.O. and Fafunso, M.A. (2006). Evaluation of the antimicrobial activity of saponins extract of *Sorghum bicolor* L. Moench. *Afr. J. Biotech.* 5, 2405-2407.

Sogabe, T., Tamura, K. and Miyakoshi, M. (2003). Natural keeping quality improving agent, food and drink having improved keeping quality and method for improving keeping quality of food and drink. *JP Patent* 2,003,009,832.

Southon, S., Johnson, I.T., Gee, J.M. and Price, K.R. (1988). The effect of Gypsophylla saponins in the diet on mineral status and plasma cholesterol concentration in the rat. *Brit. J. Nutrit.* 59, 49–55.

Sparg, S.G., Light, M.E. van Staden, J. (2004). Biological activities and distribution of plant saponins. *J. Ethnopharmacol.* 94, 219–243

Staprans, I., Rapp, J.H., Pan, X.M., Kim, K.Y. and Feingold, K.R. (1994). Oxidized lipids in the diet are a source of oxidized lipid in chylomicrons of human serum. *Arteriosclerosis and Thrombosis* 14, 1900–1905.

Steel, C.C. and Drysdale, R.B. (1988). Electrolyte leakage from plant and fungal tissues and disruption of liposome membranes by a-tomatine. *Phytochem.* 27, 1025–1030.

Steurer, S., Wurglics, M., Likussar, W., Burmistrov, K., Michelitsch, A. and Schubert-Zsilavecz, M. (1999). Lack of correlation between surface and interfacial activities of saponins and their haemolytic properties. *Pharmazie* 54, 766–767.

Stine, K.J., Hercules, R.K., Duff, J.D. and Walker, B.W. (2006). Interaction of the glycoalkaloid tomatine with DMPC and sterol monolayers studied by surface pressure measurements and Brewster angle microscopy. *J. Phys. Chem.* 110, 22220–22229.

Stolzenberg, S.J. and Parkhurst, R.M. (1976). Blastocidal and contraceptive actions by an extract and compounds from endod *(Phytolacca dodecandra). Contraception* 14, 39–51.

Sun, H.X., Xie, Y. and Ye, Y.P. (2009). Advances in saponin-based adjuvants. *Vaccine* 27, 1787–1796

Sung, W.S. and Lee, D.G. (2008a). *In vitro* candidacidal action of Korean red ginseng saponins against *Candida albicans*. *Biol. Pharm. Bull.* 31, 139–142.

Sung, W.S.and Lee, D.G. (2008b). The combination effect of Korean red ginseng saponins with Kanamycin and Cefotaxime against Methicillin-resistant *Staphylococcus aureus*. *Biol. Pharm. Bull.* 31, 1614–1617.

Takechi, M. and Tanaka, Y. (1995). Structure-activity relationship of synthetic methyl urosylate glycosides. *Phytochem.* 34, 675.

Takechi, M., Matsunami, S., Nishizawa, J., Uno, C. and Tanaka, Y. (1999). Haemolytic and antifungal activities of saponins or anti-ATPase and antiviral activities of cardiac glycosides. *Planta Medica* 65, 585–586.

Taketa, A.T.C., Schmittmann-Schlager, T., Guillaume, D., Grosmann, G. And Schenkel, E.P. (2000). Triterpenoid glycosides and a triterpene from *Ilex brevicuspis*. *Phytochem.* 53, 901–904.

Tanaka, M., Fang-I, L., Ishizaki, S. and Taguchi, T. (1995). Interaction of saponins with salt soluble proteins from walleye pollack meat. *Fisheries Sci.*, 61, 373–374.

Tanaka, O. (1987). Solubilizing properties of ginseng saponins. *Korean J. Ginseng Sci.* 11, 145–153.

Tanaka, O. and Yata, N. (1985). Promotion of absorption of drugs administered through the alimentary system. *US Patent* 4,501,734.

Tatiya A.U., Desai D.G., Surana S.J.and Patil P.H. (2007). Anti-inflammatory and nitric oxide scavenging activity of roots of *Eranthemum roseum*. *Indian Drugs* 44, 815-818

Tewary, P.V., Chaturvedi, C. and Pandey, V.B. (1973). Antifertility activity of *Costus speciosus* Sm. *Indian J. Pharmacol.* 35, 114–115.

Thompson, L.U. (1993). Potential health benefits and problems associated with antinutrients in foods. *Food Res. Int.* 26, 131–149.

Treyvaud, V., Marston, A., Dyatmiko, W. and Hostettmann, K. (2000). Molluscicidal saponins from *Phytolacca icosandra*. *Phytochem.* 55, 603–609.

Trojanowska, M.R., Osbourn, A.E., Daniels, M.J. and Threlfall, D.R. (2000). Biosynthesis of avenacins and phytosterols in roots of *Avena sativa* cv. Image. *Phytochem.* 54, 153–164.

Ueckert, J., Wray, V., Nimtz, M. and Schöpke, T., 1998. Noroleanane saponins from *Celmisia spectabilis*. *Phytochem.* 49, 2487–2492.

Uematsu, Y., Hirata, K. and Saito, K. (2000). Spectrophotometric determination of saponin in Yucca extract used as food additive. *J. AOAC Int.* 83, 1451–1454.

Ullah, N., Seebacher, W., Weis, R., Jurenitsch, J., Rauchensteiner, K. and Haslinger, E. (2000). Synthesis and hemolytic properties of glycyrrhetic acid glycosides. *Monatsh. Chem.* 131, 787-794.

Ursini, F., Zamburlini, A., Cazzolato, G., Maiorino, M, Bon. G.B. and Sevanian, A. (1998). Postprandial plasma lipid hydroperoxides: a possible link between diet and atherosclerosis. *Free Radical Biol. Med.* 25, 250–252.

Van Dyck, S., Flammang, P., Meriaux, C., Bonnel, D., Salzet, M., Fournier, I. and Wisztorski, M. (2010). Localization of secondary metabolites in marine invertebrates:

contribution of MALDI MSI for the study of saponins in cuvierian tubules of H. forskali. *PLoS One* 5, e13923.

van Putte, K.P.A.M. (2002). Process for preparing food products fortified with oleanolic acid. *US Patent* 6,338,865.

Vincken, J.P., Heng, L., de Groot, A *et al.* (2007). Saponins, classification and occurrence in the plant kingdom. *Phytochem.* 68, 275–297

Voutquenne, L., Lavaud, C., Massiot, G. and le Men-Olivier, L. (2002). Structure–activity relationships of haemolytic saponins. *Pharm. Biol.* 40, 253–262.

Wakabayashi, C., Murakami, K., Hasegawa, H., Murata, J. and Saiki, I. (1998). An intestinal bacterial metabolite of ginseng protopanaxadiol saponins has the ability to induce apoptosis in tumor cells. *Biochem. Biophy. Res. Comm.* 246, 725–730.

Walker, B.W., Manhanke, N. and Stine, K.J. (2008). Comparison of the interaction of tomatine with mixed monolayers containing phospholipid, egg sphingomyelin, and sterol. *Biochim. Biophys. Acta* 1778, 2244–2257.

Wallace, R.J., Arthaud, L. and Newbold, C.J. (1994). Influence of *Yucca shidigera* extract on ruminal ammonia concentrations and ruminal microorganisms. *Appl. Env. Microbiol.* 60, 1762–1767.

Waller, G.R., Jurzysta, M. and Thorne, R.L.Z. (1993). Allelopathic activity of root saponins from alfalfa (*Medicago sativa* L.) on weeds and wheat. *Bot. Bull. Acad. Sin.* 34, 1–11.

Walter, E.D., Van Atta, G.R., Thompson, C.R. and Maclay,W.D. (1954). Alfalfa saponin. *J. Am. Chem. Soc.* 76, 2271–2273.

Wang, Y., McAllister, T.A., Yanke, L.J. and Cheeke, P.R.. (2000) Effect of steroidal saponin from *Yucca schidigera* extract on rumen microbial protein synthesis and ruminal fermentation. *J. Sci. Food Agric.* 80, 2114–2122.

Wang, Z.-W., Gu, M.-Y. and Li, G.-Z. (2005). Surface properties of gleditsia saponin and synergisms of its binary system. *J. Disper. Sci. Technol.* 26, 341–347

Wang, Z.Y. and Nixon, D.W. (2001). Licorice and cancer. *Nutr. Cancer* 39, 1–11.

West, L.G., Greger, J.L., White, A. and Nonnamaker, B.J. (1978). *In vitro* studies on saponin-mineral complexation. *J. Food Sci.* 43, 1342–1343.

Wick, W., Grimmel, C., Wagenknecht, B., Dichgans, J. and Weller, M. (1999). Betulinic acid-induced apoptosis in glioma cells: A sequential requirement for new protein synthesis, formation of reactive oxygen species, and caspase processing. *J. Pharmacol. Exp. Ther.* 289,1306–1312.

Woldemichael, G.M. and Wink, M. (2001). Identification and biologicalactivities of triterpenoid saponins from *Chenopodium quinoa*. *J. Agric. Food Chem.* 49, 2327–2332.

Wolff, S.P. and Nourooz-Zadeh, J. (1996). Hypothesis: UK consumption of dietary lipid hydroperoxides – a possible contributory factor to atherosclerosis. *Atherosclerosis* 119, 261–263.

Xie, J.T., McHendale, S., Yuan, C.S. (2005). Ginseng and diabetes. *Amer. J. Chinese Med.* 33, 397–404.

Xu, F.Q., Zhong, H.M., Liu, H.Y. *et al* (2007.) Steroidal saponins from *Lysimachia paridiformis*. *J. Asian Nat. Prod. Res.* 9, 493–497

Xu, Z.-X., Ding, T., Haridas, V., Connolly, F. and Gutterman, J.U. (2009). Avicin D, a plant triterpenoid, induces cell apoptosis by recruitment of Fas and downstream signaling molecules into lipid rafts. *PloS One 4,* e8532.

Yamasaki, Y., Ito, K., Enomoto, Y. and Sutko, J.L. (1987). Alterations by saponins of passive calcium permeability and sodium-calcium exchange activity of canine cardiac sarcolemnal vesicles. *Biochimica et Biophysica Acta* 897, 481–487.

Yamauchi, Y., Katsunori, K. and Hideki, H. (2000). Vegetable growth regulator. *JP Patent* 2,000,119,118.

Yao, X., Li, L. and Wang N. (2005). New use of saponin compound for treating cardiovascular disease. *CN Patent* 1,562,064.

Yi, J.-S., Choo, H.-J., Cho, B.-R., Kim, H.-M., Kim, Y.-N., Ham, Y.-M. and Ko, Y.-G. (2009). Ginsenoside Rh2 induces ligand-independent Fas activation via lipid raft disruption. *Biochem. Biophys. Res. Commun.* 385, 154–159.

Yogeeswari, P. and Sriram, D. (2005). Betulinic acid and its derivatives: A review on their biological properties. *Curr. Med. Chem.*, 12, 657–666.

Yoo, B.H., Kang, B.Y., Yeom, M.H., Sung, D.S., Han, S.H., Kim, H.K. and Ju, H.K. (2003). Nanoemulsion comprising metabolites of ginseng saponin as an active component and a method for preparing the same, and a skin care composition for anti-aging containg the same. *US Patent Application*2003/0175315 A1.

Yoshikawa, M., Murakami, T., Kishi, A., Kageura, T. and Matsuda, H. (2001). Medicinal flowers. III. Marigold (1): hypoglycaemic, gastric emptying inhibitory, and gastroprotective principles and new oleanane-type triterpene oligoglycosides, calendasaponins A, B, C, and D, from Egyptian *Calendula officinalis*. *Chem. Pharm. Bull.* 49, 863–870.

Yoshikawa, K., Hirai, H., Tanaka, M. and Arihara, S. (2000). Antisweet natural products. XV. Structures of jegosaponins A–D from *Styrax japonica* Sieb. et Zucc. *Chem. Pharm. Bull.* 48, 1093–1096

Yoshiki, Y. and Okubo, K. (1995). Active oxygen scavenging activity of DDMP (2,3-dihydro-2, 5-dihydroxy-6-methyl-4H-pyran-4- one) saponin in soybean seed. *Biosc. Biotech. Biochem.* 59, 1556–1557.

Yoshiki, Y., Kudou, S. and Okubo, K. (1998). Relationship between chemical structures and biological activities of triterpenoid saponins from soybean. *Biosci. Biotechnol. Biochem.* 62, 2291–2299.

Yu, B.S. and Jo, I.-H. (1984). Interaction of sea cucumber saponins with multilamellar liposomes. *Chem. Biol. Interact.* 52, 185–202.

Yudt, M.R. and Cidlowski, J.A. (2002). The glucocorticoid receptor: coding a diversity of proteins and responses through a single gene. *Mol. Endocrinol.* 16, 1719–1726.

Yui, S., Ubukata, K., Hodono, K., Kitahara, M., Mimaki, Y., Kuroda, M., Sashida, Y and Yamazaki, M. (2001) Macrophage-oriented cytotoxic activity of novel triterpene saponins extracted from roots of *Securidaca inappendiculata. Int. Immunopharmacol.* 1, 1989–2000.

Yun, T.-K., and Choi, S.-Y. (1998). Non-organ specific cancer prevention of ginseng: a prospective study in Korea. *Int. J Epidemiol.*, 27:359–364.

Zhan, Y. (1999). Animal feed compositions and uses of triterpenoid saponin obtained from Camellia L. plants. *US Patent* 6,007,822.

Zhang, Y.-F., Fan, X.-J., Li, X., Peng, L.L., Wang, G.-H., Ke, K.-F. and Jiang, Z.-L. (2008). Ginsenoside Rg1 protects neurons from hypoxic-ischemic injury possibly by inhibiting Ca2+ influx through NMDA receptors and L-type voltage-dependent Ca^{2+} channels. *Eur. J. Pharmacol.* 586, 90–99.

Zhao, R.Z. and McDaniel, W.F. (1998). Ginseng improves strategic learning by normal and brain-damaged rats. *NeuroReport* 9, 1619–1624.

Zheng, Q.A. and Yang, C.R. (2003). Dracaenoside A and B, new C-22 steroidal lactone glycosides from the stem of *Dracaena cochinchinensis*. *Chin. Chem. Lett.* 14, 1261–1264.

Zhuang, M., Oltean, D.I., Gomez, I., Pullikuth, A.K., Soberon, M., Bravo, A. and Gill, S.S. (2002). Heliothis virescens and Manduca sexta lipid rafts are involved in Cry1A toxin binding to the midgut epithelium and subsequent pore formation. *J. Biol. Chem.* 277, 13863–13872.

Zilversmit, D.B. (1979). Atherogenesis: a postprandial phenomenon. *Circulation* 60, 473–485.

Zou, K., Tong, W.-Y., Liang, H., Cui, J.-R., Tu, G.-Z., Zhao, Y.-Y., Zhang, R.-Y., 2005. Diastereoisomeric saponins from *Albizia julibrissin*. *Carbohyd. Res.* 340, 1329–1334.

In: Saponins: Properties, Applications and Health Benefits ISBN: 978-1-62100-942-9
Editors: Rani Koh and Isaac Tay

Chapter 2

SAPONINS FROM *PANAX* SPECIES: CHEMISTRY, ISOLATION AND ANALYSIS

Jian-Bo Wan, Ying Chen, Ping Li, Wei-Hua Huang and Qing-Wen Zhang*

Institute of Chinese Medical Sciences, University of Macau, Macao SAR, China
State Key Laboratory of Quality Research in Chinese Medicine
(University of Macau), Macao SAR, China

ABSTRACT

Saponins are very important natural products that show a wide range of pharmacological activities. Ginseng saponins isolated from *Panax* species have attracted worldwide interests owing to their bioactive effects on the immune system, central nervous system, cardiovascular system, cancer and diabetes. These triterpene saponins have been generally considered to be the main bioactive components in *Panax* plants. In this review, the chemistry, isolation and analysis of saponins from *Panax* plants, mainly *P. ginseng* C.A. Mey., *P. quinquefolius* L., *P. notoginseng* (Burk) F.H. Chen were reviewed.

1. INTRODUCTION

The genus *Panax* (Araliaceae) comprises several important medicinal herbs and has been traditionally applied to clinic since ancient times. The botanic name "*Panax*" is derived from the same ancient Greek root as the term "*Panacea*", meaning a remedy for all diseases or "all-healing" reagent [1]. The *Panax* plants were first described and classified by a Swedish botanist *Carolus Linnaeus* in 1753 [2], and distributed in East and Central Asia (China, Nepal, Korea, eastern Siberia and Japan) and North America, especially in cooler climates

* Corresponding author; Dr. Qing-Wen Zhang, E-mail: qwzhang@umac.mo, Tel: +853-8397 4879, Fax: +853-2884 1358.

[1,3]. According to recent statistics, more than ten species are used as traditional Chinese medicine or folk medicine. Among them, *P. ginseng* (Asia ginseng, Chinese or Korean ginseng), *P. quinquefolius* (American ginseng) and *P. notoginseng* (Sanqi) are very well recognized worldwide (Figure 1).

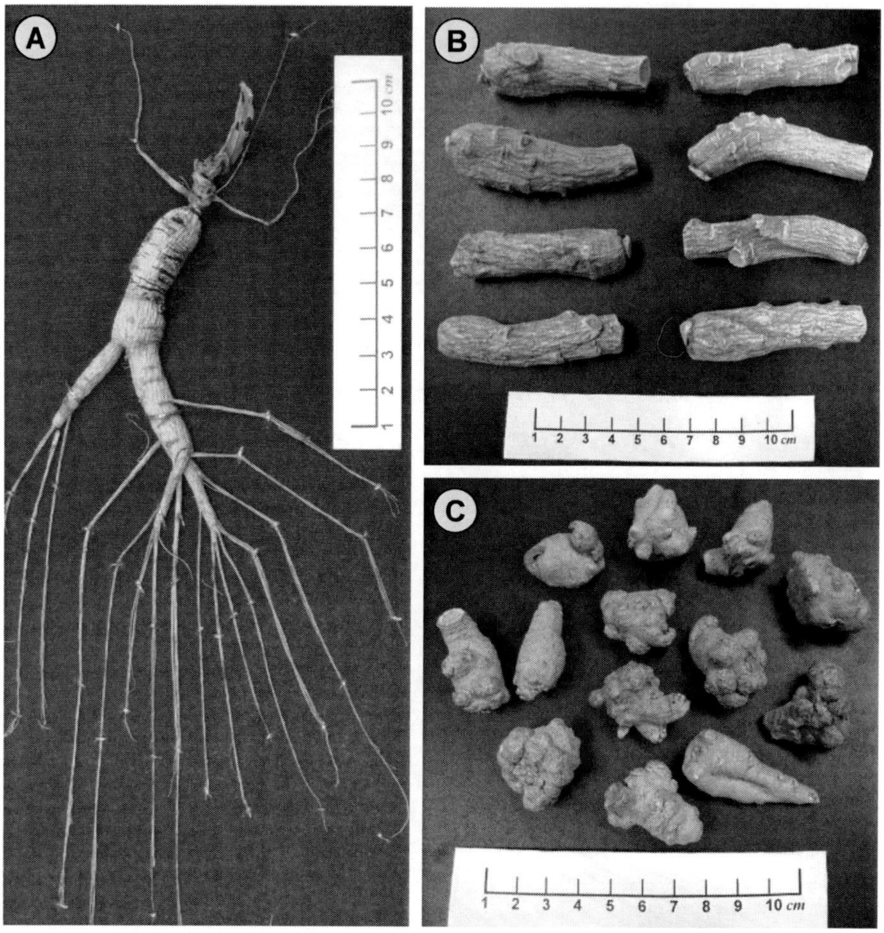

Figure 1. The dried raw medicinal material of *Panax ginseng* (A), *Panax quinquefolius* (B) and *Panax notoginseng* (C), photographed by Mr. Kun Feng from Institute of Chinese Medical Sciences, University of Macau.

Ginseng saponins (called ginsenosides) isolated from *Panax* species show widely beneficial effects on the immune system, central nervous system and cardiovascular system, cancer and diabetes [4-7]. Thus, these triterpene saponins have been generally considered to be the main bioactive components in *Panax*. To date, about 300 saponins and their derivations have been isolated and elucidated from *Panax* plants. In the past two decade, genus *Panax* has attracted more and more attention because of its diverse biological activities (Figure 2). The aim of this review is to comprehensively summarize the current knowledge on the chemical structure, isolation and analysis of the saponins from *Panax* species.

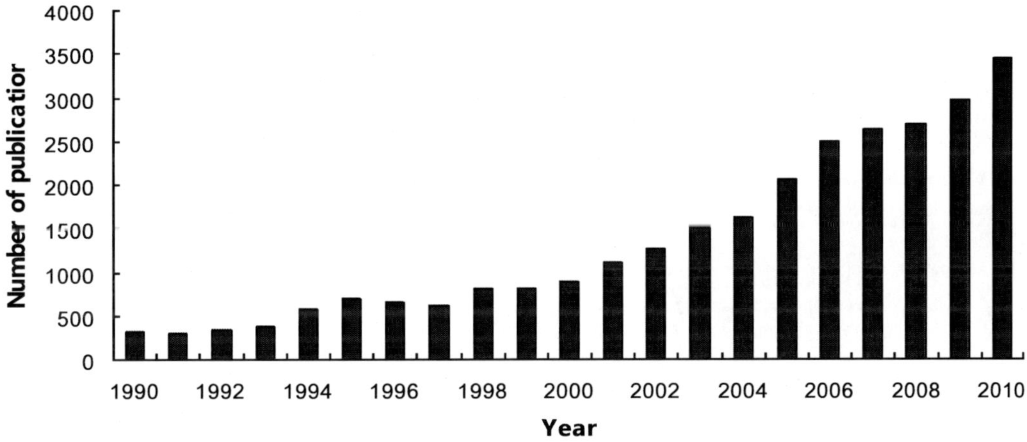

Figure 2. The numbers of literature published in last two decade on *Panax*. Source: SCI Finder scholar; keyword: *Panax*.

2. Chemical Constituents

The nomenclature of the saponins might be derived from different species and part of *Panax*. For example, ginsenoside is used to nominate for the saponins firstly isolated from *P. ginseng*, notoginsenosides or pseudo-ginsenosides for *P. notoginseng,* quinquenosides for *P. quenquifolium*, vinaginsenosides for *P. vietnamensis*, and chikusetsusaponins or yesanchinosides for *P. japonicus*. Besides, the saponins firstly obtained from the flower of *P. ginseng*, *P. notoginseng* and *P. quenquifolium* are referred to floralginsenosides, floranotoginsenosides and floralquinquenosides, respectively. According to different aglycone skeleton, the saponins from *Panax* plants could be classified into two groups as dammarane-type (4-ring triterpene) and oleanane-type (5-ring triterpene) saponins [4-16]. 20(*S*)-protopanaxadiol (PPD) [4,5,17-42] and 20(*S*)-protopanaxatriol (PPT) saponins [4,5,10,19,20,24,30-32,43-56] are two major subcategory of dammarane saponins. PPD group or its analogs have the sugar moieties at C-3 and/or C-20 positions, and PPT saponins have moieties attached to C-6 and/or C-20 positions. Up to now, about 300 saponins and derivations have been isolated from roots, leaves, stems, flower buds, fruits, berries and seeds of *Panax* plant, as well as the steaming or heating processed ginseng samples (Table 1).

Table 1. Chemical structure of saponins from *Panax* species

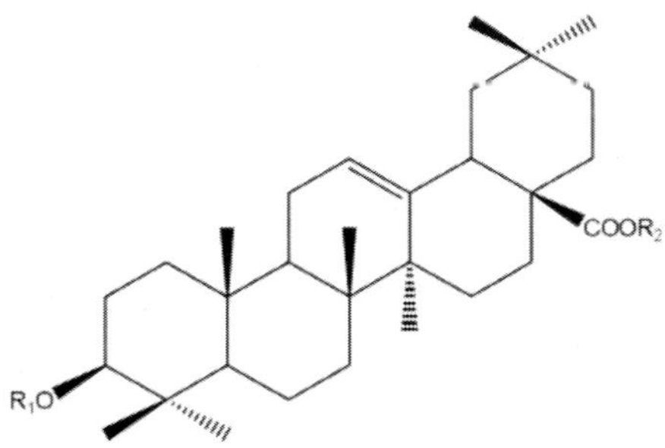

Table 1. (Continued)

No.	Name	R1	R2	Source	Ref.
1	Ginsenoside Ro	GlcA^{2}-Glc	Glc	*P. ginseng* *P. vietnamensis* *P. zingibrerensis*	[4] [5] [10]
2	Chikusetsusaponin IV	GlcA^{4}-Araf	Glc	*P. japonicus* *P. zingibrerensis*	[6] [10]
3	Chikusetsusaponin Ib	Araf -^{4}GlcA^{6}-Glc	H	*P. japonicus*	[6]
4	Ginsenoside Roa	GlcA-^{2}Glc	Glc^{6}-Glc	*P. ginseng*	[7]
5	Pseudo-ginsenoside RI3	Glc^{6}-Glc^{3}-^{2}Glc	Xyl	*P. notoginseng*	[8]
6	Pseudo-ginsenoside Rp1	GlcA^{2}-Xyl	H	*P. notoginseng*	[8]
7	Pseudo-ginsenoside RI1	GlcA^{2}-Xyl^{4}-Ac	H	*P. notoginseng*	[8]
8	Zingibroside R1	GlcA-^{3}Glc	H	*P. zingibrerensis* *P. japonicus*	[10] [57]
9	Chikusetsusaponin II	GlcA^{2}-Glc	H	*P. japonicus*	[9]
10	Chikusetsusaponin Pjs-2	GlcA^{2}-Xyl	Glc	*P. japonicas*	[15]
11	Chikusetsusaponin Pjs-4	Arap	Glc	*P. japonicus*	[15]

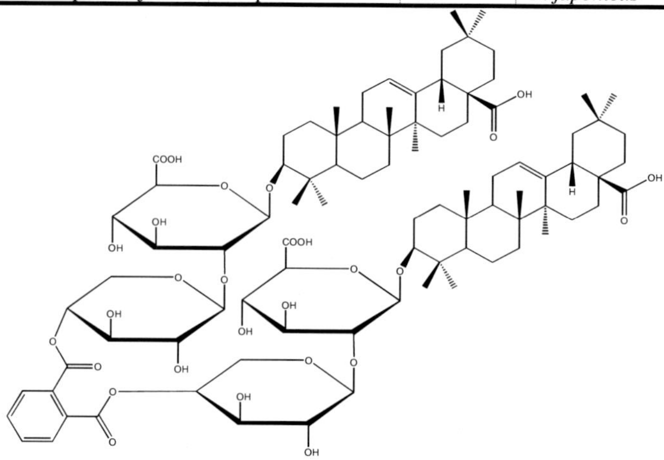

No.	Name	Source	Ref.
12	Pseudoginsenoside RI2	*P. notoginseng*	[8]

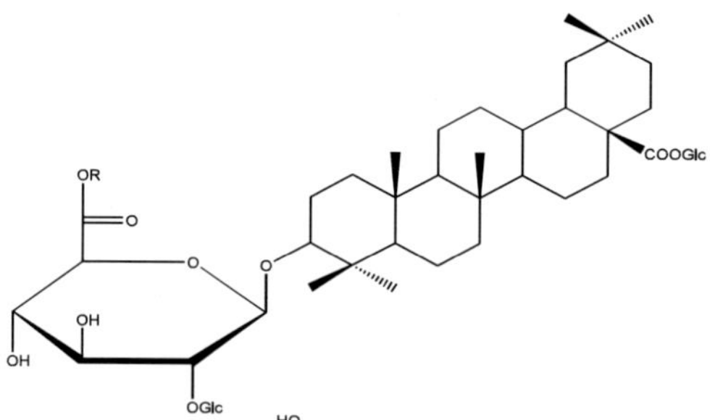

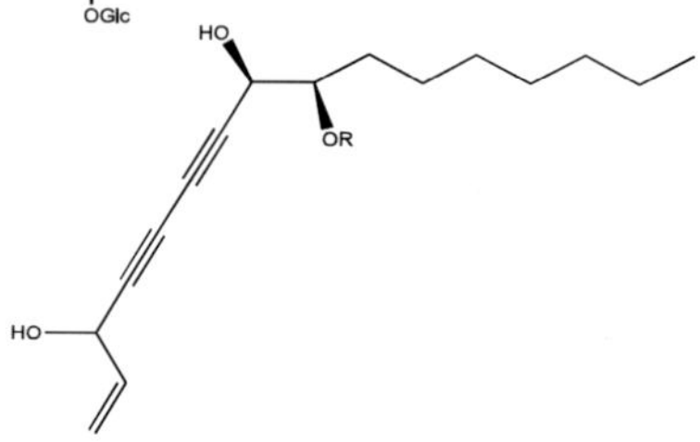

No.	Name	Source	Ref.
13	Polyacetyleneginsenoside Ro	*P. ginseng*	[13]

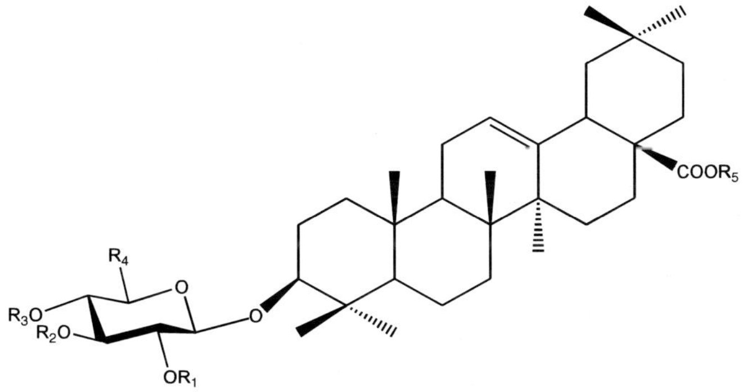

No.	Name	R1	R2	R3	R4	R5	Source	Ref.
14	Spinasaponin A methyl ester	H	Glc	H	$COOCH_3$	H	*P. stipuleanatus*	[93]
15	Pesudoginsenoside RP1 methyl ester	Xyl	H	H	$COOCH_3$	H	*P. stipuleanatus*	[93]
16	Spinasaponin A 28-O-glucoside	H	Glc	H	COOH	Glc	*P. stipuleanatus*	[93]
17	Pseudoginsenoside RT1 methyl ester	Xyl	H	H	$COOCH_3$	Glc	*P. stipuleanatus*	[93]
18	Pseudoginsenoside RT1	Xyl	H	H	COOH	Glc	*P. stipuleanatus*	[93]
19	Stipuleanoside R2 methyl ester	H	Glc	Araf	$COOCH_3$	Glc	*P. stipuleanatus*	[93]
20	Stipuleanoside R2	H	Glc	Araf	COOH	Glc	*P. stipuleanatus*	[93]
21	Araloside A methyl ester	H	H	Araf	$COOCH_3$	Glc	*P. stipuleanatus*	[93]
22	3-O-β-D-glucopyranosyl (1-3)-β-D-glucuronopyranoside-28-O-β-D-glucopyranosyl oleanolic acid methyl ester	H	Glc	H	$COOCH_3$	Glc	*P. stipuleanatus*	[93]
23	3-O-β-D-xylopyranosyl (1-2)-β-D-glucopyranosyl-28-O-β -D-glucopyranosyl oleanolic acid	Xyl	H	H	CH_2OH	Glc	*P. stipuleanatus*	[93]
24	Chikusetsusaponin IVa	H	H	H	COOH	Glc	*P. stipuleanatus* *P. zingibrerensis*	[93] [10]
25	Chikusetsusaponin V methyl ester	Glc	H	H	$COOCH_3$	Glc	*P. japonicus*	[16]
26	Oleanolic 3-O-β-D-6-methyl-pyranoglucuronyl	H	H	H	$COOCH_3$	H	*P. japonicus*	[93]

Table 1. (Continued)

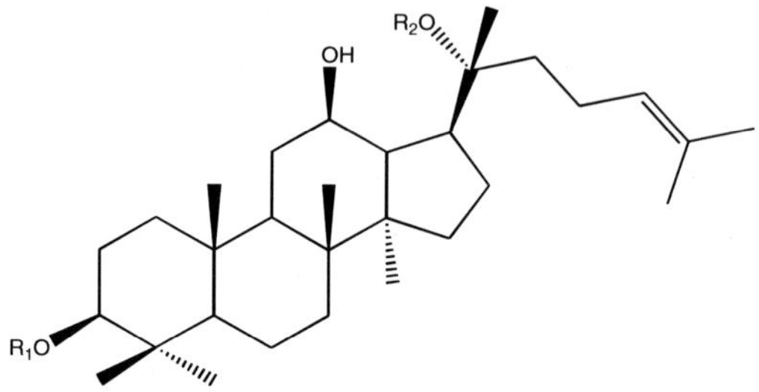

No.	Name	R1	R2	Source	Ref.
27	20R-ginsenoside Rg3	Glc²-Glc	H	*P. ginseng* *P. notoginseng*	[21] [24]
28	20R-ginsenoside Rh2	Glc	H	*P. ginseng* *P. notoginseng*	[19] [25]
29	20R-Protopanaxadiol	H	H	*P. notoginseng*	[74]

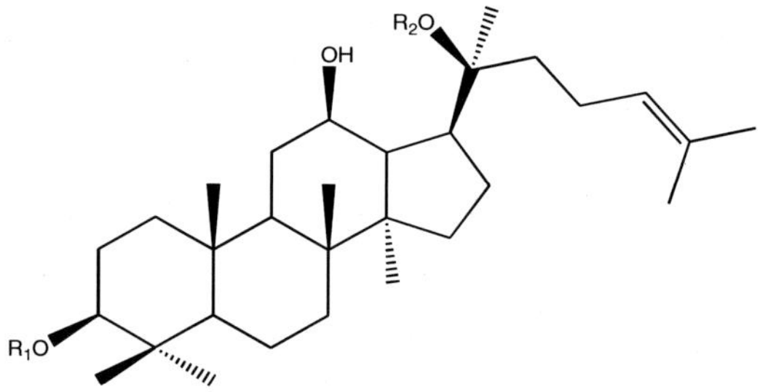

No	Name	R1	R2	Source	Ref.
30	20S-Protopanaxadiol	H	H	*P. notoginseng*	[22]
31	Ginsenoside Ra1	Glc²-Glc	Glc⁶- Arap⁴ - Xyl	*P. ginseng*	[4]
32	Ginsenoside Ra2	Glc²-Glc	Glc⁶-Araf² -Xyl	*P. ginseng*	[4]
33	Ginsenoside Ra3	Glc²-Glc	Glc⁶- Glc³-Xyl	*P. ginseng* *P. notoginseng*	[28] [17]
34	Ginsenoside Rb1	Glc²-Glc	Glc⁶- Glc	*P. ginseng* *P. quenquifolium* *P. notoginseng* *P. vietnamensis*	[19] [18] [17] [5]
35	Ginsenoside Rb2	Glc²-Glc	Glc⁶- Arap	*P. ginseng* *P. quenquifolium* *P. notoginseng* *P. vietnamensis*	[19] [18] [34] [5]
36	Ginsenoside Rb3	Glc²-Glc	Glc⁶- Xyl	*P. ginseng* *P. quenquifolium* *P. notoginseng* *P. vietnamensis*	[4] [29] [22] [5]
37	Ginsenoside Rc	Glc²-Glc	Glc⁶-Araf	*P. ginseng* *P. quenquifolium* *P. notoginseng* *p. vietnamensis*	[19] [18] [22] [30]

No	Name	R1	R2	*Source*	Ref.
38	Ginsenoside Rd	Glc^{2}-Glc	Glc	*P. ginseng* *P. quenquifolium* *P. notoginseng* *P. vietnamensis*	[19] [18] [17] [5]
39	20S-ginsenoside Rg3	Glc^{2}-Glc	H	*P. ginseng* *P. notoginseng*	[21] [24]
40	Ginsenoside F2	Glc	Glc	*P. ginseng* *P. quenquifolium*	[31] [24]
41	20S-ginsenoside Rh2	Glc	H	*P. ginseng* *P. quenquifolium* *P. notoginseng*	[19] [32] [25]
42	Ginsenoside Rs1	Glc^{2}- Glc^{6}-Ac	Glc^{6}- Arap	*P. ginseng* *P. quenquifolium*	[4] [29]
43	Ginsenoside Rs2	Glc- ^{2}Glc^{6}-Ac	Glc^{6}- Araf	*P. ginseng*	[4]
44	Ginsenoside Rs3	Glc^{2}- Glc^{6}-Ac	H	*P. ginseng*	[26]
45	Malonyl-ginsenoside Rb1	Glc^{2}- Glc^{6}-Ma	Glc^{6}- Glc	*P. ginseng* *P. quenquifolium* *P. notoginseng*	[20] [18] [17]
46	Malonyl-ginsenoside Rb2	Glc^{2}- Glc^{6}-Ma	Glc^{6}- Arap	*P. ginseng* *P. quenquifolium*	[20] [18]
47	Malonyl-ginsenoside Rc	Glc^{2}- Glc^{6}-Ma	Glc^{6}- Araf	*P. ginseng* *P. quenquifolium*	[20] [18]
48	Malonyl-ginsenoside Rd	Glc^{2}- Glc^{6}-Ma	Glc	*P. ginseng* *P. quenquifolium*	[20] [18]
49	IH-902	H	Glc^{6}-Arap	*P. quenquifolium*	[27]
50	Pseudo-ginsenoside RC1	Glc^{2}- Glc^{6}-Ac	Glc	*P. quenquifolium*	[29]
51	Pseudo-ginsenoside F8	Ac-^{6}Glc^{2}-Glc	Glc^{6}- Arap	*P. quenquifolium* *P. notoginseng*	[29] [23]
52	Quinquenoside I	Glc-^{2}Glc^{6}- Bu	Glc	*P. quenquifolium*	[20]
53	Quinquenoside II	Ac-^{6}Glc^{2}-Glc	Glc^{6}- Glc	*P. quenquifolium*	[20]
54	Quinquenoside III	Ac-^{6}Glc^{2}-Glc	Glc	*P. quenquifolium*	[20]
55	Quinquenoside V	Glc^{2}- Glc	Glc^{6}- Glc^{4}- Glc	*P. quenquifolium*	[20]
56	Quinquenoside L10	Glc	Glc^{6}- Arap	*P. quenquifolium*	[33]
57	Quinquenoside L14	Glc^{2}- Glc	Arap	*P. quenquifolium*	[33]
58	20S-protopanaxadiol	H	H	*P. notoginseng*	[22]
59	IH-901	H	Glc	*P. quenquifolium*	[27]
60	IH-903	H	Glc^{6}- Araf	*P. notoginseng*	[27]
61	Notoginsenoside R4	Glc^{2}- Glc	Glc^{6}- Glc^{6}- Xyl	*P. notoginseng*	[17]
62	Notoginsenoside D	Glc^{2}- Glc^{2}-Xyl	Glc^{6}- Glc^{6}-Xyl	*P. notoginseng*	[20]
63	Notoginsenoside Fa	Glc^{2}- Glc^{2}-Xyl	Glc^{6}- Glc	*P. notoginseng* *P. vietnamensis*	[17] [5]
64	Notoginsenoside Fc	Glc^{2}- Glc^{2}-Xyl	Glc^{6}-Xyl	*P. notoginseng*	[22]
65	Notoginsenoside Fe	Glc	Glc^{6}- Araf	*P. notoginseng*	[22]
66	Notoginsenoside L	Glc^{2}-Xyl	Glc^{6}- Glc	*P. notoginseng*	[20]
67	Notoginsenoside O	Glc	Glc^{6}-Xyl^{3}-Xyl	*P. notoginseng*	[20]
68	Notoginsenoside P	Glc	Glc^{6}-Xyl^{4}-Xyl	*P. notoginseng*	[20]
69	Notoginsenoside Q	Glc^{2}- Glc^{2}-Xyl	Glc^{6}-Xyl^{4}-Xyl	*P. notoginseng*	[20]
70	Notoginsenoside S	Glc^{2}- Glc^{2}-Xyl	Glc^{6}-Araf^{5}-Xyl	*P. notoginseng*	[20]
71	Notoginsenoside T	Glc^{2}- Glc^{2}-Xyl	Glc^{6}-Glc^{3}-Xyl	*P. notoginseng*	[17]
72	Notoginsenoside I	Glc^{2}-Glc	Glc^{6}-Glc	*P. notoginseng*	[20]
73	Notoginsenoside K	Glc^{6}- Glc	Glc	*P. notoginseng*	[17]
74	Saponin 2^{c}	Glc	Glc^{2}- Arap	*P. notoginseng*	[38]
75	Malonylginsenoside Ra3	Glc^{2}-Glc^{6}-Ma	Glc^{6}- Glc^{3}- Xyl	*P. ginseng*	[28]
76	Notoginsenoside FP2	Glc^{2}- Glc^{2}- Xyl	Glc^{6}-Araf	*P. notoginseng*	[47]
77	Notoginsenoside FT1	Glc^{2}- Glc^{2}- Xyl	H	*P. notoginseng*	[49]

Table 1. (Continued)

No	Name	R1	R2	*Source*	Ref.
78	Yesanchinoside J	Ac-^{6}Glc^{2}- Glc	Glc^{6}- Glc^{6}- Xyl	*P. japonicus*	[35]
79	Notoginsenoside Fd	Glc	Glc^{6}-Xyl	*P. notoginseng*	[38]
80	Gypenoside XVII	Glc	Glc^{6}-Glc	*P. vietnamensis* *P. notoginseng*	[30] [20]
81	Vinaginsenoside R16	Glc^{2}-Xyl	Glc	*P. vietnamensis*	[36]
82	Vinaginsenoside R17	Glc^{2}- Glc	Arap	*P. vietnamensis*	[36]
83	Vinaginsenoside R18	Glc^{2}- Glc	Xyl	*P. vietnamensis*	[36]
84	Chikusetsusaponin VI	Glc^{6}-Xyl^{2} Glc	Glc^{6}- Glc	*P. japonicus*	[6]
85	Ginsenoside RA0	Glc^{2}- Glc^{2}- Glc	Glc^{6}- Glc	*P. quenquifolium*	[7]
86	Vinaginsenoside R7	Glc^{2}- Glc^{2}-Xyl	Glc	*P. vietnamensis*	[36]
87	Chikusetsusaponin III	Glc-^{2}Glc^{6}-Xyl	H	*P. japonicus*	[41]
88	Quinquenoside R1	Glc^{2}- Glc^{6}-Ac	Glc^{6}- Glc	*P. quenquifolium*	[42]
89	Notoginsenoside I	Glc^{2}- Glc	Glc^{6}- Glc	*P. notoginseng*	[20]

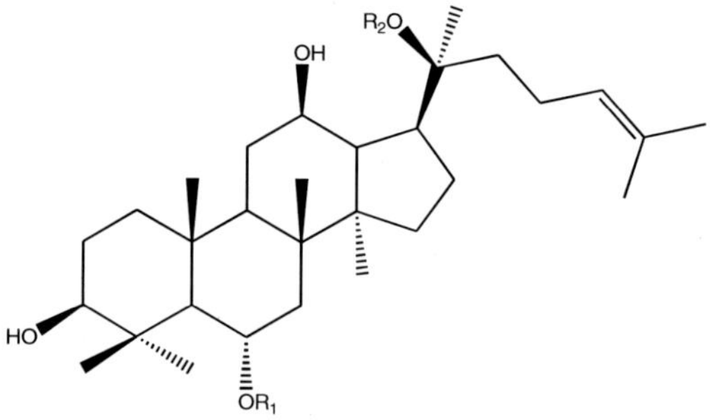

No.	Name	R1	R2	Source	Ref.
90	Ginsenoside Re	Glc^{2}-Rha	Glc	*P. ginseng* *P. quenquifolium* *P. notoginseng* *P. vietnamensis*	[4] [44] [17] [5]
91	Ginsenoside Rf	Glc^{2}- Glc	H	*P. ginseng* *P. notoginseng* *P. quenquifolium*	[4] [24] [32]
92	20-gluco-ginsenoside Rf	Glc^{2}- Glc	Glc	*P. notoginseng* *P. vietnamensis*	[4] [30]
93	Ginsenoside Rg1	Glc	Glc	*P. ginseng* *P. quenquifolium* *P. notoginseng* *P. vietnamensis* *P. zingibrerensis*	[19] [32] [17] [5] [10]
94	20S-ginsenoside Rg2	Glc^{2}-Rha	H	*P. ginseng* *P. quenquifolium* *P. notoginseng*	[4] [29] [17]
95	20S-ginsenoside Rh1	Glc	H	*P. ginseng* *P. quenquifolium* *P. notoginseng* *P. vietnamensis* *P. zingibrerensis*	[61] [32] [17] [5] [10]
96	Ginsenoside F1	H	Glc	*P. ginseng*	[54]
97	Ginsenoside F3	H	Glc^{6}- Arap	*P. ginseng* *P. quenquifolium*	[45] [29]
98	Ginsenoside F5	H	Glc^{6}- Araf	*P. ginseng*	[46]

No.	Name	R1	R2	Source	Ref.
99	Yesanchinoside D	Glc^6- Ac	Glc	*P. quenquifolium* *P. ginseng* *P. japonicas* *P. notoginseng*	[60] [43] [53] [24]
100	Floralquinquenoside E	Glc-Rha	Glc^6- Xyl	*P. quenquifolium*	[39]
101	20S-protopanaxatriol	H	H	*P. quenquifolium*	[39]
102	Notoginsenoside R1	Glc^2- Xyl	H	*P. notoginseng* *P. vietnamensis*	[17] [5]
103	Notoginsenoside R2	Glc^2-Xyl	H	*P. notoginseng*	[17]
104	Notoginsenoside R6	Glc	Glc^6- Glc	*P. notoginseng* *P. vietnamensis*	[55] [30]
105	Notoginsenoside N	Glc^4- Glc	Glc	*P. notoginseng*	[20]
106	Floralquinquenoside E	Glc^2-Rha	Glc^6-Xyl	*P. quenquifolium*	[20]
107	Floralginsenoside M	Glc^2-Rha	Glc^6-Araf	*P. ginseng*	[46]
108	Floralginsenoside N	Glc^2-Rha	Glc^6-Arap	*P. ginseng*	[46]
109	Notoginsenoside FP1	Glc	Glc^6-Arap	*P. notoginseng*	[34]
110	Notoginsenoside Rw1	Xyl	Glc^6-Xyl	*P. notoginseng*	[52]
111	Notoginsenoside T3	Glc	CH_3CH_2	*P. notoginseng*	[48]
112	Notoginsenoside U	H	Glc^6- Glc	*P. notoginseng*	[51]
113	Quinquenoside L17	Glc	Glc^6-Xyl	*P. quenquifolium*	[50]
114	Yesanchinoside E	Glc^2-Rha	Glc^6- Glc	*P. japonicas* *P. notoginseng*	[53] [59]
115	Yesanchinoside F	Ac-^{6}Glc^2-Rha	Glc^6- Glc	*P. japonicus*	[53]
116	Koryoginsenoside R1	Glc^6- Bu	Glc	*P. ginseng*	[21]
117	Pseudoginsenoside RT3	Xyl	Glc	*P. notoginseng*	[38]
118	Pseudoginsenoside RS1	Ac-^{6}Glc^2-Rha	Glc	*P. vietnamensis*	[5]
119	Notoginsenoside M	Glc^6-Glc	Glc	*P. notoginseng*	[20]
120	Chikusetsusaponin L_5	H	Glc^6-Arap^4-Xyl	*P. notoginseng* *P. japonicus*	[17] [56]
121	Notoginsenoside R3	Glc	Glc-Glc	*P. notoginseng*	[55]

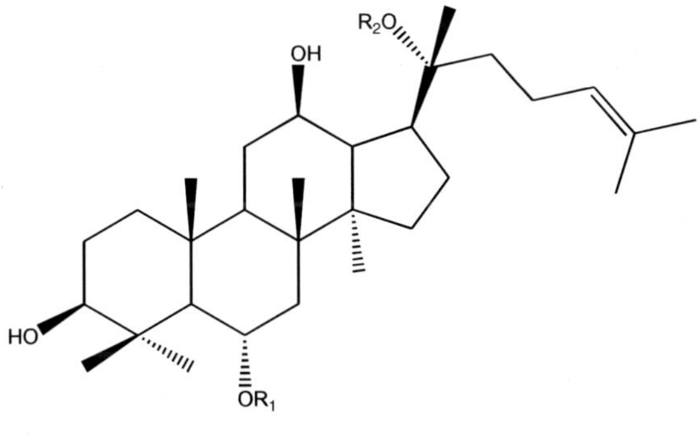

No.	Name	R1	R2	Source	Ref.
122	20R-Protopanaxatriol	H	H	*P. quenquifolium* *P. ginseng*	[39] [31]
123	20R- Ginsenoside Rh1	Glc	H	*P. ginseng* *P. quenquifolium* *P. notoginseng* *P. vietnamensis* *P. zingibrerensis*	[61] [32] [17] [5] [10]
124	20R- Ginsenoside Rg2	Glc^2-Rha	H	*P. ginseng* *P. quenquifolium* *P. notoginseng*	[4] [29] [17]

Table 1. (Continued)

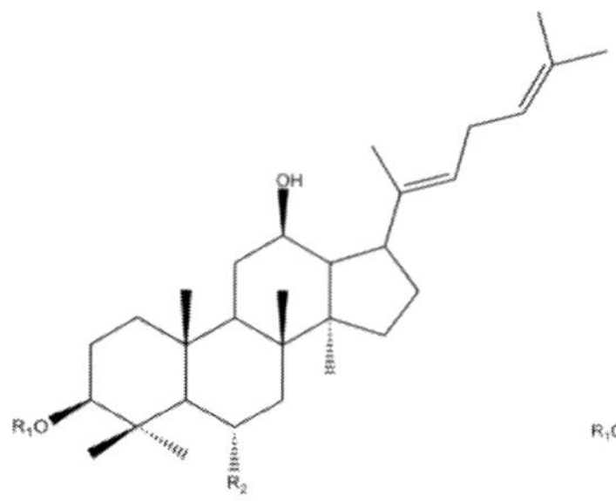

Compounds 125, 127, 130-133

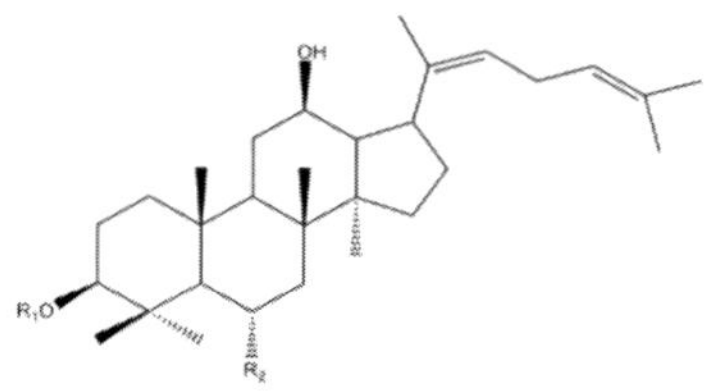

Compounds 126, 128, 129,134

No.	Name	R1	R2	Source	Ref.
125	Ginsenoside Rg5	Glc^{2}- Glc	H	*P. ginseng* *P. notoginseng*	[26] [24]
126	Ginsenoside Rh3	Glc	H	*P.ginseng* *P. notoginseng*	[19] [59]
127	Isoginsenoside Rh3	Glc	H	*P. ginseng*	[89]
128	Ginsenoside Rh4	H	O-Glc	*P. ginseng* *P. notoginseng* *P. vietnamensis*	[61] [24] [81]
129	Ginsenoside Rs4	Glc^{2}- Glc^{6}-Glc	H	*P. ginseng*	[43]
130	Ginsenoside Rs6	H	O-Glc^{6}-Ac	*P. ginseng*	[90]
131	Ginsenoside F4	H	O-Glc^{2}-Rha	*P. ginseng*	[43]
132	20S-dehydr-Protopanaxatriol	H	OH	*P. quenquifolium* *P. ginseng*	[39] [39]
133	20S-dehydr-protopanaxadiol	H	H	*P. quenquifolium*	[58]
134	Ginsenoside Rz1	Glc^{2}- Glc	H	*P. ginseng*	[68]

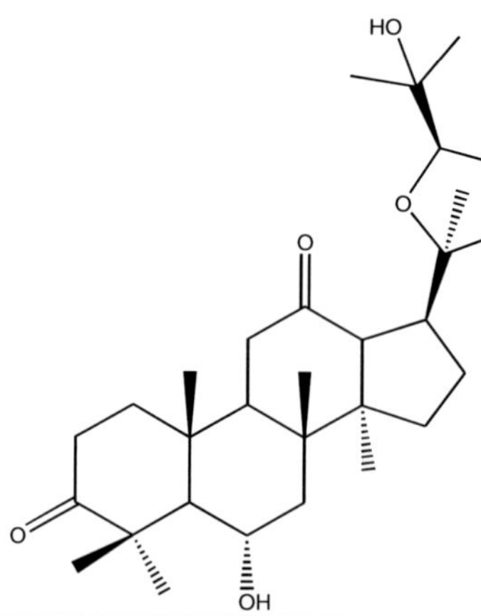

No.	Name	Source	Ref.
135	Panaxadion	*P. ginseng*	[80]

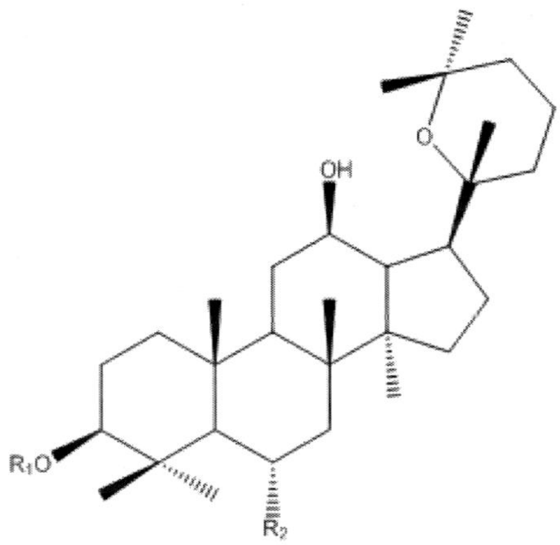

No.	Name	R1	R2	Source	Ref.
136	Notoginsenoside R7	Glc	H	*P. notoginseng*	[85]
137	Panaxatriol	H	OH	*P. ginseng*	[87]
138	6-O-β-D-Glucopyranoside	H	Glc	*P. notoginseng*	[97]
139	Panaxadiol	H	H	*P. ginseng*	[86]

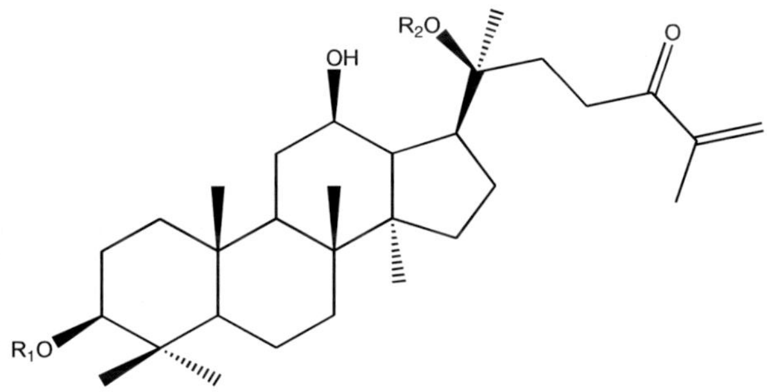

No.	Name	R1	R2	Source	Ref.
140	Notoginsenoside B	Glc^2-Glc	Glc^6-Glc	*P. notoginseng*	[20]

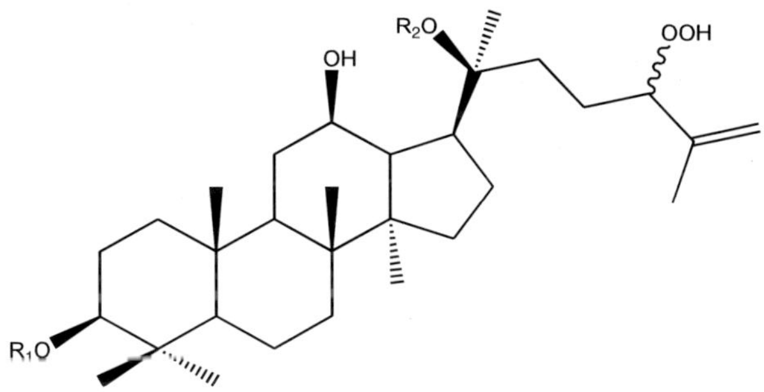

No.	Name	R1	R2	Source	Ref.
141	Notoginsenoside C	Glc^2-Glc	Glc^6-Glc	*P. notoginseng*	[20]

Table 1. (Continued)

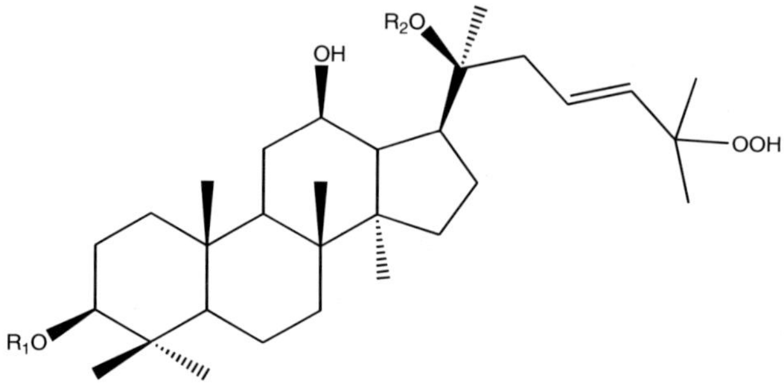

No.	Name	R1	R2	Source	Ref.
142	Notoginsenoside E	Glc^{2}-Glc	Glc	*P. notoginseng* *P. quenquifolium*	[20] [29]

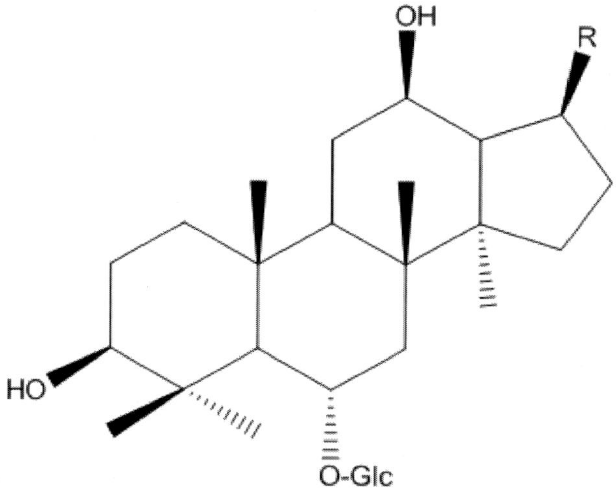

No.	Name	R	Source	Ref.
143	Notoginsenoside R10	Ac	*P. notoginseng*	[88]

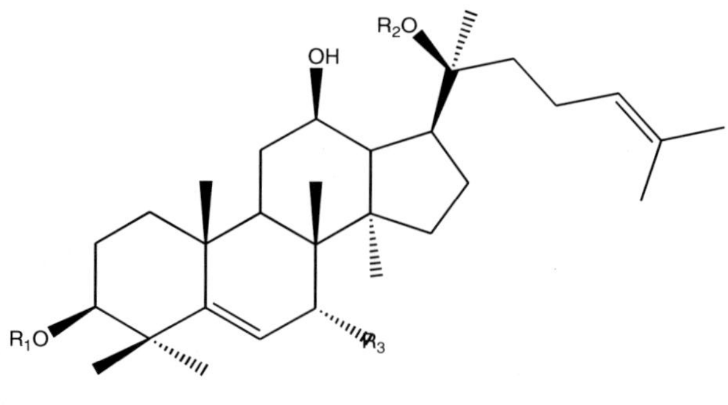

No.	Name	R1	R2	R3	Source	Ref.
144	Notoginsenoside G	Glc^{2}-Glc	Glc	OH	*P. notoginseng*	[59]
145	5,6-didehydroginsenside Rd	Glc^{2}-Glc	Glc	H	*P. notoginseng*	[17]
146	5,6-didehydroginsenside Rb1	Glc^{2}-Glc	Glc^{6}- Glc	H	*P. notoginseng*	[17]
147	Yesanchinoside G	Glc^{2}-Glc	Glc-Xyl	OH	*P. japonicus*	[53]

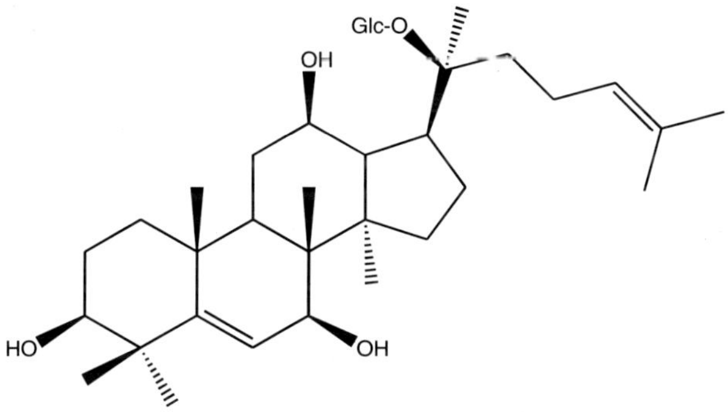

No.	Name	Source	Ref.
148	Ginsenoside Rh7	*P. ginseng*	[79]

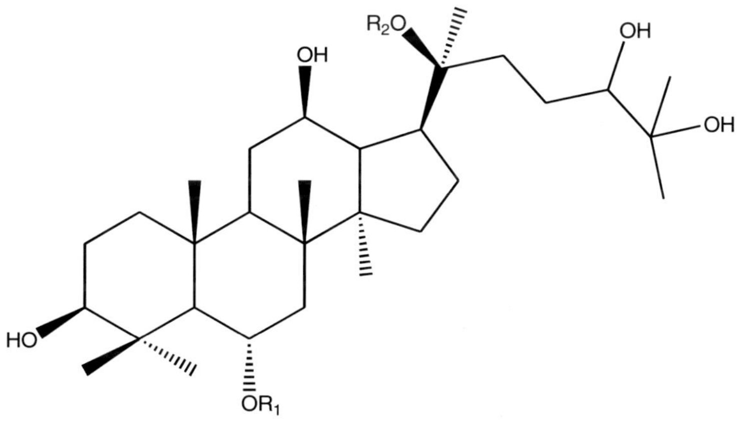

No.	Name	R1	R2	Source	Ref.
149	Vinaginsenoside R22 OH R	Glc	Glc	*P. vietnamensis*	[36]
150	Vinaginsenoside R21OH S	Glc	Glc	*P. vietnamensis*	[36]
151	Vinaginsenoside R12	H	Glc	*P. vietnamensis*	[36]

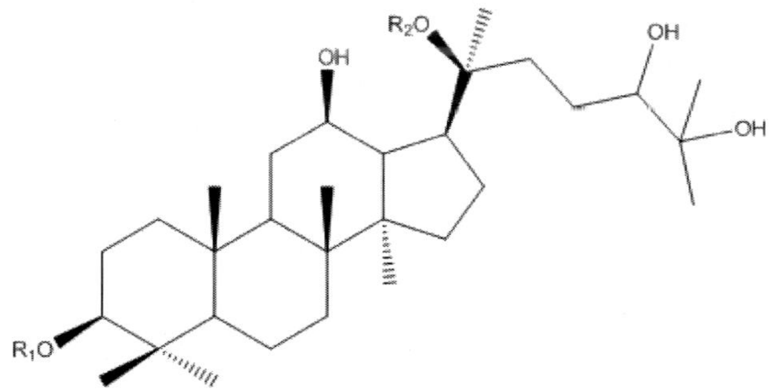

Table 1. (Continued)

No.	Name	R1	R2	Source	Ref.
152	Quinquenoside F1	Glc²-Glc	H	*P. vietnamensis* *P. quinquenfolium*	[30] [101]
153	Vinaginsenoside R13	Glc²-Glc	Glc	*P. vietnamensis*	[36]

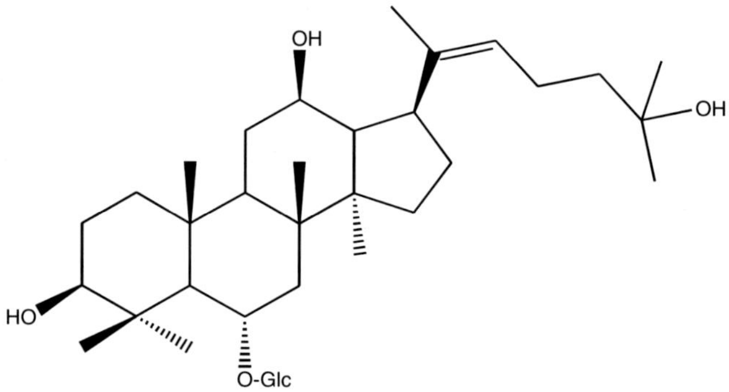

No.	Name	Source	Ref.
154	Sanchinoside B1	*P. notoginseng*	[24]

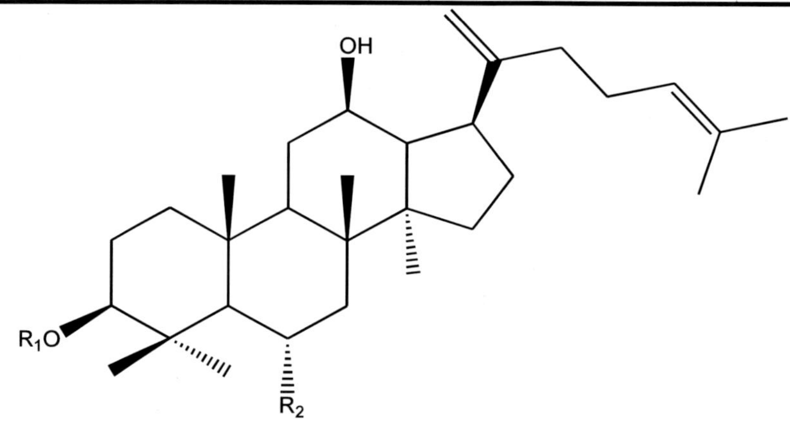

No.	Name	R1	R2	Source	Ref.
155	Ginsenoside Rg6	H	O-Glc²-Rha	*P. ginseng*	[45]
156	Ginsenoside Rk1	Glc²- Glc	H	*P. notoginseng* *P. ginseng*	[24] [71]
157	Ginsenoside Rk2	Glc	H	*P. ginseng* *P. notoginseng*	[70] [24]
158	Ginsenoside Rk3	H	O- Glc	*P. ginseng* *P. notoginseng*	[61] [24]
159	Ginsenoside Rs5	Glc²- Glc⁶-Ac	H	*P. ginseng*	[69]
160	Ginsenoside Rs7	H	O- Glc⁶- Ac	*P. ginseng*	[90]
161	Notoginsenoside T5	H	O-Glc²- Xyl	*P. notoginseng*	[91]

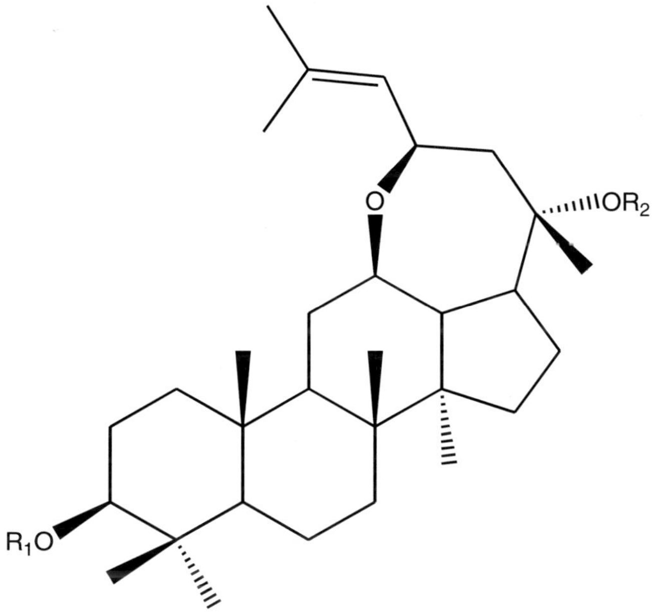

No.	Name	R1	R2	Source	Ref.
162	Ginsenoside La	Glc	Glc	*P. ginseng*	[66]

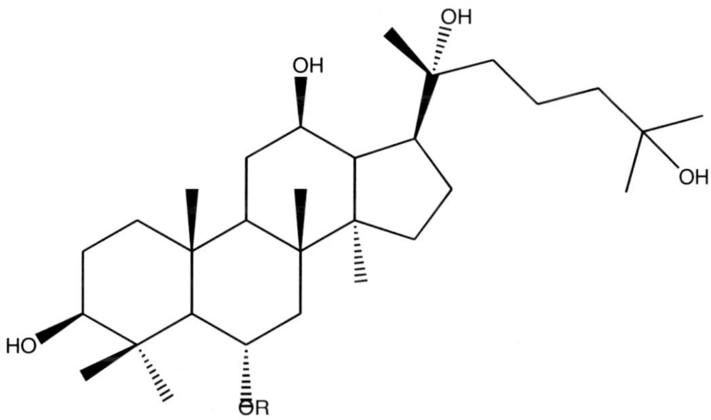

No.	Name	R	Source	Ref.
163	Ginsenoside Rf2	Glc^2-Rha	*P. ginseng*	[26]

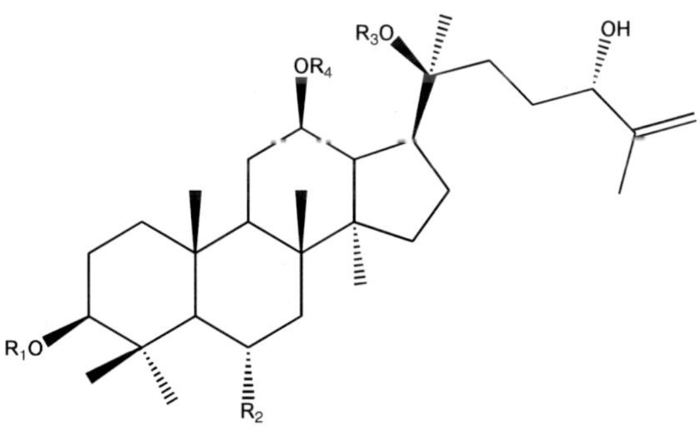

Table 1. (Continued)

No.	Name	R1	R2	R3	R4	Source	Ref.
164	Ginsenoside Rg7	Glc	H	Glc	H	*P. ginseng*	[79]
165	Chikusetsusaponin L9bc	H	OH	H	Glc	*P. notoginseng*	[76]
166	Ginsenoside M7cd	H	OH	Glc	H	*P. ginseng*	[46]

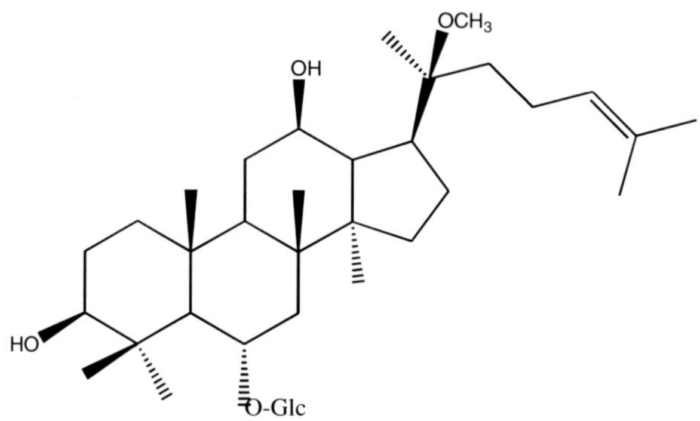

No.	Name	Source	Ref.
167	Ginsenoside Rh5	*P. ginseng*	[79]
		P. vietnamensis	[81]

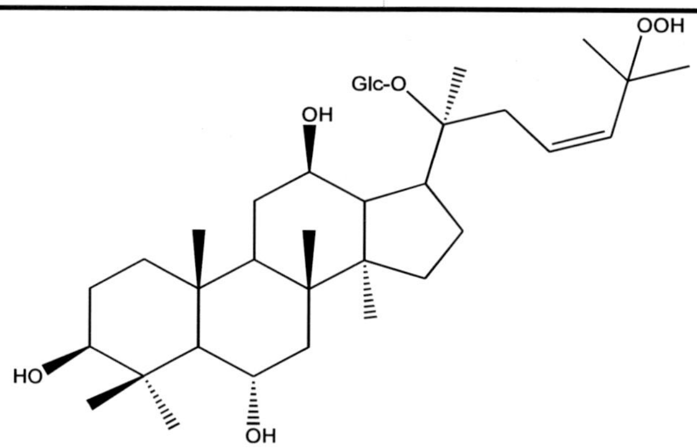

No.	Name	Source	Ref.
168	Ginsenoside Rh6	*P. ginseng*	[79]

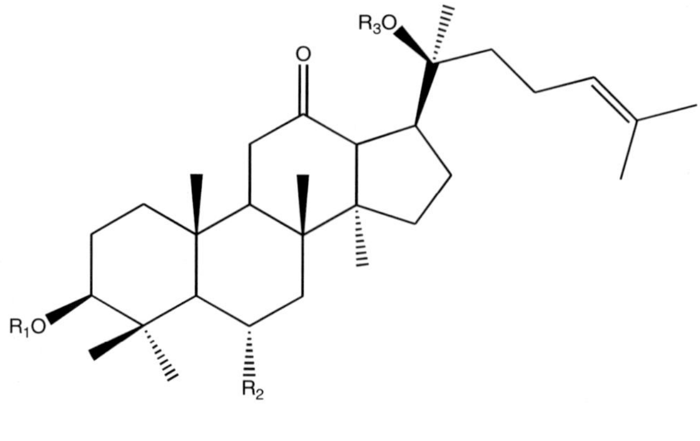

No.	Name	R1	R2	R3	Source	Ref.
169	Ginsenoside Rh8	H	OH	Glc	*P. ginseng*	[79]
170	Chikusetsusaponin LT5	Glc	H	Glc^{6}- Glc	*P. japonicus*	[100]
171	Chikusetsusaponin LT8	Glc	H	Glc	*P. japonicus*	[99]
172	Chikusetsusaponin LN4	Glc^{6}-Xyl	H	Glc^{6}-Arap	*P. japonicus*	[100]

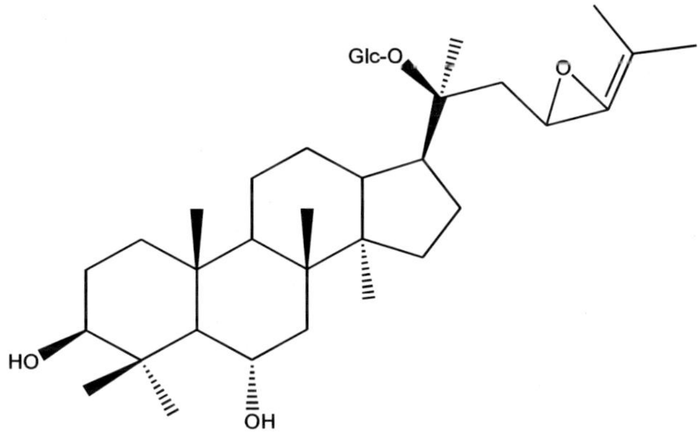

No.	Name	Source	Ref.
173	Ginsenoside Rh9	*P. ginseng*	[79]

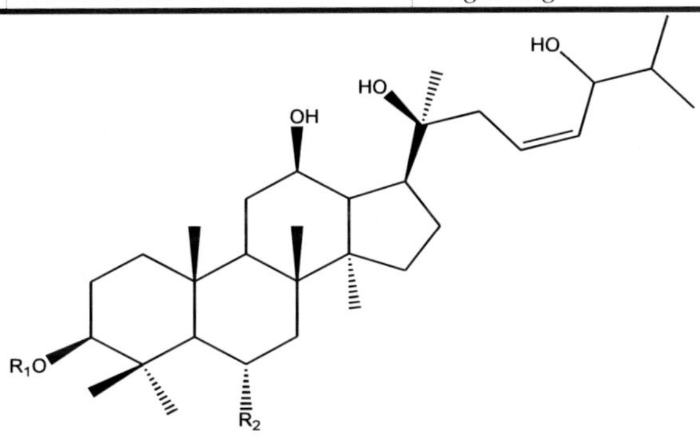

No.	Name	R1	R2	R3	Source	Ref.
174	Majoroside F5	H	O-Glc^{2}-Rha	Glc	*P. japonicus*	[63]
175	Majoroside F3	Glc	H	Glc	*P. japonicus*	[63]

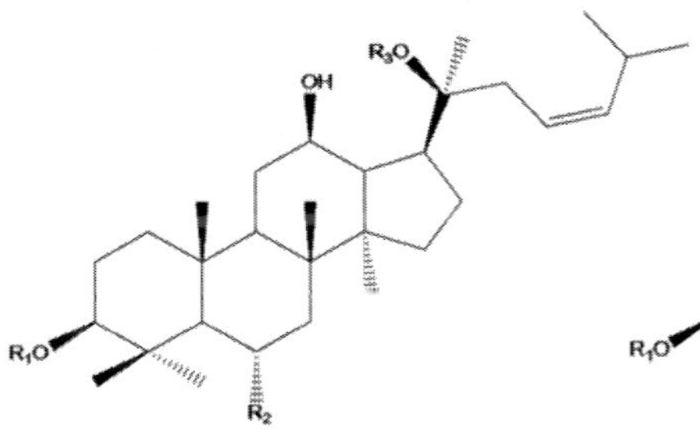

Compound 176

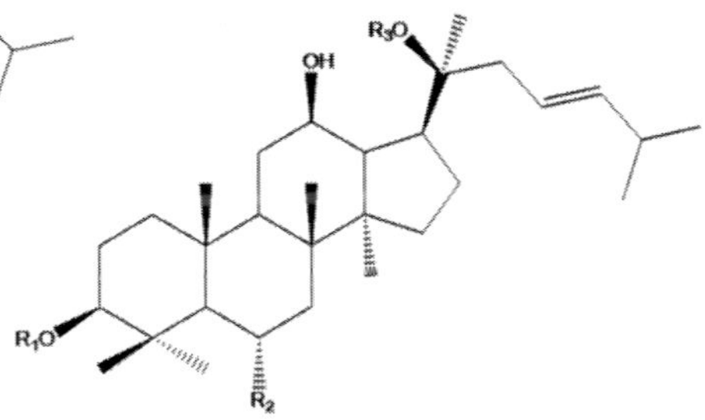

Compound 177

Table 1. (Continued)

No.	Name	R1	R2	R3	Source	Ref.
176	Ginsenoside Rs9	Glc[6]-Ac	OH	H	*P. ginseng*	[78]
177	Vinaginsenoside R8	Glc[2]- Glc	H	Glc	*P. vietnamensis*	[36]

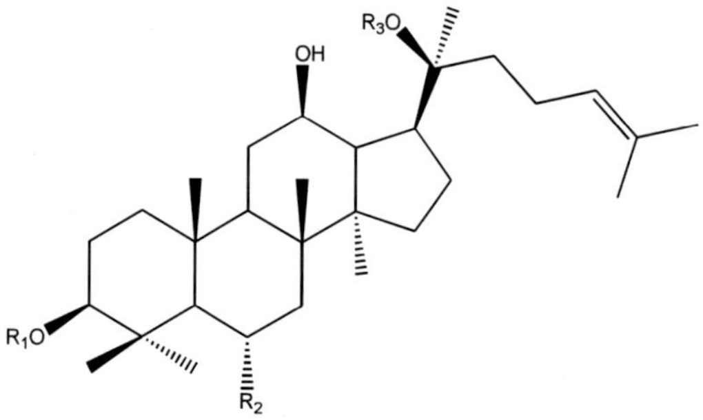

No.	Name	R1	R2	R3	Source	Ref.
178	Ginsenoside Ia	Glc	OH	Glc	*P. ginseng*	[54]
179	Floralginsenoside P	Glc[2]- Glc	OH	Glc[6]-Arap	*P. ginseng*	[73]
180	Vinaginsenoside R4	Glc[2]-Glc	OH	Glc	*P. vietnamensis*	[36]
181	Pseudo-ginsenoside F8	Ac-[6]Glc[2]-Glc	H	Glc[6]-Xyl	*P. notoginseng*	[23]

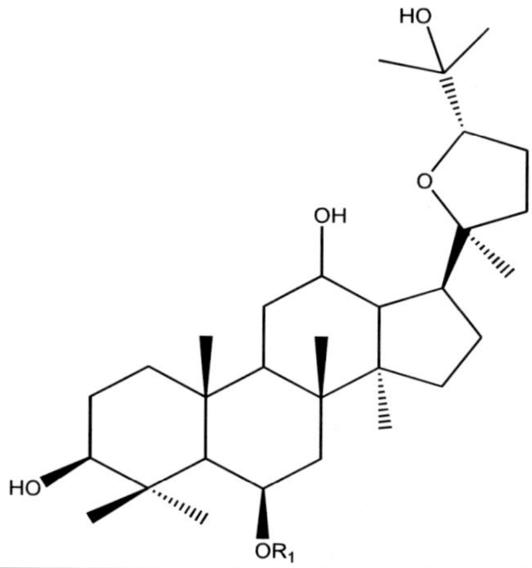

No.	Name	R	Source	Ref.
182	24R-pseudo- Ginsenoside F11	Glc[2]-Rha	*P. quenquifolium* *P. notoginseng* *P.japonicus*	[29] [4] [57]
183	Pseudo-ginsenoside RT5	Glc	*P. quenquifolium* *P. notoginseng*	[29] [102]
184	24R-vina-ginsenoside R1	Ac-[6]Glc[2]-Rha	*P. quenquifolium* *P. vietnamensis*	[29] [5]
185	24R-vina-ginsenoside R2	Ac-[6]Glc[2]-Xyl	*P. vietnamensis*	[36]
186	Vinaginsenoside R14	Glc[2]-Xyl	*P. vietnamensis*	[36]
187	Pseudo-ginsenoside RT2	Glc[2]-Xyl	*P. notoginseng*	[102]

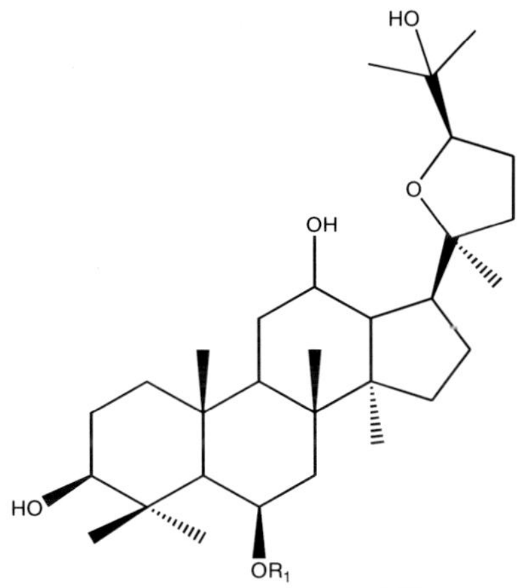

No.	Name	R	Source	Ref.
188	Pseudo-ginsenoside RT4	Glc	*P. vietnamensis*	[5]
			P.notoginseng	[102]
189	24S-Vina-ginsenoside R2	Ac-^{6}Glc^{2}-Rha	*P. vietnamensis*	[36]
190	24S-Pseudo-ginsenoside F11	Glc^{2}-Rha	*P. quenquifolium*	[29]
			P. notoginseng	[23]
			P. vietnamensis	[5]
191	Vina-ginsenoside R6	Xyl-^{2}Glc^{6}-Glc	*P. vietnamensis*	[36]
192	Majonoside R1	Glc^{2}- Glc	*P.japonicus*	[63]
193	Vina- Ginsenoside R5	Glc^{2}-Xyl^{4}- Glc	*P. vietnamensis*	[36]
194	Majonoside R2	Glc^{2}-Xyl	*P.japonicus*	[63]

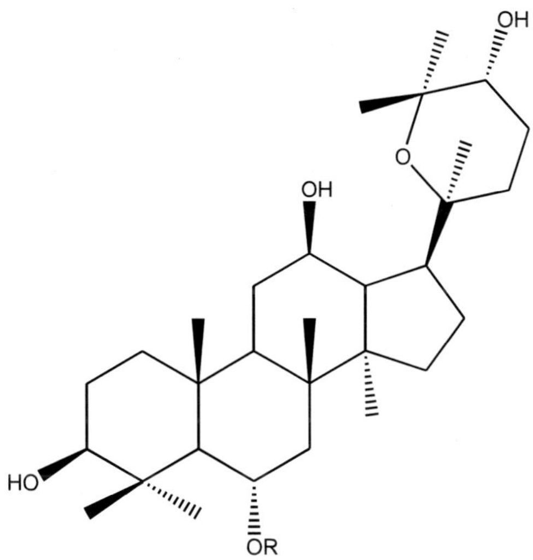

No.	Name	R	Source	Ref.
195	Vina-ginsenoside R10	Glc	*P. vietnamensis*	[36]
196	Vina-ginsenoside R11	Glc^{2}-Xyl	*P. vietnamensis*	[36]

Table 1. (Continued)

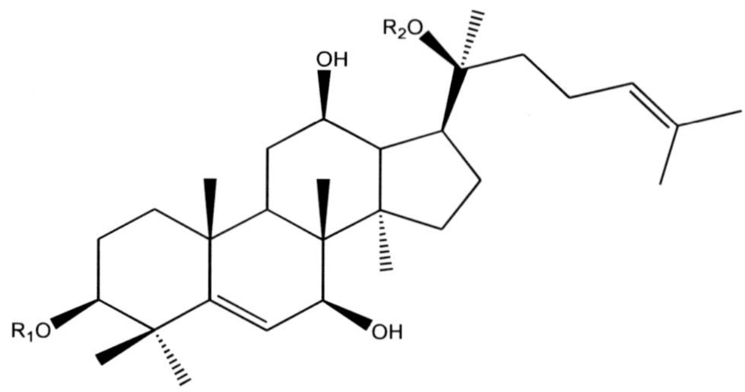

No.	Name	R1	R2	Source	Ref.
197	Quinquenoside IV	Glc^{2}-Glc	Glc^{6}-Glc	*P. quenquifolium*	[60]

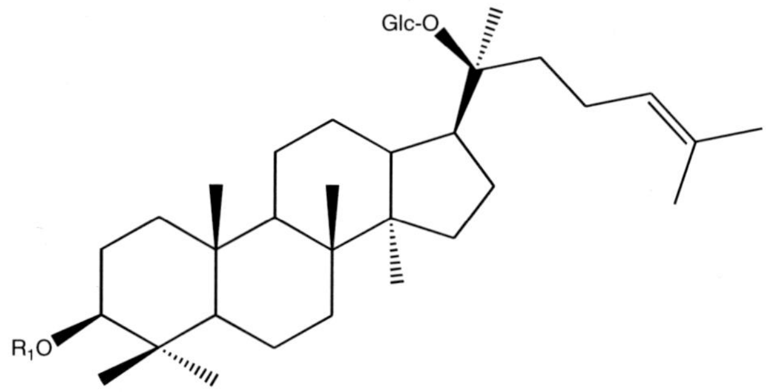

No.	Name	R	Source	Ref.
198	Vina-ginsenoside R3	Glc^{2}-Glc	*P. quenquifolium*	[44]
			P. vietnamensis	[30]

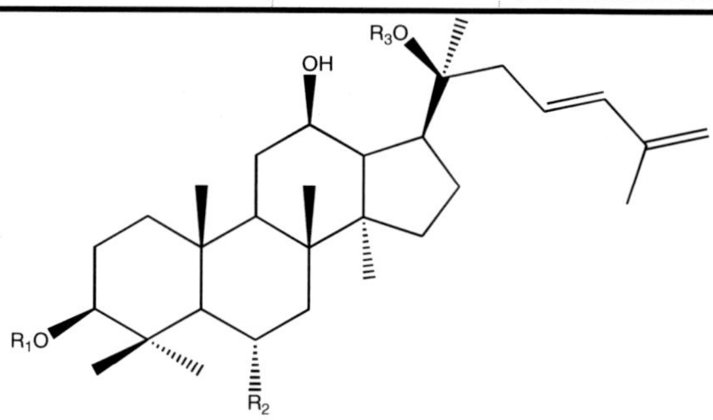

No.	Name	R1	R2	R3	Source	Ref.
199	Quinquenoside L1	Glc^{2}-Glc	H	Glc	*P. quenquifolium*	[83]
200	Quinquenoside L8	Glc	H	Glc^{6}-Xyl	*P. quenquifolium*	[92]

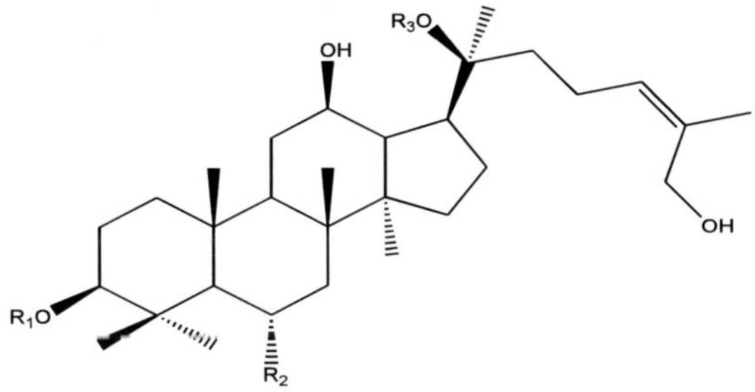

No.	Name	R1	R2	R3	Source	Ref.
201	Quinquenoside L2	Glc^2-Glc	H	Glc	*P. quenquifolium*	[83]
202	Quinquenoside L11	H	O-Glc^2-Rha	H	*P. quenquifolium*	[92]

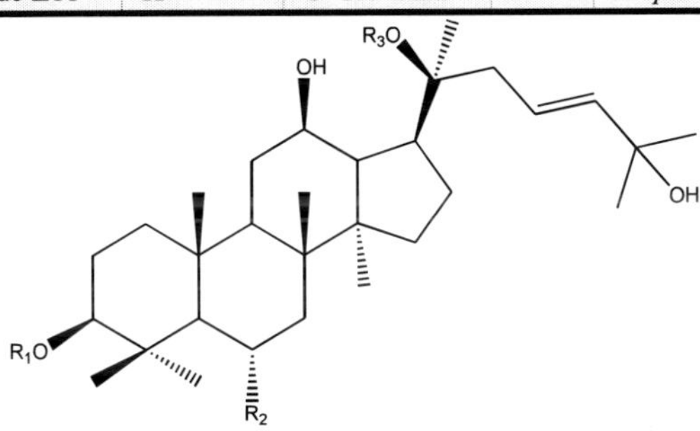

No.	Name	R1	R2	R3	Source	Ref.
203	Quinquenoside L3	Glc	H	Glc^6-Xyl	*P. quenquifolium*	[84]
204	Quinquenoside L7	Glc^2-Glc	H	Glc^6-Xyl	*P. quenquifolium*	[92]
205	Vina-Ginsenoside R8	Glc^2-Glc	H	Glc	*P. vietnamensis*	[30]
206	Quinquenoside L9	H	O-Glc^2-Rha	H	*P. quenquifolium*	[29]
207	Quinquenoside L16	Glc^2-Glc	H	Glc^6- Glc	*P. quenquifolium*	[33]

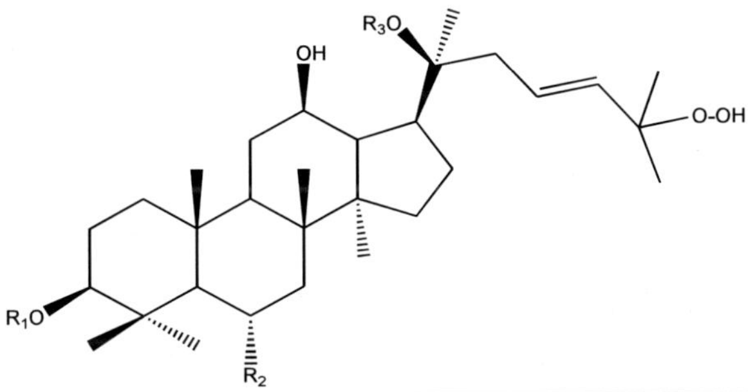

No.	Name	R1	R2	R3	Source	Ref.
208	Floralquinquenoside A	H	O- Glc	H	*P. quenquifolium*	[39]
209	Floralginsenoside B	H	O- Glc	Glc	*P. ginseng*	[72]
210	Floralginsenoside D	H	OH	Glc^6-Araf	*P. ginseng*	[72]
211	Floralginsenoside E	Glc^2-Glc	H	H	*P. ginseng*	[72]
212	Floralginsenoside F	Glc	H	Glc	*P. ginseng*	[72]
213	Floralginsenoside G	Glc^2-Glc^6- Ac	H	Glc	*P. ginseng*	[20]
214	Floralginsenoside I	H	O- Glc^2-Rha	Glc	*P. ginseng*	[20]
215	Floralginsenoside K	Glc^2- Glc	H	Glc	*P. ginseng*	[20]
216	Floralginsenoside O	Glc^2- Glc	H	Glc^6-Araf	*P. ginseng*	[73]
217	Floralquinquenoside C	H	O- Glc^2-Rha	H	*P. quenquifolium*	[39]

Table 1. (Continued)

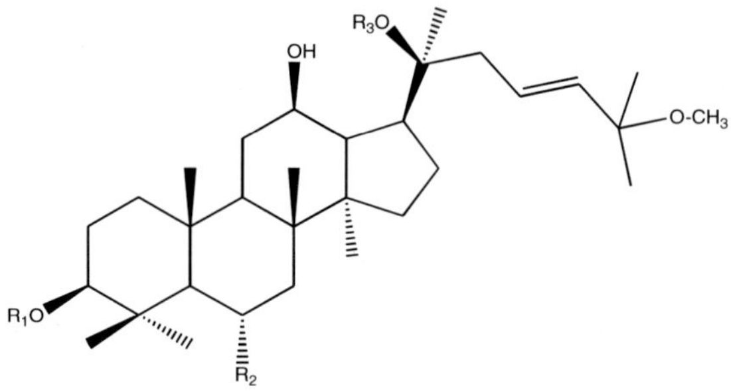

No.	Name	R1	R2	R3	Source	Ref.
218	Quinquefoloside La	Glc^{2}-Glc	H	Glc^{6}-Arap	*P. quenquifolium*	[44]
219	Quinquefoloside Lc	Glc^{2}-Glc	H	Glc^{6}-Xyl	*P. quenquifolium*	[44]

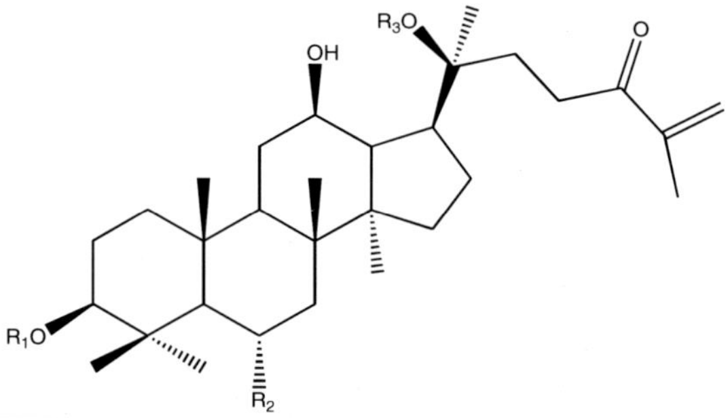

No.	Name	R1	R2	R3	Source	Ref.
220	Ginsenoside III	Glc^{2}-Glc	H	Glc	*P. quenquifolium* *P. ginseng*	[39] [103]

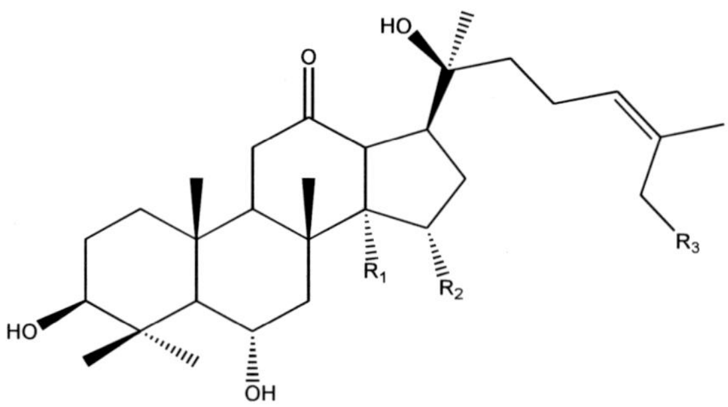

No.	Name	R1	R2	R3	Source	Ref.
221	12-OXO-26-hydroxyl-20S- Protopanaxatriol	H	H	OH	*P. quenquifolium*	[39]
222	12-OXO-15α-hydroxyl-20S- Protopanaxatriol	CH_3	OH	H	*P. quenquifolium*	[39]
223	12-OXO-27-hydroxyl-20S- Protopanaxatriol	CH_3	H	OH	*P. quenquifolium*	[39]

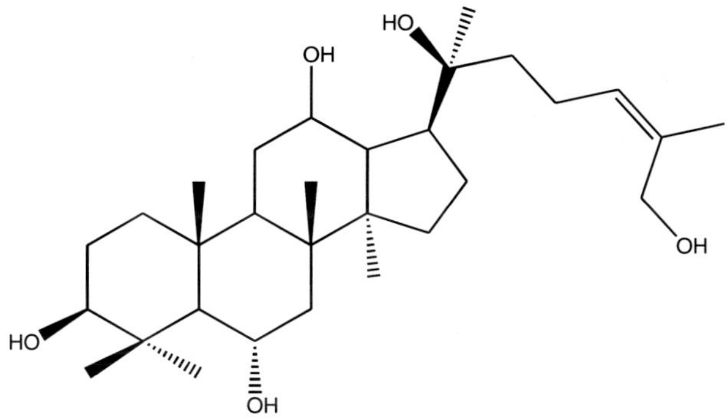

No.	Name	Source	Ref.
224	27-hydroxyl-20s- Protopanaxatriol	*P. quenquifolium*	[39]

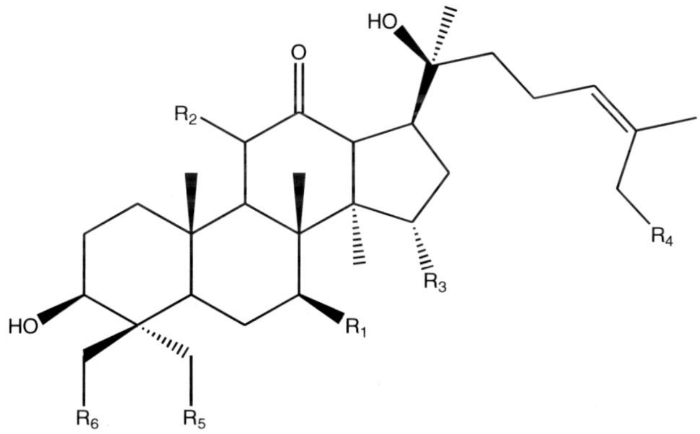

No.	Name	R1	R2	R3	R4	R5	R6	Source	Ref.
225	12-oxo-15α,27-dihydroxyl-20s- Protopanaxadiol	H	H	OH	OH	H	H	*P. quenquifolium*	[39]
226	12-oxo-7β,28-dihydroxyl-20s- Protopanaxadiol	OH	H	H	H	OH	H	*P. quenquifolium*	[39]
227	12-oxo-7β,11α,28-dihydroxyl-20s- Protopanaxadiol	OH	H	H	H	OH	H	*P. quenquifolium*	[39]
228	12-oxo-15α,29-dihydroxyl-20s- Protopanaxadiol	H	H	OH	H	H	OH	*P. quenquifolium*	[39]
229	12-oxo-7β, 15α -dihydroxyl-20s- Protopanaxadiol	OH	H	OH	H	H	H	*P. quenquifolium*	[39]
230	12-oxo-7β,11β-dihydroxyl-20s- Protopanaxadiol	OH	OH	H	H	H	H	*P. quenquifolium*	[39]
231	12-OXO-15α-hydroxyl-20s-Protopanaxadiol	H	H	OH	H	H	H	*P. quenquifolium*	[39]
232	12-OXO-7β-hydroxyl-20s-Protopanaxatriol	OH	H	H	H	H	H	*P. quenquifolium*	[39]

Table 1. (Continued)

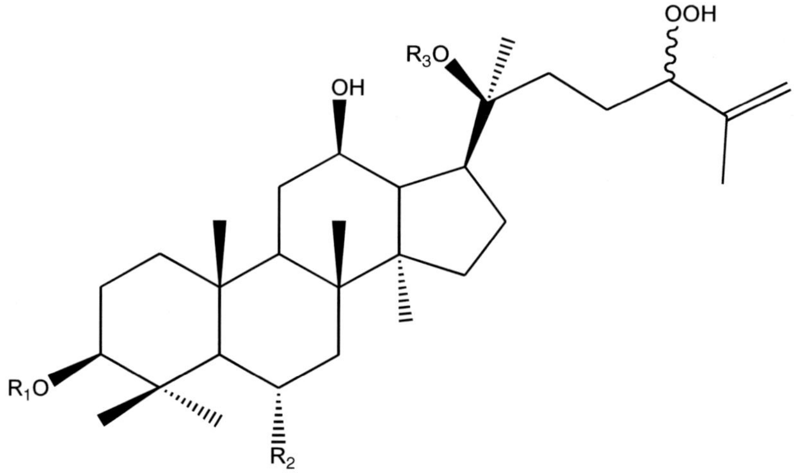

No.	Name	R1	R2	R3	Source	Ref.
233	Floralginsenoside A	H	O-Glc	Glc	*P. ginseng*	[72]
234	Floralginsenoside C	H	OH	Glc^{6}-Arap	*P. ginseng*	[72]
235	Floralginsenoside H	Glc^{2}-Glc^{6}-Ac	H	Glc	*P. ginseng*	[20]
236	Floralginsenoside J	H	O- Glc^{2}-Rha	Glc	*P. ginseng*	[20]
237	Floralginsenoside Ka	H	OH	Glc	*P. ginseng*	[46]
238	Floralginsenoside Tc	Glc^{2}-Glc	H	Glc^{6}-Arap	*P. ginseng*	[94]
239	Floralquinquenoside B	H	O- Glc^{2}-Rha	H	*P. quenquifolium*	[29]
240	Floralquinquenoside D	Glc	H	Glc	*P. quenquifolium*	[29]
241	Floranotoginsenoside B	Glc^{2}-Glc	H	Glc^{6}-Xyl	*P. notoginseng*	[47]
242	Floranotoginsenoside C	Glc^{2}-Glc	H	Glc^{6}-Araf	*P. notoginseng*	[47]
243	24R-Ginsenoside I	Glc^{2}-Glc	H	Glc	*P. ginseng*	[46]
244	24S-Ginsenoside II	Glc^{2}-Glc	H	Glc	*P. ginseng*	[46]
245	Ginsenoside SL1	H	O- Glc	H	*P. ginseng*	[95]
246	Quinquenoside I	Bu-^{6}Glc^{2}-Glc	H	Glc	*P. quenquifolium*	[29]
247	Notoginsenoside C	Glc^{2}-Glc	H	Glc^{6}-Glc	*P.notoginseng*	[20]

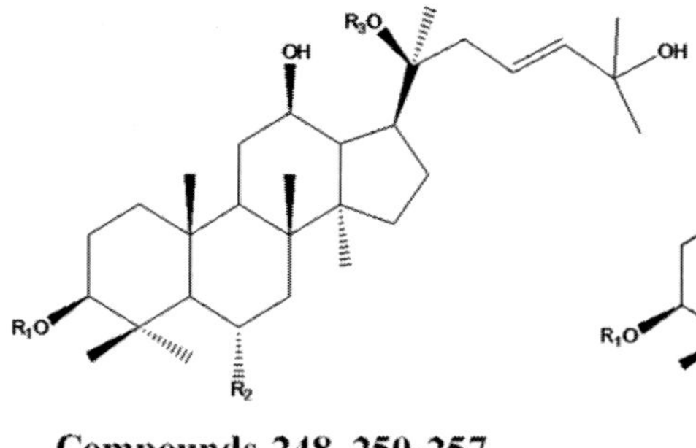

Compounds 248, 250-257

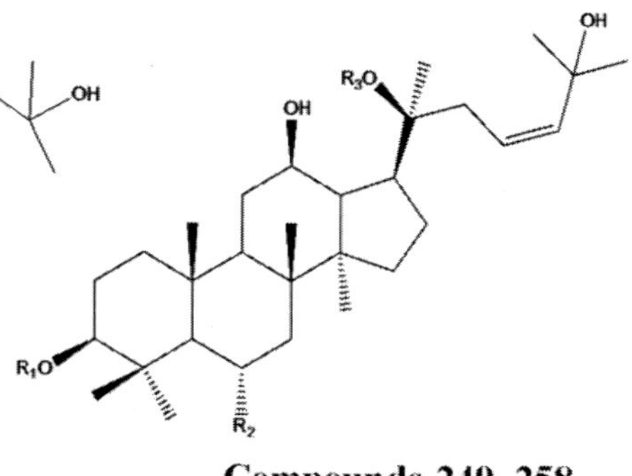

Compounds 249, 258

No.	Name	R1	R2	R3	Source	Ref.
248	Saponin 3b	H	O-Glc	Glc	*P. notoginseng*	[38]
249	Notoginsenoside H	H	O-Glc^2-Xyl	Glc	*P. notoginseng*	[20]
250	Floranotoginsenoside A	Glc^2- Glc	H	Glc^6-Araf	*P. notoginseng*	[47]
251	Ginsenoside ST2	H	O-Glc	H	*P. ginseng*	[96]
252	Notoginsenoside Rw2	H	O-Glc^2-Xyl	H	*P. notoginseng*	[52]
253	Notoginsenoside ST5	Glc^2- Glc^2-Xyl	H	H	*P. notoginseng*	[24]
254	Yesanchinoside H	Glc^2- Glc	H	Glc^6-Xyl	*P .japonicus* *P. notoginseng*	[35] [59]
255	Notoginsenoside A	Glc^2- Glc	H	Glc^6- Glc	*P. notoginseng*	[59]
256	Majoroside F4	Glc	OH	Glc	*P. japonicus*	[63]
257	Ginsenoside M6a	Glc^2- Glc	H	Glc	*P. japonicus*	[104]
258	Majoroside F6	H	O-Glc^2-Rha	Glc	*P. japonicus*	[105]

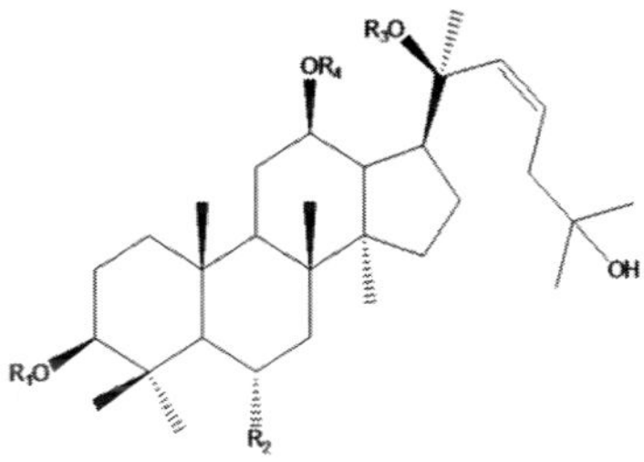

Compounds 259,261,262

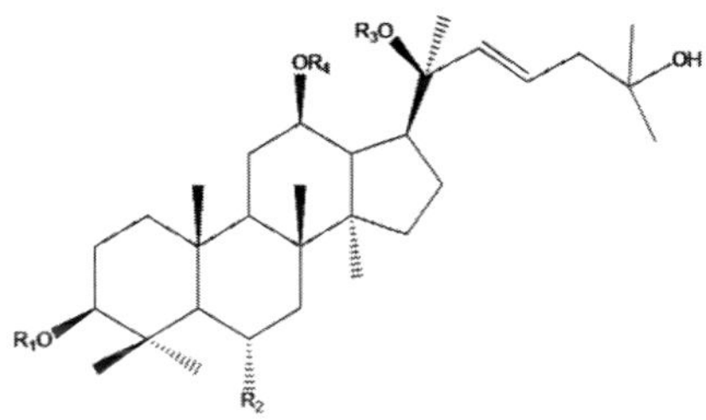

Compound 260

No.	Name	R1	R2	R3	R4	Source	Ref.
259	Notoginsenoside R8	H	O-Glc	H	H	*P. notoginseng*	[74]
260	Notoginsenoside R9	H	O-Glc	H	H	*P. notoginseng*	[74]
261	Chikusetsusaponin L9a	H	OH	H	Glc	*P. notoginseng* *P. japonicus*	[74] [56]
262	Koryoginsenoside Rg2	Glc2-Glc	H	Glc6-Glc	H	*P. ginseng*	[21]

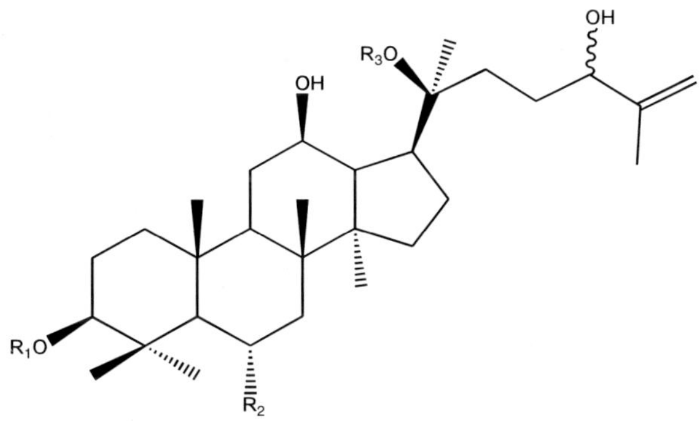

No.	Name	R1	R2	R3	Source	Ref.
263	24R Floralginsenoside La	H	O- Glc^2-Rha	Glc	*P. ginseng*	[73]
264	24S-Floralginsenoside Lb	H	O- Glc^2-Rha	Glc	*P. ginseng*	[73]
265	Floranotoginsenoside D	Glc^2- Glc	H	Glc^6-Araf	*P. notoginseng*	[47]
266	Notopanaxoside A	H	O- Glc	H	*P. notoginseng*	[76]
267	Notoginsenoside FT3	Glc^2- Glc^2-Xyl	H	H	*P. notoginseng*	[49]
268	Gypenoside LXXI	Glc-Glc	H	Glc^6-Xyl	*P. quenquifolium*	[44]
269	Majoroside F1	Glc^2- Glc	H	Glc	*P. japonicus* *P. vietnamensis*	[63] [5]
270	Majoroside F2	Glc	H	Glc	*P. japonicus*	[63]

Table 1. (Continued)

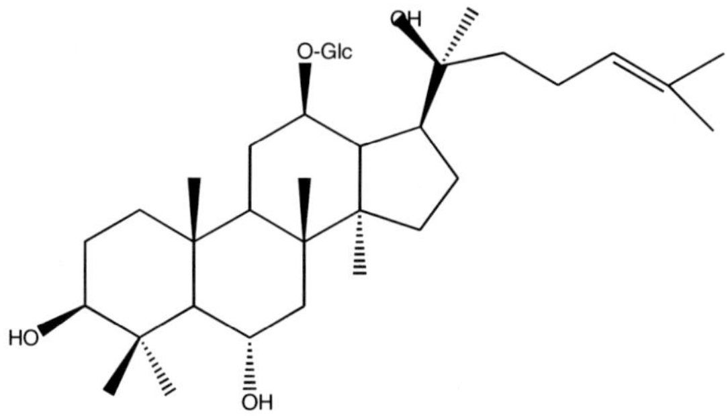

No.	Name	Source	Ref.
271	Chikusetsusaponin L_{10}	*P. japonicus*	[56]

No.	Name	R	Source	Ref.
272	Floralginsenoside Kb	Glc^2-Glc	*P. ginseng*	[46]

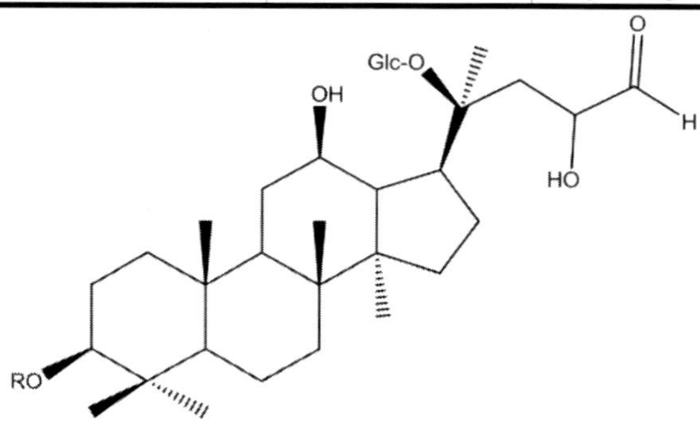

No.	Name	R	Source	Ref.
273	Floralginsenoside Kc	Glc^2-Glc	*P. ginseng*	[46]

No.	Name	R	Source	Ref.
274	Floralginsenoside Ta	OH	*P. ginseng*	[64]
275	Vina-ginsenoside R25	O-Glc	*P. ginseng* *P. vietnamensis*	[46] [81]

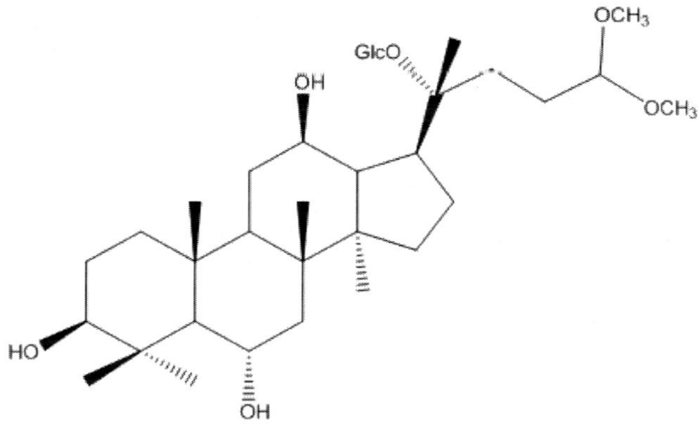

No.	Name	Source	Ref.
276	Floralginsenoside Tb	*P. ginseng*	[64]

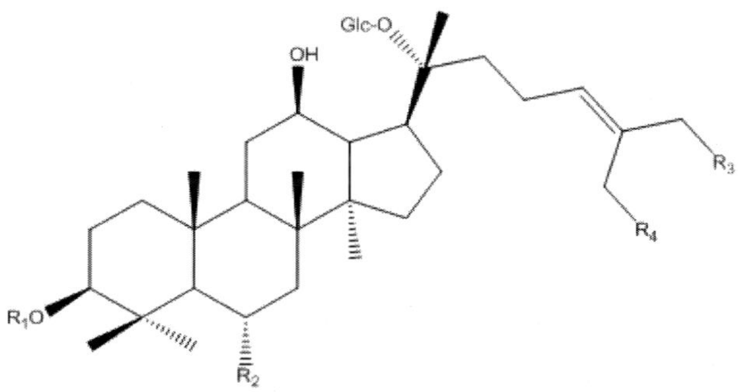

No.	Name	R1	R2	R3	R4	Source	Ref.
277	Ginsenoside Ki	H	OH	CH_3	OH	*P. ginseng*	[54]
278	Ginsenoside Km	H	OH	OH	H	*P. ginseng*	[54]
279	Quinquenoside L2	Glc^{2}Glc	H	H	OH	*P. quenquifolium*	[39]

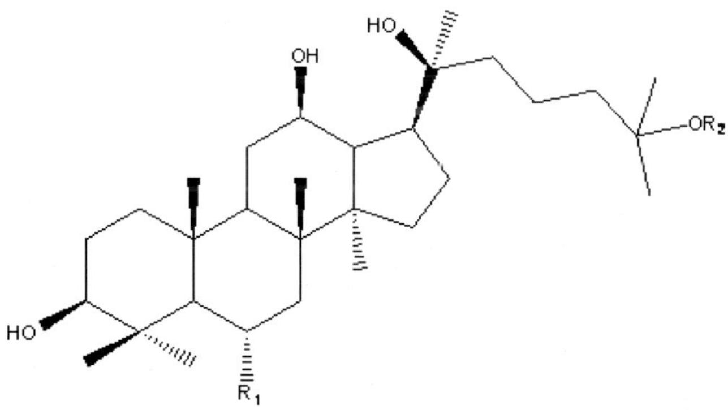

Table 1. (Continued)

No.	Name	R1	R2	Source	Ref.
280	25-OCH_3-Protopanaxadiol	H	CH_3	*P. notoginseng*	[62]
281	25-OH-Protopanaxadiol	H	H	*P. ginseng*	[19]
282	25-OH-Protopanaxatriol	OH	H	*P. ginseng*	[19]

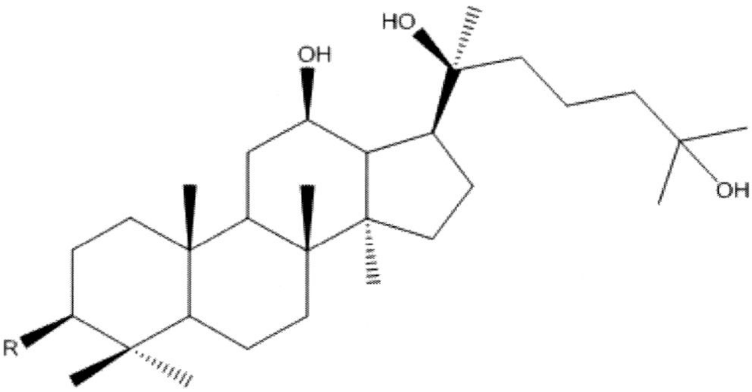

No.	Name	R	Source	Ref.
283	Notoginsenoside FT2	Glc^2-Glc^2-Xyl	*P. notoginseng*	[49]

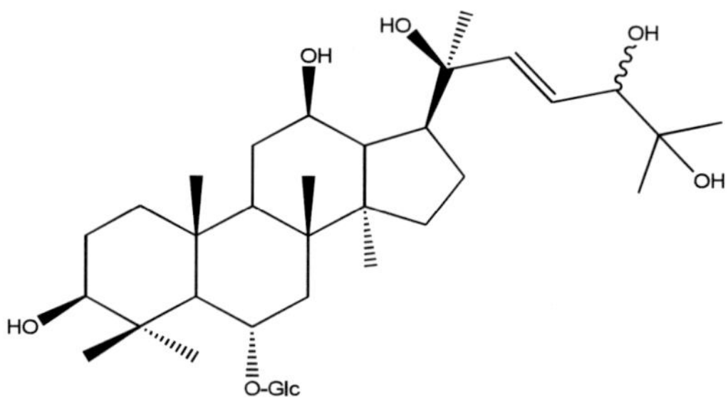

No.	Name	Source	Ref.
284	Notoginsenoside T4	*P. notoginseng*	[48]

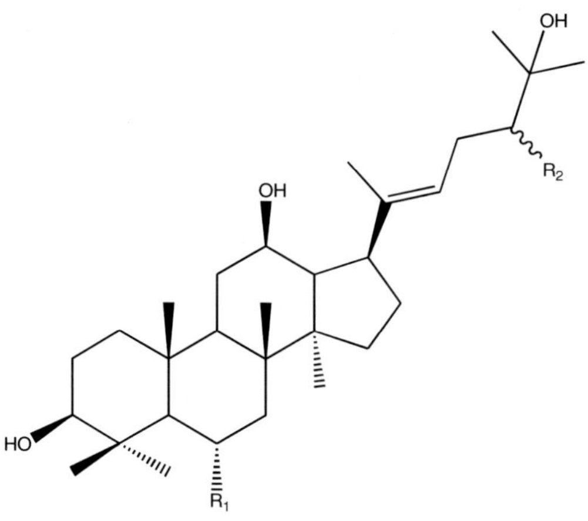

No.	Name	R1	R2	Source	Ref.
285	Notoginsenoside ST1	O-Glc	H	*P. notoginseng*	[24]

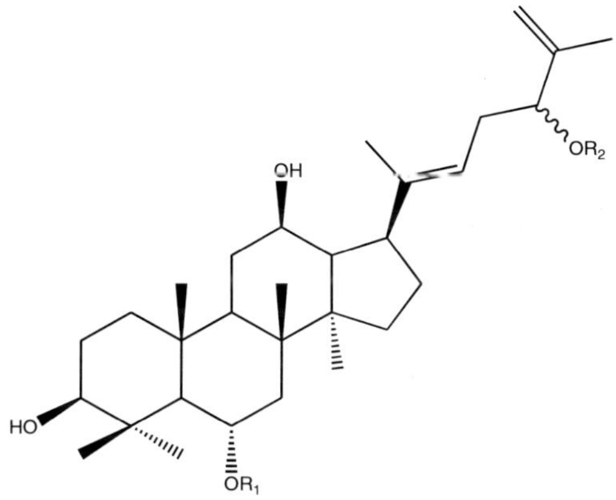

No.	Name	R1	R2	Source	Ref.
286	Ginsenoside SL2	Glc^2-Rha	OH	*P. ginseng*	[70]
287	Ginsenoside ST1	Glc	OH	*P. ginseng*	[70]

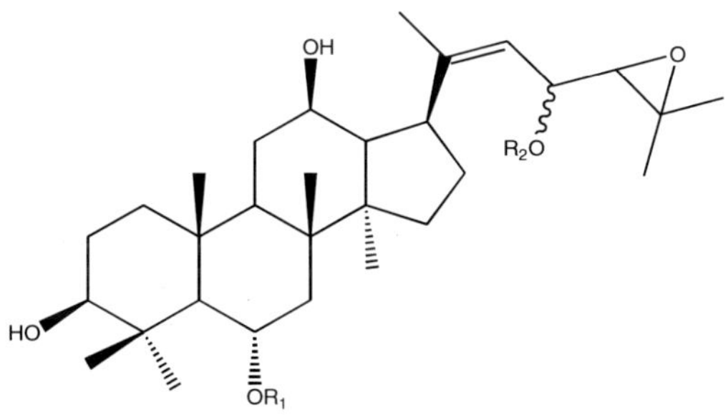

No.	Name	R1	R2	Source	Ref.
288	Ginsenoside Rg8	Glc^2-Rha	H	*P. ginseng*	[67]
289	Notoginsenoside T1	Glc	H	*P. notoginseng*	[82]
290	Notoginsenoside T2	Glc	CH_3	*P. notoginseng*	[82]

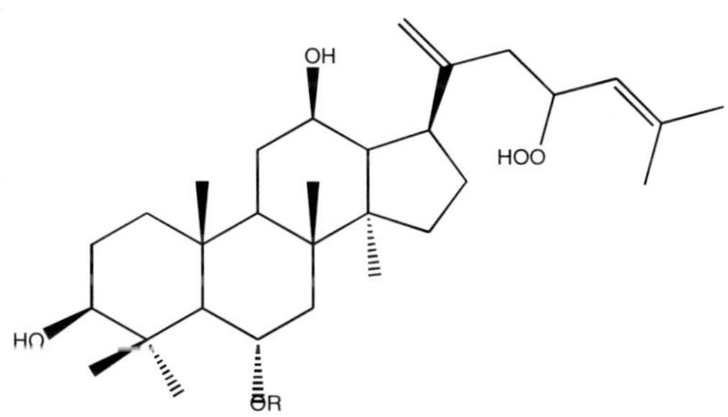

No.	Name	R	Source	Ref.
291	Ginsenoside SL3	Glc^2-Rha	*P. ginseng*	[70]

Table 1. (Continued)

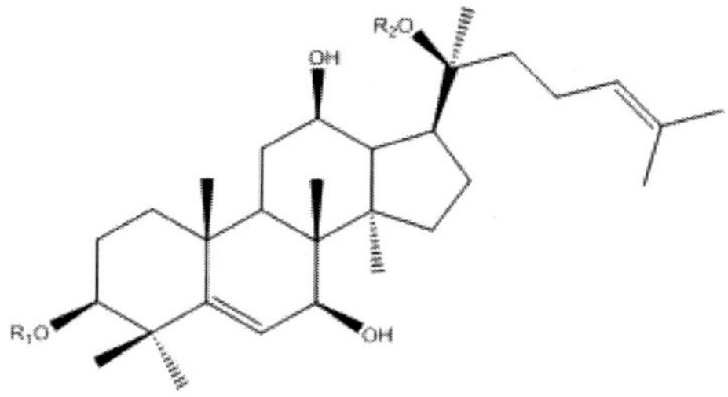

No.	Name	R1	R2	Source	Ref.
292	Yesanchinoside G	Glc^{2}-Glc	Glc^{2}-Xyl	*P. japonicus*	[35]

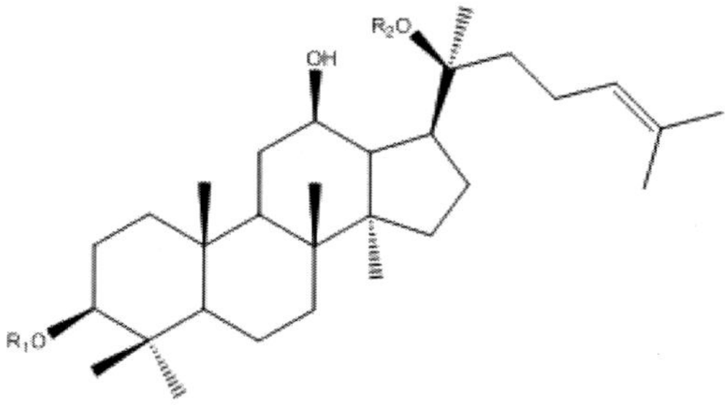

No.	Name	R1	R2	Source	Ref.
293	Yesanchinoside I	Glc^{2}-Glc	Glc^{6}- Glc^{6}-Xyl	*P. japonicus*	[35]

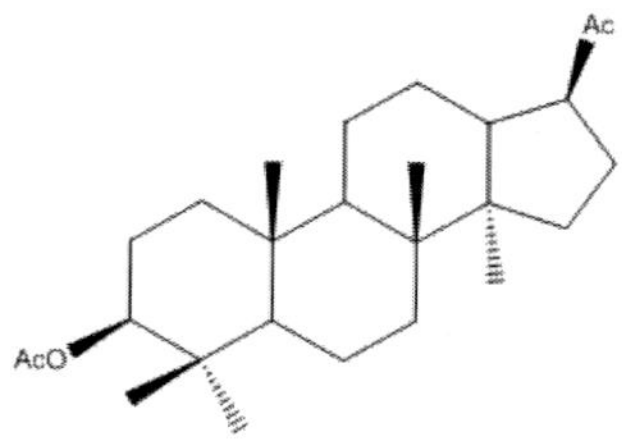

No.	Name	Source	Ref.
294	Hexanordammaran	*P .ginseng*	[75]
		P. notoginseng	[77]

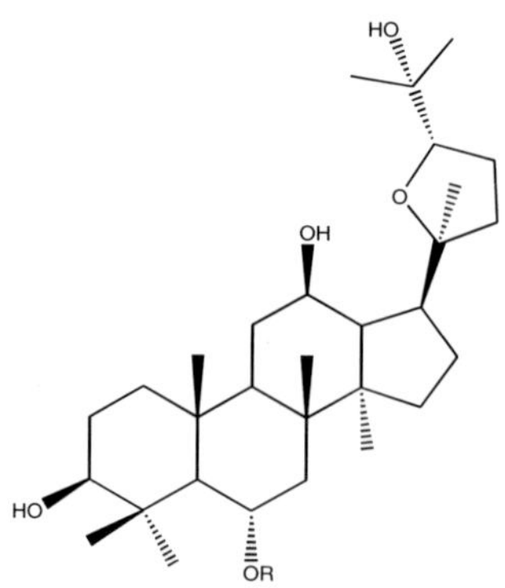

No.	Name	R	Source	Ref.
295	Yesanchinoside A	Ac-[6]Glc[2]-Glc	*P .japonicus*	[53]
296	Yesanchinoside B	Glc-[6]Glc[2]- Glc	*P .japonicus*	[53]
297	Yesanchinoside C	Glc[2]- Glc[2]-Xyl	*P .japonicus*	[53]

Ac, acetyl; Araf, α-L-arabinofuranosyl; Arap, α-L-arabinopyranosyl; Bu, Butenoyl; Glc, β-D-glucopyranosyl; GlcA, β-D-Glucuronopyranosyl; Ma, malonyl; Oc, Octenoyl Rha, mannopyranosyl; Xyl, β-D-xylopyranosyl.

Besides the saponins, some triterpenes are also listed in the table since they possess structural similarities and might contribute similar pharmacological activities.

3. Isolation and Purification

Highly purified chemical compounds and fractions of ginsenosides are absolutely necessary for the pharmacological test, structure-activity relationship study and quality control of *Panax* plants. It's interesting that the bioactivities of several ginsenosides are mutual antagonic [10,11]. Therefore, it is highly valuable to separate ginsenosides on a large scale for the further pharmacological studies. The repeated-column chromatography is the most common method for separation and purification of ginsenosides from genus *Panax* [106]. However, this conventional method is time-consuming, labor intensive and inefficient. In the past decade, with the development of novel isolation methods, many new technologies have been developed and applied to the isolation and purification of ginsenosides from *Panax* plants.

3.1. Macroporous Resins

Macroporous resins is a type of adsorbent possessing distinguishing features, including high separation efficiency, less labor intensiveness, low cost, and easy regeneration [12,13]. In whole process, only aqueous ethanol is used to desorb target compounds. Therefore, macroporous resins also has been considered to be an environmental-friendly absorbent [107]. Technically, the affinity between compounds and resin is influenced by molecular weight, polarity or configuration of different molecules. Thus, the target compounds can be enriched and purified due to the differences in the affinity for the adsorbent [108]. Macroporous resins has been widely used in the isolation of the total saponins from *P. ginseng* [109], *P. quinquefolius* [110], *P. notoginseng* [111] and *P. japonicus* [112], as well as group separation of protopanaxadiol and protopanaxatriol saponins from *P. notoginseng* [113] and *P. ginseng* [114,115].

Comparing with the polar macroporous resins, the non-polar and weak-polar absorbents (e.g. D-101, HPD-100 and DS-401) towards ginsenosides showed the better adsorption characteristics, such as higher adsorption and desorption capacities, higher desorption ratio and preferable separation behaviors [16-18,20]. Typically, ginseng samples are extracted with distilled water [110,115], ethanol [111,112] or methanol [113] using reflux [17-19], ultrasonication [115] or pressurized liquid extraction [113] once or several times, then the crude extracts are combined and concentrated *in vacuo* to dryness. The residue is suspended in water and subjected to macroporous resins column. High polar components are eluted by distilled water. Subsequently, the total saponins in ginseng samples are always desorbed by 60% - 80% (*v/v*) aqueous ethanol. In addition, PPT and PPD saponins could be successfully separated by 30% and 80% ethanol, respectively, due to their different adsorption force to resin (Figure 3). After the treatment of optimum resins and chromatographic conditions, the contents of PPT and PPD saponins were increased from 4.65% and 3.40% in the roots of *P. notoginseng* to 88.2% and 92.6% in the final products with the recoveries of 80.2% and 82.3%, respectively [113]. In order to increase desorption efficiency, microwave-assisted process (MAP), a technology that relates to extract soluble products into a fluid from wide rang of materials using microwave energy [116], was used to desorb the target compounds. PPT and PPD saponins were desorbed under different microwave condition with their desorption efficiency of more than 90% [114]. Compared with conventional methods for separating the two groups of saponins such as liquid-liquid extraction [117], silica gel column chromatography [118] and dialysis [119], macroporous resins possesses obvious merits, such as less solvent, less separation time and high separation efficiency.

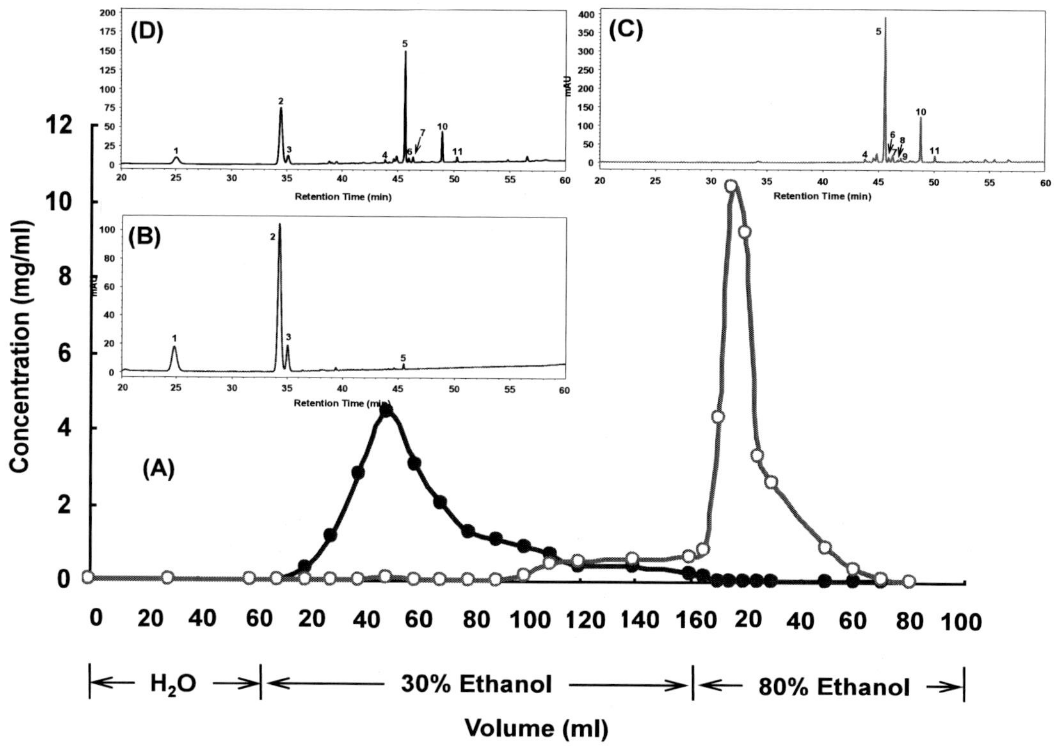

Figure 3. Dynamic desorption curves of PTS (•) and PDS (○) from *P. notoginseng* extract on DS-401 resin (A). The column packed with saturate DS-401 resin was gradually flushed with water, 30% and 80% aqueous ethanol (*v/v*) for respective different volumes. HPLC profiles of 20(*S*)-protopanaxtriol type (B) and 20(*S*)- protopanaxadoil type (C) saponin solution and feeding solution of *Panax* notoginseng extract (D). 1, notoginsenoside R1; 2-10, ginsenoside Rg1, Re, Rf; Rb1, Rg2, Rc, Rb2, Rb3 and Rd; 11, Notoginsenoside K, respectively. Reproduced with permission of Elservier Sciences from Ref. [113].

3.2. Preparative High Performance Liquid Chromatography (Prep-HPLC)

Prep-HPLC has become a principal method for the isolation and purification of interesting components from complex samples, such as extract of medicinal herbs, benefit by its online detection, parallel collection, high separation efficiency and short separation time [120]. There are various separation modes for prep-HPLC, such as normal-phase, reversed-phase and ion exchange chromatography, which have been employed to purify most types of natural products [121].

A number of studies reported the isolation of high purity ginsenosides from crude extracts of *P. ginseng* [122,123] and *P. notoginseng* [31-33] using pre-HPLC. Reversed phase C_{18} column [32-34] are widely used for separation of ginsenosides, besides, normal-phase column [124] is casually applied. Several mobile phase systems, such as n-butanol-ethyl acetate-water [124], methanol-water [123,125], acetonitrile-water [122,126] and ethanol-water [127] are used for large-scale preparation of ginsenosides. However, in most of studies, only one or two ginsenosides were separated and purified [30-32,34]. Moreover, before the pre-HPLC separation, the crude extracts need to be pre-treated and enriched by silica gel column [32,34], macroporous resin [124] or semi-preparative LC [122]. A simple pre-HPLC method was established to simultaneously isolate large quantity of pure notoginsenoside R1, ginsenosides Rg1, Re, Rb1 and Rd from the commercial total saponins or root of *P. notoginseng* [127], the separation of these 5 ginsenosides was achieved on an Zorbax ODS C18 preparative column using a special binary elution system: 40% (A) and 60% aqueous ethanol (B). The purity of each ginsenoside was more than 95% assessed by analytical HPLC-DAD.

3.3. Counter-Current Chromatography and Centrifugal Partition Chromatography

High-speed counter current chromatography (HSCCC), firstly introduced by Ito in the early 1970s [128], is a liquid-liquid partition chromatographic separation technique. Due to the absence of solid stationary phase, HSCCC eliminates the irreversible adsorption of samples on the support matrix, and enhances the sample loading capacity [129]. HSCCC has been successfully applied to the preparative separation of various ginsenosides from *Panax* species [37-42]. In order to enrich ginsenoside fraction, the crude extracts were usually pre-treated with normal phase chromatography, medium-pressure liquid chromatography [130], reversed-phase C18 column [131] and macroporous resin column [37,41,42], before loading to HSCCC. In addition, there is also a report of direct HSCCC separation of ginsenosides from crude extracts without pretreatment [132]. Ginsenosides always have few chromophores in their chemical structures, resulting in very poor ultraviolet (UV) absorption. Therefore, the evaporative light scattering detection (ELSD), a universal and nonspecific detector, is widely applied through the split valve to track separation results [37-42].

The two-phase solvent system of HSCCC is one of the critical important factors and greatly affects the separation results [133]. The composition of a two-phase solvent system can be optimized according to the partition coefficient (K) of the target ginsenosides that relied on their solubility in two immiscible phases [133]. Their K value should lie in the range 0.5 ~2.0 for the efficient separation. The separation of diverse ginsenosides has been achieved using preferable solvent systems, such as ethyl acetate–isopropanol –0.1% formic acid (3:1:5, *v/v*) [130], methylene chloride–methanol–water– isopropanol (6:6:4:1, *v/v*) [131], n-hexane–n-butanol–water (3:4:7, *v/v*/v) [132], ethylene chloride–methanol–5mM aqueous ammonium acetate–isopropanol (6:2:4:3, *v/v*) [134] and chloroform–methanol– water–isopropanol (4:3:2:1, *v/v*) [135].

To date, notoginsenoside R1, ginsenosides Rb1, Rb2, Rg1, Re, Rd, Rf, R0, Rg3, Rk1, Rg5, F4, Rh1 and Rc have been isolated on a large scale from *Panax* species using HSCCC technique with high purity and recovery, their structures also have been identified and confirmed by electrospray ionization mass spectrometry (ESI-MS) and/or nuclear magnetic resonance spectroscopy (NMR) [37-42].

Like HSCCC, centrifugal partition chromatography (CPC) is also a support-free liquid–liquid partition chromatographic separation method [136]. CPC combined with ELSD was employed for preparative separation of notoginsenoside R1, ginsenosides Rg1, Re and Rb1 from *P. notoginseng* using two-phase solvent system composed of ethyl acetate-n-butanol-water (1:1:2, *v/v*/v), and the purities of the products in a single run were over 98% [137]. Therefore, liquid-liquid isolation techniques, including HSCCC and CPC, were the fast and efficient methods for preparative separation of high purity ginsenosides from *Panax* species.

3.4. Immunoaffinity Chromatography

Immunoaffinity chromatography (IAC) provides a specific and sensitive method to isolate and purify target components from complicated sample matrices. Due to specific and reversible interaction between compounds of interest and their antibodies, single-step isolation and purification of components from herbal extracts will be possible [138]. IAC has been applied to isolate ginsenoside Rb1 from a crude extract of *P. ginseng* using anti-ginsenoside Rb1 monoclonal antibody [139]. In order to produce ginsenoside Re knock-out extracts for bioactivity studies, ginsenoside Re was removed from the berry of *P. quinquefolius* using its monoclonal antibody [140]. IAC method has many apparent merits, such as effective, rapid, specific and simple. However, a large amount of polyclonal or monoclonal antibody for target small molecule compound is required for preparative separation by IAC. In addition, instability of the immune-affinity column also limits its application.

4. Quality Control

Ginsenosides, processing various pharmacological activities, are generally considered to be the main bioactive principles of *Panax* species [141,142]. Thus, these saponins are the focus of quality control studies in *Panax* species. Given the fact that several species, such as *P. ginseng*, *P. quinquefolium* and *P. notoginseng*, are very popular botanic medicine worldwide, their quality control is particularly important to ensure safe and appropriate use of these herbs. During the last decade, considerable efforts have been made to develop qualitatively and quantitative methods to control the quality of the raw materials, extracts and commercial products.

4.1. Sample Preparation

Sample preparation is an essential step that greatly influences all the later assay procedure, it typically takes 70-80% of the total analysis time [143]. The aim of sample preparation is to isolate and/or concentrate as much as possible the desired chemical compounds from herbal material, and make the analytes more suitable for separation and detection [144]. The conventional sample preparation methods, such as ultrasound-assisted extraction (USE) [51-55], soxhlet extraction [56-58], heat reflux extraction (HRE) [145], immersion [60,61] have been widely used for extraction of ginsenosides from *Panax* species using various solvents, including methanol, ethanol, their aqueous mixtures and water-saturated n-BuOH.

However, these conventional sample preparation methods consisting of many steps are highly labor intensive, time-consuming and lack efficiency. Over the past decade, many new extraction approaches, such as pressurized liquid extraction (PLE) [60,62-64], ultrahigh pressure extraction (UPE) [56,65], pulsed electric field extraction (PEF) [146] and microwave- assisted extraction (MAE) [56,65], have been developed to obtain high yield ginsenosides with high efficiency.

PLE accelerates the extraction process by using solvent at elevated temperature and pressure. Pressure is applied to the sample extraction cell to maintain the heated solvent in a liquid state during the extraction process [147]. PLE has been applied to extract ginsenosides from *Panax* genus [60,62-64,67], and was compared with other extraction methods, including USE, soxhlet extraction and immersion. The results showed that the extraction efficiency of PLE was the highest one [60].

PEF extraction is an novel technique that use high the electric pressure, induce cell membrane permeability at room temperature, and thereby improve extraction efficiency [148]. A comparative study on sample preparation of *P. ginseng* using 6 extraction methods, including PEF, PLE, UPE, MAE, USE and HRE, was carried out, the results indicated that the whole extraction process of PEF takes less than 1 s with the highest yield of the ginsenosides [146]. These new sample preparation techniques have the obvious advantages of short extraction time, less solvent and energy consumption, high extraction efficiency and automatic operation compared to conventional extraction methods.

In order to eliminate the contaminants interference, thereby increase the detection sensitivity, sample clean-up is very important and necessary for further enrich the compounds of interest from complex matrices. Reversed-phase solid-phase extraction (SPE) has been commonly used to remove interfering substances and purify ginsenosides for subsequent analysis from raw material [149] and biological specimens, such as rat tissues [150], serum [151], urine [151] and feces [152].

4.2. High Performance Liquid Chromatography (HPLC)

HPLC is one of the most common analytical methods for separating non-volatile and polar components in a mixture using a solid stationary phase and a liquid mobile phase [153]. Due to low cost, readily available and versatile, HPLC has been widely applied for the analysis of ginsenosides in *Panax* plants and their products (Table 2). Generally, several chromatographic parameters, such as column, mobile phase, flow rate and elution program, greatly affect the separation results. Reverse phase C18 column is most commonly used to separate the ginsenoside. Besides, only one paper report to use NH_2 columns [154].

Table 2. Application of HPLC coupled with conventional detectors in analysis of ginsenosides

Analytes	Sample	Sample preparation	Column	Mobile phase	Flow rate (ml/min)	Detection	Ref
Rg1, Re, Rb1, Rc, Rb2 and Rd	*P. ginseng*	pulsed electric field; HER; PLE; HER; UPE, USE, MAE	YMC C18	ACN- water, gradient	1.2	UV, 203 nm	[146]
Rg1, Re, Rf, Rg2, Rb1, Rc, Rb3, Rd	*P. ginseng*	water saturation n-BuOH, USE	Agilent TC-C18	ACN-0.05% aqueous phosphoric acid	1.0	UV, 203 nm	[159]
Rg1, Re, Rf, Rg2, Rb1, Rc, Rb2, Rb3 and Rd	*P. ginseng* (root, leaf)	methanol, PLE	Prevail C18 rocket	ACN-water, gradient	2.5	UV, 203 nm APCI-MS(-)	[160]
Rg2, Rg3, Rh1, Rh2, Rg5 and Rk1	Red ginseng	Ethanol, USE	Unison UK-C18	30%(v/v) ACN-80% ACN, gradient	0.2	PAD	[161]
Rb1,Rd, F2, K	Process of biotransfor-mation of Rb1	NA	Eclipse XDB C18	ACN-water, gradient	1.0	UV, 203 nm	[162]
NR1, Rg1, Re, NR4, NFa, Rb1, NR2, Rg2, Rh1, Rd and NK	*P. notoginseng*	Water, USE	Zorbax Bonus-RP	ACN-water, gradient	1.5	UV, 203 nm ESI-MS(-)	[163]
NR1, Rg1 and Rb1	Fufang Danshen tablet	70% methanol, USE	Zorbax Extend C18	ACN-0.1% aqueous phosphoric acid	1.0	UV, 203 nm	[164]
NR1, F11, Rg1, Re, Rf, Rb1, Rg2, Rc, Rb2, Rb3, Rd, and Rg3	*P. ginseng* *P. notoginsen* *P. quinquefolius*	Methanol, PLE	Zorbax ODS C18	ACN-water, gradient	1.5	ELSD	[165]
Rg1, Re, Rf, Rh1, Rg2, Rb1, Rc, Rb2, Rb3, Rd, Rg3,Rk1, Rg5, and Rh2	Red ginseng powder and its concentrate	100% methanol after wetting samples in water for 2 h, USE, then SPE	Zorbax SB-Aq C18	ACN-water, gradient	1.0	ELSD	[166]
20 (R)-Rg2 and 20(S)-Rg2	Plasma after iv	SPE	Diamonsil™ ODS C18	MeOH-4% phosphoric acid (65:35, v/v)	1.0	UV, 203 nm	[167]
Rg1, Re, Rb1, Rc, Rb2 and Rd	*P. ginseng*	pulsed electric field; HER; PLE; HER; UPE, USE, MAE	YMC C18	ACN- water, gradient	1.2	UV, 203 nm	[146]
Rg1, Re, Rf, Rg2, Rb1, Rc, Rb3, Rd	*P. ginseng*	water saturation n-BuOH, USE	Agilent TC-C18	ACN-0.05% aqueous phosphoric acid	1.0	UV, 203 nm	[159]
Rg1, Re, Rf, Rg2, Rb1, Rc, Rb2, Rb3 and Rd	*P. ginseng* (root, leaf)	methanol, PLE	Prevail C18 rocket	ACN-water, gradient	2.5	UV, 203 nm APCI-MS(-)	[160]
Rg2, Rg3, Rh1, Rh2, Rg5 and Rk1	Red ginseng	Ethanol, USE	Unison UK-C18	30%(v/v) ACN-80% ACN, gradient	0.2	PAD	[161]
Rb1,Rd, F2, K	Process of biotransfor-mation of Rb1	NA	Eclipse XDB C18	ACN-water, gradient	1.0	UV, 203 nm	[162]
NR1, Rg1, Re, NR4, NFa, Rb1, NR2, Rg2, Rh1, Rd and NK	*P. notoginseng*	Water, USE	Zorbax Bonus-RP	ACN-water, gradient	1.5	UV, 203 nm ESI-MS(-)	[163]
NR1, Rg1 and Rb1	Fufang Danshen tablet	70% methanol, USE	Zorbax Extend C18	ACN-0.1% aqueous phosphoric acid	1.0	UV, 203 nm	[164]
NR1, F11, Rg1, Re, Rf, Rb1, Rg2, Rc, Rb2, Rb3, Rd, and Rg3	*P. ginseng* *P. notoginsen* *P. quinquefolius*	Methanol, PLE	Zorbax ODS C18	ACN-water, gradient	1.5	ELSD	[165]
Rg1, Re, Rf, Rh1, Rg2, Rb1, Rc, Rb2, Rb3, Rd, Rg3,Rk1, Rg5, and Rh2	Red ginseng powder and its concentrate	100% methanol after wetting samples in water for 2 h, USE, then SPE	Zorbax SB-Aq C18	ACN-water, gradient	1.0	ELSD	[166]
20 (R)-Rg2 and 20(S)-Rg2	Plasma after iv	SPE	Diamonsil™ ODS C18	MeOH-4% phosphoric acid (65:35, v/v)	1.0	UV, 203 nm	[167]

Analytes	Sample	Sample preparation	Column	Mobile phase	Flow rate (ml/min)	Detection	Ref
Rg1, Re, Rb1, Rc, Rb2 and Rd	*P. ginseng*	pulsed electric field; HER; PLE; HER; UPE, USE, MAE	YMC C18	ACN- water, gradient	1.2	UV, 203 nm	[146]
Rg1, Re, Rf, Rg2, Rb1, Rc, Rb3, Rd	*P. ginseng*	water saturation n-BuOH, USE	Agilent TC-C18	ACN-0.05% aqueous phosphoric acid	1.0	UV, 203 nm	[159]
Rg1, Re, Rf, Rg2, Rb1, Rc, Rb2, Rb3 and Rd	*P. ginseng* (root, leaf)	methanol, PLE	Prevail C18 rocket	ACN-water, gradient	2.5	UV, 203 nm APCI-MS(-)	[160]
Rg2, Rg3, Rh1, Rh2, Rg5 and Rk1	Red ginseng	Ethanol, USE	Unison UK-C18	30%(v/v) ACN-80% ACN, gradient	0.2	PAD	[161]
Rb1,Rd, F2, K	Process of biotransformation of Rb1	NA	Eclipse XDB C18	ACN-water, gradient	1.0	UV, 203 nm	[162]
NR1, Rg1, Re, NR4, NFa, Rb1, NR2, Rg2, Rh1, Rd and NK	*P. notoginseng*	Water, USE	Zorbax Bonus-RP	ACN-water, gradient	1.5	UV, 203 nm ESI-MS(-)	[163]
NR1, Rg1 and Rb1	Fufang Danshen tablet	70% methanol, USE	Zorbax Extend C18	ACN-0.1% aqueous phosphoric acid	1.0	UV, 203 nm	[164]
NR1, F11, Rg1, Re, Rf, Rb1, Rg2, Rc, Rb2, Rb3, Rd, and Rg3	*P. ginseng* *P. notoginsen* *P. quinquefolius*	Methanol, PLE	Zorbax ODS C18	ACN-water, gradient	1.5	ELSD	[165]
Rg1, Re, Rf, Rh1, Rg2, Rb1, Rc, Rb2, Rb3, Rd, Rg3,Rk1, Rg5, and Rh2	Red ginseng powder and its concentrate	100% methanol after wetting samples in water for 2 h, USE, then SPE	Zorbax SB-Aq C18	ACN-water, gradient	1.0	ELSD	[166]
20 (R)-Rg2 and 20(S)-Rg2	Plasma after iv	SPE	Diamonsil^{TM} ODS C18	MeOH-4% phosphoric acid (65:35, v/v)	1.0	UV, 203 nm	[167]
Rb1, Rb2, Rc, Rd, Re, and Rg1	*P. quinquefolium*	UPE, USE, HRE, MAE, Soxhlet, Supercritical CO2 extraction	Diamonsil C18	ACN-0.05% aqueous phosphoric acid	1.0	UV, 203 nm	[168]
Rb1, Rb2, Rb3, Rc, Rd, Re, Rg1, Rg2, 20(R)-Rg2, Rg3, Rh1, and Rh2. Rh1,Rg2, and 20(R)-Rg2	*P. quinqueforlius* (roots, rootlets, leaf and berry)	Methanol, Soxhlet, then SPE	Prodigy ODS(2) Gemini C18	ACN-water, gradient	1.0	UV, 202 nm	[149]
NR1, Rg1, Re, Rb1, Rc, Rb2, Rb3 and Rd	*P. notoginseng* (root, fibre root, rhizome, leaf, flower and seed)	Methanol, PLE	Zorbax ODS C18	ACN-water, gradient	1.5	ELSD	[169]
NR1, Rg1, Re, Rf, Rb1, Rc, Rb2, Rb3 and Rd	*P. notoginseng*	PLE, USE, Soxhlet, Immersion	Zorbax ODS C18	ACN-water, gradient	1.5	UV, 203 nm ESI-MS(-)	[60]
Rg1, Re,Rb1, Rc,Rb2, and Rd	*P. quinquefolium* *P. ginseng*	70% methanol, USE	Phenomenex Luna 3μm C18(2)	90% 10mM NH4CO2 + 10%ACN - 90%ACN + 10%100mM NH4CO2, gradient	1.0	UV, 205 nm ESI-MS(+)	[74]
Rg1, Re, Rb1, Rc and Rd	*P. quinquefolium*	Methanol–H2O(4:1), HRE	Bondapak C18	ACN-water, gradient	1.2	UV, 203 nm	[145]
Rg1, Rb1 and Rd	Rat tissues (kidney, liver, heart, spleen and lung) after the administration of PNS	SPE	Zorbax ODS C18	ACN-water, gradient	0.8	UV, 203 nm	[150]
NR1, Rg1, Rb1, Rg2, Rh1 and Rd	*P. notoginseng*	80% aqueous methanol, USE	Zorbax SB-C18	ACN-0.001% aqueous formic acid, gradient	0.8	UV, 203 nm	[156]
NR1, Rg1, Rb1, Rd	*P. notoginseng*	Immersion	NOVA-PAK C18	ACN-50mM KH2PO4, gradient	1.0	UV, 203 nm	[155]
Rb1, Rb2, Rc, Rd, Re, and Rg1	*P. quinquefolium*	HRE, USE	end-capped Purosphere C18	ACN-water, gradient	1.0	UV, 203 nm	[170]

Rb1, Rc, Rd, Re, Rg1, NR2, R0, Majonoside R2, Chikusetsusaponin III, IV, IVa	12 *Panax* taxa	70% Ethanol, USE	YMC-Pack ODS-AQ 303	10Mm K-phosphate buffer (pH 5.80)-ACN, gradient	1.0	UV, 196 nm	[171]
NR1, Rg1, Rb1 and Rd	Rat serum after oral and iv administration of PNS	SPE	Zorbax SB-C18	ACN-water, gradient	0.8	UV, 203 nm	[151]
Rb1, Rc, Rd, Re and Rg1	*P. ginseng*, *P. quinquefolium*, *P. japonicus* and *P. noteginseng*	80% methanol, USE	Li Chrosorb RP-18	ACN–0.5% H3PO4 (20 : 80 for Rg1 and Re, 31 : 69 for others)	1.0	UV, 203 nm	[172]
NR1, Rg1, Rb1 and Rd	*P. notoginseng*	70% methanol, Soxhlet	NOVA-PAK C18	ACN-50 mM KH2PO4, gradient	1.0	UV, 203 nm	[173]
Rg1, Rb1	Serum	Reacts with FMOC-hydrazine, then SPE	NOVA-PAK C18	50%MeOH (0.1% TFA)-90% MeOH (0.1% TFA)	0.8	Fluorescence detector (λex=270nm, λem=310nm)	[174]
R1, Rg1, Rb1, Rd	Urine after oral and iv administration of PNS	SPE	Zorbax SB-C18	ACN-water, gradient	0.8	UV, 203 nm	[151]

ACN, acetonitrile; APCI, atmospheric-pressure chemical ionization; BuOH, butanol; ELSD, evaporative light-scattering detector; HRE, heat reflux extraction; iv, intravenous; MAE; microwave-assisted extraction; NA, not available; PAD, pulsed amperometric detection, PLE, pressurized liquid extraction; PNS, total saponin of *P. notoginseng*; SPE, solid phase extraction; UPE, ultrahigh pressure; USE; ultrasonic-assisted extraction.

Acetonitrile-water system with gradient elution program has been used to separate ginsenosides as the mobile phase in most studies. In order to improve the separation results, several chemical additives, such as KH_2PO_4 [155], H_3PO_4 [54,73], NH_4CO_2 [74] and HCOOH [156], were also added to mobile phase. For example, the concentration of the phosphate buffer greatly affects the separation of 12 ginsenosides in white ginseng [157]. Due to the similar chemical structure and retention characteristics, ginsenoside Rg1 and Re could not be fully resolved in several studies [57,61,77].

However, their desired resolution can be obtained using low percentage (18%~19%) of acetonitrile in the initial 30min [20,33,60,63,64]. Moreover, flow rate is important factor for the separation of ginsenoside Rg1 and Re [158]. The separations are achieved using the flow rate of 0.8-2.5ml/min.

Another advantage of HPLC is versatility of detection, numerous detectors, including ultraviolet (UV), evaporative light scattering (ELSD), fluorescence, refractive index (RI) and more recently, mass spectrometry (MS), have been employed to detect the ginsenosides.

4.2.1. Ultraviolet (UV)

Among the various detection techniques, UV or diode array detection (DAD) is most commonly used to analyze the ginsenosides, because it is prevailing detector in most phytochemical laboratories. Ginsenosides are a group of triterpene saponins and show very weak UV absorption, the detection of ginsenosides is limited between 196 and 205 nm [73,74] with limit of detection (LOD) of 0.2–0.3 μg on column. Therefore, this feature also limits the choice of solvents and mobile-phase additives, they should no or very low UV absorption in detection wavelength. Otherwise, the detection of ginsenosides will be greatly influenced, especially using gradient elution program. HPLC-UV/DAD has been developed for simultaneous detection of 11 saponins in *P. notoginseng* [163], 15 ginsenosides in different parts of *P. quinqueforlius* (including roots, rootlets, leaf and berry) [149], and 11 saponins in 47 samples of ginseng drugs derived from 12 *Panax* taxa [171]. Pseudo-ginsenoside F11, an ocotillol type triterpene, is unique component in *P. quinquefolium*, could be used as the chemical marker to distinguish *P. quinquefolium* from other *Panax* species [165]. However, due to the lack of chromophore in chemical structure, pseudo-ginsenoside F11 could not be detected by UV, but by the universal detection method, such as ELSD or MS detector.

4.2.2. Evaporative Light Scattering Detection (ELSD)

ELSD is a mass detector and an alternative method for determination of non-chromophoric compounds, its signal only rely on the concentration/ amount of the solute in the effluent, rather than its optical characteristics [175]. ELSD provides a stable baseline even with steep gradient elution, which resolves the main problem in UV detection of ginsenosides [176].

Furthermore, many volatile mobile phase additives, including ammonium hydroxide, ammonium acetate, formic acid and acetic acid, have been used for improving the separation results and detection selectivity. The flow rate of the nebulizer gas and drift tube temperature is two important adjustable parameters and significantly affects the signal response of ELSD. In order to obtain the better sensitivity of detection, these parameters should be optimized systematically [158].

HPLC-ELSD method has been widely used for simultaneous determination of 11 saponins in *P. notoginseng* [158], 8 saponins in different parts of *P. notoginseng* (including root, fibre root, rhizome, leaf, flower and seed) [169], 14 ginsenosides in powder and concentrate of red ginseng [166], and 12 saponins, including pseudo-ginsenoside F11, in *P. ginseng*, *P. notoginseng* and *P. quinquefolius* [165]. The sensitivity of ELSD was found to be greatly higher than that of UV with the LOD of 18–300ng. However, ELSD is still not much in use for the routine quality control of ginseng sample, HPLC-UV remains the recommended method because of easier handling and greater availability.

4.2.3. Mass Spectrometry (MS)

MS is another mass detector and provides higher selectivity and sensitivity for the determination of minor components without chromophore groups in the herbs.

In the past years, HPLC coupled with different type of MS detector has been extensively applied to qualitatively and quantitatively assay the ginsenosides in raw materials [85-87], ginseng products [88,89] and biological specimens [90-93].

Most of the quantitative analysis of ginseng samples is performed by HPLC–UV/MS, MS information is used to assign peaks or identify ginsenosides [53,60,62,74]. Several types of ion sources or interfaces, including electrospray ionization (ESI) [88,94,95], fast-atom-bombardment (FAB) [177], thermospray (TSP) [178], fourier transform ion cyclotron resonance (FTICR) [179], atmospheric pressure chemical ionization (APCI) [180] and surface enhanced laser desorption (SELD) [98], were also used for ionization of ginsenosides. Two types of mass analyzer, including ion trap [86,87,94], time-of-flight (TOF) [85,98,99] are widely used to assay ginseng samples.

In order to a gain stable and maximal signal to noise, several factors should be optimized, such as ion source, detective mode (positive or negative ion mode), and the composition of mobile phase. Typically, negative ion mode is more sensitive, and provides straightforward structural information of ginsenosides [87,88], but more structural information on the ginsenosides was obtained in the positive ion mode [181].

The mobile phase modifier, such as ammonium acetate [88,100], ammonium formate [177] and acetic acid [87,96], were used to improve the separation results and enhance the ion intensity. Deprotonated molecular ion of ginsenosides could be observed along with its molecular weight by LC-MS, and the product ions from these deprotonated molecular ions were further analyzed by LC-MS/MS. The glycosidic linkages, core and attached sugar of the ginsenosides are obtained by collision-induced dissociation (CID) from the deprotonated molecular ion. Thereby, the ginsenosides could be identified.

Therefore, HPLC coupled with MS is a powerful tool for analysis of saponins in *Panax* species.

Table 3. Application of liquid chromatography in analysis of ginsenosides

Analytes	Sample	Sample preparation	Column	Mobile phase	Analytical time and flowrate	Detection	Ref
Rf, F11	*P. ginseng* *P. quinquefolium*	70% (v/v) MeOH, USE	BEH C18 (50mm× 2.1mm i.d.,1.7μm)	H_2O–HCOOH (100:0.2) : ACN–THF(10:1)=70:30, isocratic	2min 0.4 ml/min	Q-TOF-MS	[183]
Re, Rg1	Human serum after iv Shen-Fu injection	MeOH extraction	BEH C18 (100mm× 2.1mm i.d., 1.7μm)	H_2O:ACN:MeOH=45:22:33, isocratic	4min NA	ESI-MS/MS RMR model	[184]
Re, Rg1, Rh1	Mouse serum after iv and oral administration of Re or ginseng berry extract	After removing protein, MeOH extraction	BEH C18 (50mm× 2.1mm i.d.,1.7μm)	5mM NH_4CO_2 (pH 3.3) and ACN, gradient	6.5 min 0.45 ml/min	ESI-MS/MS SIR model (-)	[105]
NR1, Rg1, Re, Rb1	rat plasma after oral administration of Qi-luo- tong-qiao tablets	After removing protein, MeOH extraction	HSS T3 C18 (100mm× 2.1mm i.d., 1.8μm)	ACN - 0.5nM aqueous NH_4Cl, gradient	9min 0.2ml/min	ESI-MS/MS SIR model (-)	[185]
Rg1, Re, Rf, Rb1, Rg2, Rc, Rb2, Rb3, Rd and Rg3	*P. notoginseng*	MeOH, PLE	BEH C18 (50mm× 2.1mm i.d.,1.7μm)	H_2O:ACN, gradient	12min 0.35 ml/min	UV, 203nm	[182]
metabolite profiling	Raw and steamed *P. notoginseng*	70% (v/v) MeOH, USE	BEH C18 (100mm× 2.1mm i.d., 1.7μm)	H_2O (0.1% HCOOH) – ACN(0.1% HCOOH), gradient	12min 0.5 ml/min	TOF-MS	[186]
metabolite profiling	*P. ginseng P. notoginseng, P. Japonicus, P quinquefolium*	70% (v/v) methanol, USE	BEH C18 (100mm× 2.1mm i.d., 1.7μm)	10–70% ACN(0.05% HCOOH)- H_2O (0.05% HCOOH), gradient	20min 0.35 ml/min	TOF-MS	[187]

Q-TOF-MS, Quadrupole time-of-flight mass spectrometry; USE, ultrasonic-assisted extraction; THF, tetrahydrofuran; iv, intravenous ACN, acetonitrile.

4.3. Ultra Performance Liquid Chromatography (UPLC)

One of the most common problems encountered in performing HPLC analyses of ginseng sample is long analytic time of more than 45 min [53,55,58,63,67].

In order to well separate ginsenosides Rg1 and Re, the low percentage (18%~19%) of acetonitrile in the initial 30 min has been used, hereby, the total analytic time extended largely [60,67]. UPLC utilizes the smaller particles (1.7μm~1.8μm) as stationary phases and causes the high operating pressures ranging 6000–15,000 psi, which obtain the higher peak capacity, greater resolution, increased sensitivity and efficiency together with short times of analysis [101,102].

Recently, UPLC has been extensively used to determine the ginseng samples in less than 20 min (Table 3). Guan *et al* developed an UPLC method for simultaneous determination of 11 saponins in *P. notoginseng* using an Acquity UPLC^{TM} BEH C_{18} column (50mm× 2.1mm i.d., 1.7μm) and gradient elution of water-acetonitrile system in only 12min, and the LOD of analytes were lower to 0.1-1.8 ng on the column [182]. UPLC coupled with MS detector, such as ESI-MS, TOF-MS, has also been used for analysis of ginsenosides in serum and plasma after administration of ginseng-related products [104-106].

In addition, UPLC holds promising attributes in metabolite profiling and metabolomics, especially, for large-scale untargeted metabolic profiling due to its enhanced reproducibility [108,109]. UPLC has been applied in metabolite profiling studies of raw and steamed *P. notoginseng* [186], and 5 medicinal *Panax* species [187]. Currently, due to high cost of equipment and consumables, UPLC hampers to apply to analysis of ginseng sample.

4.4. Capillary Electrophoresis (CE)

CE is a means of separating electrically charged materials according to their different electrophoretic mobility under the influence of an electric field. CE became a very popular and effective analytical technique due to high efficiency, fast analysis, low cost, and minimal waste consumption [188]. Due to the absence of charge in neutral ginsenosides, conventionally, could not be suitable to detect by capillary zone electrophoresis (CZE), but micellar electrokinetic chromatography (MEKC). In MEKC separation model, the low molecular mass surfactants are added to the buffer, aggregates and forms micelle, neutral analytes can be separated according to the partitioning of analytes between the ionic micelle and the surrounding aqueous mobile phase [189]. Therefore, MEKC has been applied to determine the ginsenosides in *P. ginseng* [190], *P. quinquefolius* [191] and *P. notoginseng* [114,115]. For example, 10 saponins, such as notoginsenoside R1, ginsenoside Rb1, Rg1, Rh1, Rg2, Rf, Re Rd, Rc and Rb3, in *P. notoginseng* were simultaneously determined by MEKC with LOD of 1.7–6.3 μg/ml [192]. Recently, another separation model, microemulsion electrokinetic chromatography (MEEKC) was also employed to analyze ginsenosides [116,117]. MEEKC is very similar to MEKC in separation principle, and the main difference is that the microemulsion has a core of tiny droplets of oil inside the micelles. In order to improve the sensitivity of MEKC or MEEKC, several on-line preconcentration techniques, including field-enhanced sample injection with reverse migrating micelles [192], dual sweeping via complexation and organic solvent field enhancement [117,118], pressure and electrokinetic injections of long sample plugs with simultaneous stacking [193], have developed and applied in the analysis of ginseng saponins.

4.5. Others

Besides the analytical methods mentioned above, thin layer chromatography (TLC) [194], gas chromatography (GC) [195], near infrared (NIR) spectroscopy [196], Raman spectroscopy [197], nuclear magnetic resonance (NMR) spectroscopy [198], HPLC coupled with Charged aerosol detector (CAD) [199] or fluorescence detector [174], and Enzyme-linked immunosorbent assay (ELISA) [200] have also been used for quantitative and qualitative analysis of ginsenosides from *Panax* plants. However, all of these methods have their own disadvantages and still are not extensively applied to determination of ginseng samples.

Conclusion

The saponins isolated from *Panax* species have attracted worldwide interests due to their extensive benefits to human beings. Current pharmacological studies revealed that the extracts and individual saponins from *Panax* plants possessed protective effect against cardiovascular and cerebrovascular diseases, immunomodulatory, anticarcinogenic and anti-diabetes activities. About 300 tritrepene saponins and derivations have been isolated from *Panax* plants, and are an abundant source of chemical diversity. Saponins are generally considered as active compounds, which is the focus of quality control of raw materials and relative products of *Panax* species.

References

[1] Lu Q, Fu L, Li XG. *J. Jilin. Agr. Univ.* 1992, 14, 107-111.
[2] Ambrose CT. *Pharos Alpha Omega Alpha Honor Med. Soc.* 2010, 73, 4-10.
[3] Tanaka O. *Pure Appl. Chem.* 1990, 62, 1281-1284.
[4] Shibata S. *J Korean Med Sci. 2001*, 16, 28-37.
[5] Duc MN, Nham NT, Aiko KR *et al. Chem. Pharm. Bull.* 1993, 41, 2010-2014.
[6] Noriko LT, Junzo S. *Chem. Pharm. Bull.* 1976, 24, 253-261.
[7] Liu SY, Shang WF, Xu LZ *et al. J. Asian Nat. Prod. Res.* 2005, 7, 643-648.
[8] Shukla Y, Raghunath S, Pachaly P. *Phytochemistry* 1992, 31, 1046-1048.
[9] Junzo L. *J. Chin. Chem. Soc.* 1979, 26, 29-35.
[10] Yang Z, Wu M, Zhou O. *Yaoxue Xuebao* 1984, 19, 232-236.
[11] Shukla Y, Raghunath S. *Phytochemistry* 1990, 29, 239-241.
[12] Hu Y, He Y, Wang H *et al. Zhongguo Zhong Yao Za Zhi* 2010, 35, 1009-1013.
[13] Zhang HL, Tan Z, Qiu GT *et al.Tetrahedron Lett.* 2002, 43, 973-977.
[14] Noriko K, Junzo S. *Chem. Pharm. Bull.* 1971, 19, 1103-1107.
[15] Li H, Qi LW, L Yi *et al. Anal. Chim. Acta* 2007, 596, 264-272.
[16] Zhao HH, Yuan Y, Zhang D *et al. Agri. Sci. Tech.* 2010, 11, 126-129.
[17] Wan JB, Zhang QW, Hong SJ *et al. Molecules* 2010, 15, 8169-8176.
[18] Du XW, Wills RBH, Stuart DL. *Food Chem.* 2004, 86, 155-159.
[19] Lee SY, Park N, Kim CS et al. *J. Med. Plants Res.* 2010, 4, 349-353.
[20] Sugimoto S, Matsuda H, Kitagawa N et al. *Chem. Pharm. Bull.* 2009, 57, 283-287.
[21] Kim DS, Ye JC, Zedk U *et al. Phytochemistry 1995*, 40, 1493-1497.
[22] Yang TR, Kasaia R, Zhu J *et al. Phytochemistry* 1983, 22, 1473-1478.
[23] Tanakaa O. *Phytochemistry* 1978, 17, 1353-1358.
[24] Liao PY, Wang D, Zhang YJ *et al. J. Agric. Food Chem.* 2008, 56, 1751-1756.
[25] Li HZ, Ying J, Yan C. *Tianran Chanwu Yanjiu Yu Kaifa* 2006, 18, 549-554.
[26] Park JD, Kim DS, Kwon HY *et al. Arch. Pharm. Res.* 1998, 21, *615-617.*
[27] Kim DH, Jung JS, Moon YS *et al. Biol. Pharm. Bull.* 2003, 26, 1035-1038.

[28] Ruan CC, Liu Z, Li X *et al. Molecules* 2010, 15, 2319-2325.
[29] Nakamura S, Sugimoto S, Matsuda H *et al. Chem. Pharm. Bull.* 2007, 55, 1342-1348.
[30] Duc MN, Kasai RO, Kazuhiro IA *et al. Chem. Pharm. Bull.* 1994, 42, 115-122.
[31] Dou D, Wen Y, Weng M *et al. Zhongguo Zhongyao Zazhi* 1997, 22, 35-37.
[32] Qu C, Bai Y, Jin X *et al. Food Chem.* 2009, 115, 340-346.
[33] Chen J, Zhao R, Zeng YM, *et al. J. Asian Nat. Prod. Res.* 2009, 11, 195-201.
[34] Wang XY, Wang D, Ma XX *et al. Helvetica Chim. Act.* 2008, 91, 195-199.
[35] Zou K, Zhu S, Meselhy MR *et al. J. Nat. Prod.* 2002, 65, 1288-1292.
[36] Duc NM, Kasai R, Yamasaki K *et al. Studies in Plant Sci.* 1999, 6, 77-82.
[37] Hasegawa H. *J. Pharmacol. Sci.* 2004, 95, 153-157.
[38] Wang CZ, McEntee E, Wicks S. *J Nat. Med.* 2006, 60.97-106.
[39] Qi LW, Wang CZ, Yuan CS *et al. Phytochemistry* 2011, 72, 689-699
[40] Xu S, Cai Y, Cai Z Yao *et al.Yaoxue Xuebao* 1987, 22, 750-755.
[41] Kanamori H, Terauchi M, Fuse J *et al. Med* 1995, 49, 293-297.
[42] Besso H, Kasai R, Wei J *et al.Chem. Pharm. Bull.* 1982, 30, 4534-4538.
[43] Tung NH, Kim JA, Song GY *et al. Bull. Korean Chem.* 2010, 3,3423-3426.
[44] Qiu YK, Dou DQ, Cai LP. *Fitoterapia* 2009, 80, 219-223.
[45] Tung NH, Kim JA, Song GY *et al. Bull. Korean Chem.* 2010, 31, 1381-1385.
[46] Tung NH, Song GY, Nhiem NX *et al. J. Agric. Food Chem.* 2010, 58, 868-874.
[47] Wang JR, Yamasaki Y, Tanaka T *et al. Molecules* 2009, 14, 2087-2094.
[48] Teng RW, Li HZ, Wang DZ *et al. Helvetica Chim. Acta* 2004, 87, 1270-1278.
[49] Chen JT, Li HZ, Wang D *et al. Helvetica Chim. Acta* 2006, 89, 1442-1448.
[50] Li GY, Zeng YM, He M *et al. Chin. Chem. Lett.* 2009, 20, 1207-1210.
[51] Sun H, Ye Y. *Int Immunopharmacol* 2006, 6, 14 - 25.
[52] Cui XM, Zhang ZY, Zeng J *et al. J. Asian Nat. Prod. Res.* 2008, 10, 845-849.
[53] Zou KZ, Shu CT, Cai S *et al. J. Nat. Prod.* 2002, 65, 346-351.
[54] Tung NH, Park YJ, Kim YH. *Chem. Pharm. Bull.* 2009, 57, 1412-1414.
[55] Matsuura H, Kasai R, Tanaka O *et al. Chem. Pharm. Bull.* 1983, 31, 2281-2287.
[56] Yahara S, Kim R, Tanaka O *et al. Chem. Pharm. Bull.* 1977, 25, 2041-2047.
[57] D Wang, J Fan, S Liu *et al.* Jiaxun. *Yunnan Zhiwu Yanjiu* 1988, 10, 101-104.
[58] Lu F, Sun D, Yu X *et al. Zhongcaoyao* 2001, 32, 619-621.
[59] Liu J, Wang X, Cai S *et al. J Chin Pharm Sci* 2004, 13, 225-237.
[60] Yoshikawa M, Murakami T, Yashiro K *et al. Chem. Pharm. Bull.* 1998, 46, 647-654.
[61] Yamabe N, Lee JG, Lee YJ *et al. J. Ginseng Res.* 2011, 35, 60-68.
[62] Wang K, Zhang Y. *Zhongguo Yaowu Huaxue Zazhi* 2008, 18, 288-290.
[63] Feng B, Wang X, Wang D et al. *Yunnan Zhiwu Yanjiu* 1987, 9, 477-484.
[64] Tung NH, Song GY, Kim JA et al. *Bioorg. Med. Chem. Letters* 2010, 20, 309-314.
[65] Han B, Ming Q, Li Q *et al. Arzneimittel Forschung* 2011, 61, 148-152.
[66] Hang S, Yang X, Chen Y *et al. Chem. Pharm. Bull.* 1989, **37**, 1966-1968.
[67] Dou D, Guo N, Fu R *et al. Chem. Pharm. Bull.* 2006, 54, 751-753.
[68] Lee SM, Shon HJ, Choi CS *et al. Chem. Pharm. Bull.* 2009, 57, 92-94.
[69] Kim SH, Hyun SH, Yang SO *et al. J. Food Sci.* 2010, 75, 577-581.
[70] Nguyen HT, Quang TH, Son JH *et al. Arch. Pharm. Res.* 2011, 34, 681-685.
[71] Kwon SW, Han SB, Park IH *et al. J. Chromatogr. A* 2001, 921, 335-339.
[72] Yoshikawa M, Sachiko S, Nakamura S *et al. Chem. Pharm. Bull.* 2007, 55, 571-576.
[73] Nakamura S, Sugimoto S, Matsuda H *et al. Chem. Pharm. Bull.* 2007, 55. *1342-1348.*

[74] Zhao P, Liu YQ, Yang CR. *Phytochemistry* 1996, 41, *1419-1422,*.
[75] Wu L, Wang L, Gao H *et al. Fitoterapia* 2007, 78, 556-560.
[76] Komakine N, Okasaka M, Takaishi Y *et al. J Nat. Med.* 2006, 60,135-137..
[77] Li HZ, Teng RW, Yang CR *et al. Chin. Chem. Lett.* 2001, 12, 59-62.
[78] Tang X, Song X, Huang J *et al. Asian J. Trad. Med.* 2007, 2, 124-126.
[79] Dou DQ, Cong YJ, Liang LH *et al. Chem. Pharm. Bull.* 2001, 49, 442-446.
[80] Iwasaki H, Nomura M, Suzuki N *et al. Jpn Kokai Tokkyo Koho* 2011, 15,67-69.
[81] Quan LT; Ketut AI, Yasuhiro T *et al. J. Nat. Prod.* 2001, 64, 456-461.
[82] Rong W, Teng HZ, Zhang XM *et al. Chin. Chem. Lett.* 2001, 12, 239-242.
[83] Chen J, Zhao R, Zeng YM *et al. J .Asian Nat. Prod. Res.* 2001, 3, 123-130.
[84] Wang J, Liu W, Li X *et al. J Asian Nat.* Prod. Res. 1998, 1, 93-97.
[85] Zhao P, Liu Y, Yang C. Yunnan Zhiwu Yanjiu 1993, 15, 409-412.
[86] Shibata S, Fujita M, Itokawa H et al. Chem. Pharm. Bull. 1963, 11, 759-764.
[87] Shibata S, Tanaka O, Soma K *et al. Tetrahedron Lett* 1965, 42, 207-213.
[88] Li HZ, Wei RT, Yang CR *et al. Chin. Chem. Lett.* 2001, 12, 59-62.
[89] Wang JY, Li XG, Zheng YN *et al. J. Asian Nat. Prod. Res.* 2004, 6, 289-293.
[90] Park IH, Han SB, Kim JM *et al. Arch harm Res* 2002, 25, 837-841.
[91] W Rong, HZ Teng, XM Zhang *et al Helvetica Chim. Acta* 2004, 87, 1270-1278.
[92] Cong Y, Li W, Liu C *et al. Asian J Traditional Med* 2008, 6, 24-27.
[93] Liang C, Ding Y, Nguyen HT *et al. Bioorg. Med. Chem. Lett.* 2010, 20, 7110-7115.
[94] Tung NH, Song GY, Kim JA *et al. Bioorg. Med. Chem. Lett.* 2010, 20, 309-314.
[95] Tung NH, Song GY, Mihn CV *et al. Chem. Pharm. Bull.* 2010, 58, 1111-1115.
[96] Tung NH, Song GY, Kang HK *et al. Bull Korean Chem. Soc.* 2010, 31, 2094-2096.
[97] Yuan Y, Gao H, Wu B *et al. Asian J. Trad. Med.* 2006, 1, 91-93.
[98] Park JD, Kim DS, Kwon HY *et al. Arch. Pharm. Res.* 1996, 19, 213-218.
[99] Atopkina LN, Denisenko VA. *Chem. Nat. Compd.* 2006, 42, 55-60.
[100] Yahara S, Tanaka O, Nishioka I *et al. Chem. Pharm. Bull.* 1978, 26, 3010-3016.
[101] X Hao, P Li, X Li, Y Liu *et al. Zhongcaoyao* 2000, 31, 801-803.
[102] O Tanaka, T Morita, R Kasai *et al. Chem. Pharm. Bull.* 1985, 33, 2323-2330.
[103] Qiu F, Ming ZZ, Pei YP *et al.Chin. Chem. Lett.* 1998, 9, 643-645.
[104] Takemoto Y, Ueyama T, Saito H *et al. Chem. Pharm. Bull.* 1984, 32, 3128-3133.
[105] Wang DQ, Feng BS, Wang XB *et al. Acta pharm. Sin.* 1989, 24, 633-636.
[106] Wei JX, Du YC. *Panax notoginseng*: Modern Scientific Investigation and Application. Yunnan Science and Technology Press, Kunming 1993.
[107] Liu L, Li YF, Cheng YY. *J. Chromatogr. B. Analyt. Technol. Biomed. Life Sci* 2008, 862, 196-204.
[108] Bernardin FE: Experimental design and testing of adsorption and adsorbates. In: Adsorption Technology. Slejko FL (Ed), Marcel Dekker Inc., New York 1985:1-35.
[109] Xie LL, Ren L, Lai XS *et al. Zhong Yao Cai* 2009, 32, 1602-1605.
[110] Wang ZH, Liu JH, Wei JF. *Hebei Med* 2001, 7, 851-852.
[111] Zheng Y, Lu H, Du GM. *J. Jiling Inst. Tech.* 2008, 24, 76-78.
[112] Liang Q, Lu Z, Han Q *et al. J. Jilin. Med. Coll.* 2009, 30, 319-322.
[113] Wan JB, Zhang QW, Ye WC *et al. Sep Pur Tech* 2008, 60, 198-205.
[114] Zhao Y, Chen B, Yao S. *Sep. Pur. Tech.* 2007, 52, 533-538.
[115] Zhao Y, Chen B, Luo XB *et al. Nat. Prod. Res. Dev.* 2004, 16, 235-238.
[116] Jocelyn Pare JR, Belanger JMR. *Trends Anal. Chem.* 1994, 13, 176-184.

[117] Chen YP, Meng Q, Song CC *et al. Chin. Pharm. J.* 2007, 32, 273-275.
[118] Ma XQ, Yu HS, Tian B *et al. J. Dalian Inst. Light Ind.* 1999, 18, 39-43.
[119] Zhou J, Wu MZ, Taniyasu S *et al. Chem. Pharm. Bull.* 1981, 29, 2844-2850.
[120] Jin Y, Xue X, Liu Y *et al. J. Chromatogr. A.* 2008, 1183, 76-86.
[121] Latif Z: Isolation by Preparative High-Performance Liquid Chromatography. In: *Natural Products Isolatio.* Sarker SD, Latif Z, Gray AI (Eds), Humana Press, New York 2005:213-232.
[122] Paik NH, Park MK, Choi KJ *et al. Arch Pharm Res* 1982, 5, 7-12.
[123] Zhang W, Lin BC, Li Q. *Special Wild Eonomic Animal and Plant Res* 2008, 60-63.
[124] Han JY, Liu C, Wang H *et al. J. Chem. Engin. Chin. Univ.* 2005, 19, 192-196.
[125] Liu JN, Zhu JB, Yan HQ *et al. J. Dalian Polytech. Univ.* 2010, 29, 18-20.
[126] Chen B, Pan ZQ, Feng JL *et al. Practical Preventive Med.* 2001, 8, 333-335.
[127] Wang YT, Wan JB, Zhang QW: A method for separation of notoginsenoside R1, ginsenoside Rg1, Re, Rb1 and Rd. In: 200810096148.4. Macau uo (Ed) China (2008).
[128] Ito Y, Bowman RL. *Science* 1970, 167, 281-283.
[129] Sutherland IA, Fisher D. *J. Chromatogr. A.* 2009, 1216, 740-753.
[130] Cheng Y, Liang Q, Hu P *et al. Sep. Pur. Tech.* 2010, 73, 397-402.
[131] Ha YW, Lim SS, Ha IJ *et al. J. Chromatogr. A.* 2007, 1151, 37-44.
[132] Du Q, Jerz G, Waibel R *et al. J. Chromatogr. A.* 2003, 1008, 173-180.
[133] Marston A, Hostettmann K. *J. Chromatogr. A.* 2006, 1112, 181-194.
[134] Qi X, Ignatova S, Luo G *et al. J. Chromatogr. A.* 2010, 1217, 1995-2001.
[135] Shehzad O, Jin Ha I, Park Y *et al. J. Sep. Sci.* 2011, 34, 1116-1122.
[136] Marchal L, Legrand J, Foucault A. *Chem. Rec.* 2003, 3, 133-143.
[137] Wang J, Liu CM, Li L *et al. Phytochem. Anal.* 2011, 22, 263-267.
[138] Hage DS. *J. Chromatogr. B. Biomed. Sci. Appl.* 1998, 715, 3-28.
[139] Fukuda N, Tanaka H, Shoyama Y. *J Nat Prod* 2000, 63, 283-285.
[140] Yuan CS, Tanaka H. *Curr. Drug Discov. Technol.* 2011, 8, 32-41.
[141] Wan JB, Wang YT, Li SP: Panax notoginseng (Sanqi). In: *Pharmacological Activity-Based Quality Control of Chinese Herbs.* Li SP, Wang YT (Eds), Nova Science Publishers, New York 2008:179-203.
[142] Leung KW, Wong AS. *Chin. Med.* 2010, 5, 20.
[143] Chen Y, Guo Z, Wang X *et al. J. Chromatogr. A.* 2008, 1184, 191-219.
[144] Deng C, Liu N, Gao M *et al. J. Chromatogr. A.* 2007, 1153, 90-96.
[145] Schlag EM, McIntosh MS. *Phytochemistry* 2006, 67, 1510-1519.
[146] Hou J, He S, Ling M *et al. J. Sep. Sci.* 2010, 33, 2707-2713.
[147] Alonso-Salces RM, Korta E, Barranco A *et al. J. Chromatogr. A.* 2001, 933, 37-43.
[148] Turk MF, Baron A, Vorobiev E. *J. Agric. Food Chem.* 2010, 58, 9611-9616.
[149] Wang CZ, Wu JA, McEntee E *et al. J. Agric. Food Chem.* 2006, 54, 2261-2266.
[150] Li L, Sheng YX, Zhang JL *et al. Biomed. Chromatogr.* 2006, 20, 327-335.
[151] Li L, Sheng Y, Zhang J *et al. Biomed. Chromatogr.* 2004, 18, 849-856.
[152] Li L, Sheng Y, Zhang J *et al. J. Chromatogr. Sci.* 2005, 43, 421-425.
[153] Newton R. *Monogr. Endocrinol.* 1988, 30, 1-31.
[154] Zhou YC, Zhao HQ, Liang N *et al. J. shenyang Pharm. Univ.* 2003, 20, 27-31.
[155] Dong TT, Zhao KJ, Huang WZ *et al. Phytother. Res.* 2005, 19, 684-688.
[156] Li L, Zhang JL, Sheng YX *et al. J. Pharm. Biomed. Anal.* 2005, 38, 45-51.
[157] Chuang WC, Sheu SJ. *J. Chromatogr. A.* 1994, 685, 243-251.

[158] Wan JB, Li P, Li S *et al. J. Sep. Sci.* 2006, 29, 2190-2196.
[159] Gao J, Zhai Y, Wang R *et al. Zhongguo Zhong Yao Za Zhi* 2010, 35, 989-991.
[160] Qian ZM, Lu J, Gao QP *et al. J. Chromatogr. A.* 2009, 1216, 3825-3830.
[161] Kim YK, Yoo DS, Xu H *et al. Nat. Prod. Commun.* 2009, 4, 903-906.
[162] Zhou W, Li J, Li X *et al. J. Sep. Sci.* 2008, 31, 921-925.
[163] Qian ZM, Wan JB, Zhang QW *et al. J Pharm. Biomed. Anal.* 2008, 48, 1361-1367.
[164] Wei YJ, Li SL, Li P. *Biomed Chromatogr* 2007, 21, 1-9.
[165] Wan JB, Li SP, Chen JM *et al. J. Sep. Sci.* 2007, 30, 825-832.
[166] Kim SN, Ha YW, Shin H *et al. J. Pharm. Biomed. Anal.* 2007, 45, 164-170.
[167] Gui FJ, Yang XW, Li LY *et al. J. Chromatogr. B Analyt Technol Biomed Life Sci* 2007, 850, 1-6.
[168] Zhang S, Chen R, Wu H *et al. J. Pharm. Biomed. Anal.* 2006, 41, 57-63.
[169] Wan JB, Yang FQ, Li SP *et al. J. Pharm. Biomed. Anal.* 2006, 41, 1596-1601.
[170] Corbit RM, Ferreira JF, Ebbs SD *et al. J. Agric. Food Chem.* 2005, 53, 9867-9873.
[171] Zhu S, Zou K, Fushimi H *et al. Planta Med* 2004, 70, 666-677.
[172] Washida D, Kitanaka S. *Chem. Pharm. Bull. (Tokyo)* 2003, 51, 1314-1317.
[173] Dong TT, Cui XM, Song ZH *et al. J. Agric. Food Chem.* 2003, 51, 4617-4623.
[174] Shangguan D, Han H, Zhao R *et al. J. Chromatogr. A.* 2001, 910, 367-372.
[175] Harlesworth JM. *Anal. Chem.* 1978, 50, 1414-1420.
[176] Oleszek W, Bialy Z. *J. Chromatogr. A.* 2006, 1112, 78-91.
[177] Luchtefeld R, Kostoryz E, Smith RE. *J. Agric. Food Chem.* 2004, 52, 4953-4956.
[178] Li L, Tsao R, Dou J *et al. Anal. Chim. Acta* 2004, 536, 21-28.
[179] Dan M, Xie G, Gao X *et al. Phytochem Anal* 2009, 20, 68-76.
[180] Wang X, Sakuma T, Asafu-Adjaye E *et al. Anal. Chem.* 1999, 71, 1579-1584.
[181] Miao XS, Metcalfe CD, Hao C *et al. J. Mass Spectrom.* 2002, 37, 495-506.
[182] Guan J, Lai CM, Li SP. *J. Pharm. Biomed. Anal.* 2007, 44, 996-1000.
[183] Li L, Luo GA, Liang QL *et al. J. Pharm. Biomed. Anal.* 2010, 52, 66-72.
[184] Li X, Tang MH, Zhang F *et al. Sichuan Da Xue Xue Bao Yi Xue Ban* 2009, 40, 912-917.
[185] Deng GF, Wang DL, Meng MX *et al. J. Chromatogr. B Analyt. Technol. Biomed. Life Sci.* 2009, 877, 2113-2122.
[186] Chan EC, Yap SL, Lau AJ *et al. Rapid. Commun. Mass Spectrom.* 2007, 21, 519-528.
[187] Xie G, Plumb R, Su M *et al. J. Sep. Sci.* 2008, 31, 1015-1026.
[188] Altria KD: *Capillary Electrophoresis Guidebook : Principles, Operation and Applications.* Humana, New York (1995).
[189] Terabe S. *Annu. Rev. Anal. Chem.* 2009, 2, 99-120.
[190] Glockl I, Veit M, Blaschke G. *Planta Med.* 2002, 68, 158-161.
[191] Yang WF, Zhao WL. *Zhongguo Zhong Yao Za Zhi* 2003, 28, 1135-1137.
[192] Wang S, Ye S, Cheng Y. *J. Chromatogr. A.* 2006, 1109, 279-284.
[193] Cao J, Qi LW, Chen J *et al. Electrophoresis* 2008, 29, 4422-4430.
[194] Wan JB, Li SP, Jian JR *et al. Chin. J. Nat. Med.* 2004, 2, 214-218.
[195] Cui JF. *Eur. J. Pharm. Sci.* 1995, 3, 77-85.
[196] Chen Y, Sorensen LK. *Fresenius J. Anal. Chem.* 2000, 367, 491-496.
[197] Edwards HG, Munshi T, Page K. *Anal. BioAnal. Chem.* 2007, 389, 2203-2215.
[198] Kang J, Lee S, Kang S *et al. Arch. Pharm. Res.* 2008, 31, 330-336.

[199] Bai CC, Han SY, Chai XY *et al. J. Liq. Chromatogr. Relat. Technol.* 2009, 32, 242-260.

[200] Sritularak B, Morinaga O, Yuan CS *et al. J. Nat. Med.* 2009, 63, 360-363.

In: Saponins: Properties, Applications and Health Benefits ISBN: 978-1-62100-942-9
Editors: Rani Koh and Isaac Tay

Chapter 3

TRITERPENOID SAPONINS FROM GENUS *GYPSOPHILA* L. (*CARYOPHYLLACEAE*)

M. Yotova, I. Krasteva and S. Nikolov
Department of Pharmacognosy, Faculty of Pharmacy,
Medical University, Sofia, Bulgaria

ABSTRACT

Saponins are widespread in medicinal plants and very often are responsible for their pharmacological effects. The genus *Gypsophila,* family *Caryophyllaceae*, is well known to contain triterpenoid saponins with medicinal, industrial and decorative applications. Some species are broadly used as a drug with extensive medical importance, such as an expectorant and diuretic, and are used in treatments of hepatitis, gastritis and bronchitis. *Gypsophila* saponins have anticarcinogenic properties, including direct cytotoxicity, immunomodulating effects, normalization of carcinogen induced cell proliferation, and a cytoprotective effect over hepatocytes, etc.

Various triterpene saponins have been reported in *Gypsophila* species including gypsogenin as the major aglycone and other aglycones as quillaic, echinocystic, hederagenin and oleanolic acids. Recently, sulfated triterpene saponins have been reported to occur in the genus.

This review deals with the chemistry, methods of purification, structure elucidation and biological activity of triterpene saponins from genus *Gypsophila*.

INTRODUCTION

Genus *Gypsophila* L. (*Caryophyllaceae*) comprises about 150 species, annual to perennial herbs, distributed in temperate regions of the world, such as Asia, Europe, Africa, Pacific Islands, Australia and has been introduced in South America. The common name of *Gypsophila* is Baby's Breath. Much of the species are naturalized and cultivated. *Gypsophila* species don't like acid soils and are found on calcium rich soils that are high in gypsum which also served as an origin of the name of the genus.

Gypsophila species are well known by their medicinal, decorative and industrial application. *G. paniculata* and *G. elegans* are grown commercially and used as cut flowers in floral arrangements or as fillers in flower bouquets [25]. Saponin (E. Merck No. 7695), also known as Saponin album, is a crude saponin fraction obtained from roots and rhizomes of *G. paniculata* L. and *G. arrostii* Guss.

It has been extensively used in the past as a standard for hemolytic tests in most saponin determinations [17, 34]. Some *Gypsophila* species are broadly used in traditional medicine such as: expectorant, diuretic, purgative and contraceptive and for the treatments of hepatitis, gastritis and bronchitis [26, 40, 85, 89].

The most important classes of abundant secondary metabolites in genus *Gypsophila* are saponins. They are widely found in the roots of the species [37, 40]. Various triterpene saponins have been reported in *Gypsophila* including both monodesmosidic and bidesmosidic triterpene saponins of gypsogenin, oleanolic acid, quillaic acid, etc. [18-19, 37, 40, 50-53, 58-59]. *Gypsophila* saponins possess many biological effects such as: anticholesteremic, hepatoprotective, spermicidal, antidiabetic, etc. [8, 20, 52-53, 72, 75].

Recent studies have illustrated useful pharmacological properties of saponins, including anticancer, immunomodulatory and cytotoxicity activities [34-35, 63, 78-83]. They have considerable adjuvant activity and are used in production of vaccines [55].

The conditions under which different *Gypsophila* species can be cultivated *in vitro* cultures were explored; their growth behavior and accumulation of saponins were also investigated [32, 33, 61].

In this review are described the structure of triterpene saponins from genus *Gypsophila*, their biological activity and methods of purification and structure elucidation according to literature and data prior to 2010.

TRITERPENOID SAPOGENINS AND SAPONINS ISOLATED FROM GENUS *GYPSOPHILA*

Triterpeniod saponins are widespread in the plant kingdom. Their structures are described in many reviews [15-16, 37]. The saponins which were isolated from *Gypsophila* species are predominantly pentacyclic triterpene of the oleanane and lupane group.

Triterpenes can be found rarely in the genus and they occur usually as glycosides. There are some reports for the isolation of lupan-type triterpene from *G. struthium* [7] and *G. repens* [18]. The isolated saponins can be monodesmosides and bidesmosides according to the number of the sugar chains attached to the aglycone [37, 40, 18-19; 50-54, 58-59].

The first studies of *Gypsophila* constituents date back to 1930[s] [40, 65]. Later many researchers investigated the saponins from *Gypsophila* and they reported the contents of gypsogenin as an aglycone, but no detailed phytochemical study was described [38-39, 43, 49, 56, 60]. Tagiev et al. [70] identified a gypsogenin lactone, obtained from the acid hydrolysis of saponin.

Table 1. Sapogenins from genus *Gypsophila*

- Oleanane-type

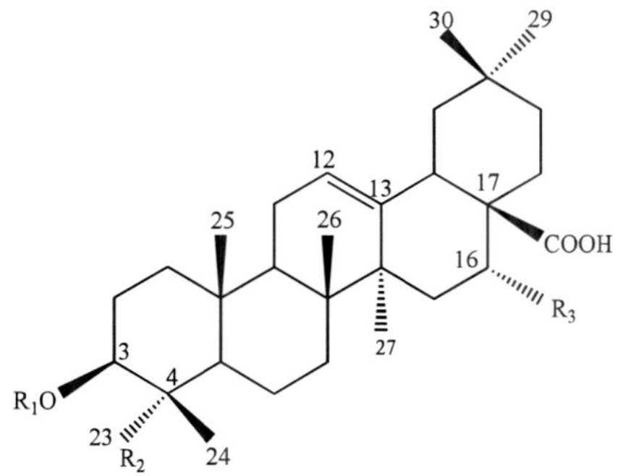

№	Name	Structure	R_1	R_2	R_3	Species [Ref]
1	oleanolic acid	3*β*-hydroxy-olean-12-en-28-oic acid	H	CH_3	H	*G. struthium* L. [7], *G. oldamiana* Miq. [68]
2	hederagenin	3*β*,23-dihydroxyolean-12-en-28-oic acid	H	CH_2OH	H	*G. odhamiana* Miq. [52]
3	gypsogenin	3*β*-hydroxy-23-oxoolean-12-en-28-oic acid	H	CHO	H	*G. oldhamiana* Miq. [84]
4	quillaic acid	3*β*,16*α*-dihydroxy-23-oxoolean-12-en-28-oic acid	H	CHO	OH	*G. oldhamiana* Miq. [52]
5	echinocystic acid	3*β*,16*α*-dihydroxy-23-oxoolean-12-en-28-oic acid	H	CH_3	OH	*G. oldhamiana* Miq. [52]
6	gypsogenic acid	3*β*-hydroxyolean-12-en-23,28-dioic acid	H	COOH	H	*G. oldhamiana* Miq. [52]
7	collinsogenin	3*β*,16*α*,23-trihydroxyolean-12-en-28-oic acid	H	CH_2OH	OH	*G. oldhamiana* Miq. [52,68]
8	**No common name*	3*β*-sulfate ester of gypsogenin	SO_3H	CHO	H	*G. bermejoi* G. [2]
9	*No common name*	hederagenin-3-*O*-sulfate	SO_3H	CH_2OH	H	*G. oldhamiana* Miq. [52]
№	Name	Structure	R_1	R_2	R_3	Species [Ref]
10	**No common name*	23-sulfate ester of hederagenin	H	CH_2OSO_2H	H	*G. bermejoi* G. López [2]
11	**No common name*	3-*O*-sulfooleanolic acid	SO_3H	CH_3	H	*G. trichotoma* Wend. [44]
12	**No common name*	3-*O*-sulfoquillaic acid	SO_3H	CHO	OH	*G. trichotoma* Wend. [44]
13	**No common name*	3-*O*-sulfoechinocystic acid	SO_3H	CH_3	OH	*G. trichotoma* Wend. [44]
14	*vaccaric acid	3*β*,4*α*-dihydroxy-23-norolean-12-en-28-oic acid	H	OH	H	*G. oldhamiana* Miq. [51]
15	*segetalic acid	3*β*,4*α*,16*α*-trihydroxy-23-norolean-12-en-28-oic acid	H	OH	OH	*G. oldhamiana* Miq. [53]

*Aglycone of saponin.

Table 1. (Continued)

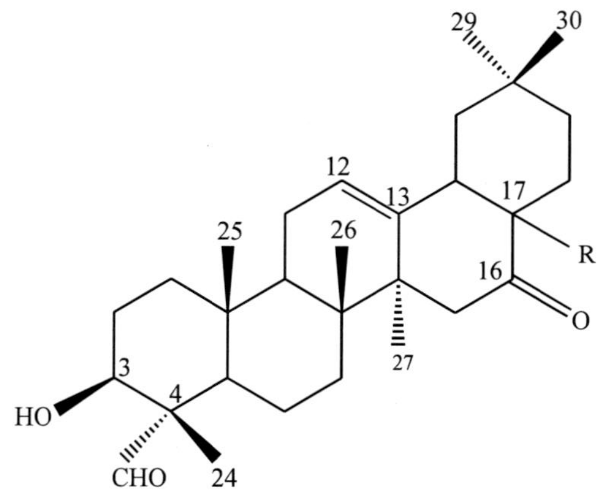

№	Name	Structure	R	Plant [Ref]
16	neogypsogenin A	(3β,17α)-3-hydroxy-28-norolean-12-ene-16,23-dione	α-H	*G. oldhamiana* Miq. [50]
17	neogypsogenin B	(3β,17β)-3-hydroxy-28-norolean-12-ene-16,23-dione	β-H	*G. oldhamiana* Miq. [50]

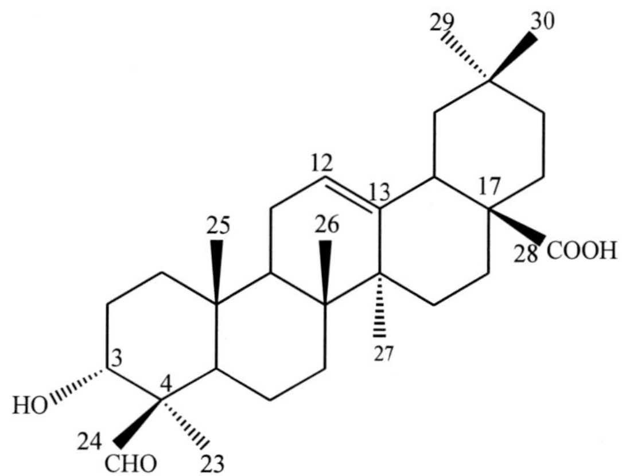

№	Name	Structure	Plant [Ref]
18	*No common name*	3α-hydroxyepigypsogenin	*G. oldhamiana* Miq. [52]

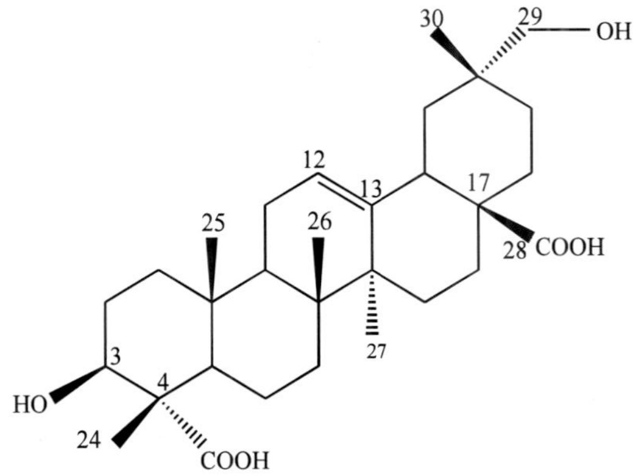

№	Name	Structure	Plant/Ref
19	**No common name*	29*α*-hydroxygipsogenic acid	*G. capillaries* Forssk. [24]

*Aglycone of saponin.

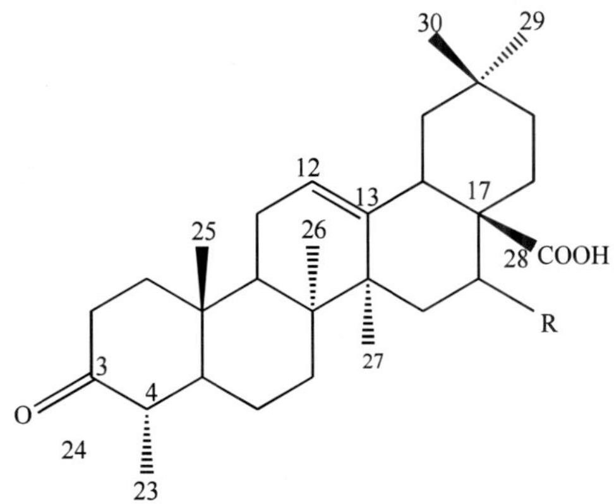

№	Name	Structure	R	Plant [Ref]
20	hederagonic acid	3-oxo-24-norolean-12-en-28-oic acid	H	*G. oldhamiana* Miq. [52]
21	**No common name*	3-keto-16-*α*-hydroxy-24-noroleanolic acid	OH	*G. oldhamiana* Miq. [53]

*Aglycone of saponin.

Table 1. (Continued)

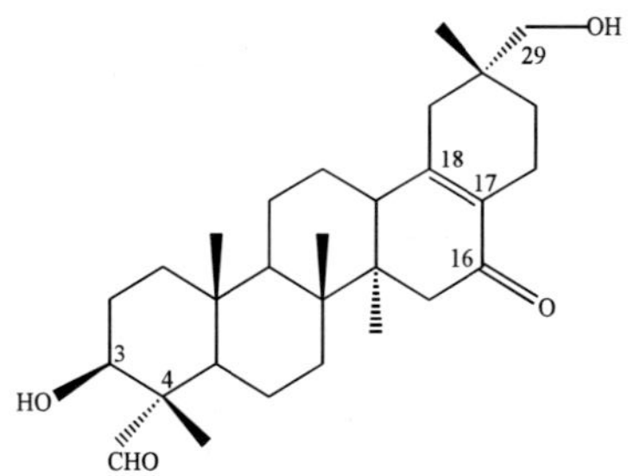

№	Name	Structure	Plant/Ref
22	**No common name*	$3\beta,4\alpha,20\alpha$-3,29-dihydroxy-16,23-dioxo-28-norolean-17-en-3-yl	*G. paniculata* L. [86]

*Aglycone of saponin.

- Lupane-type

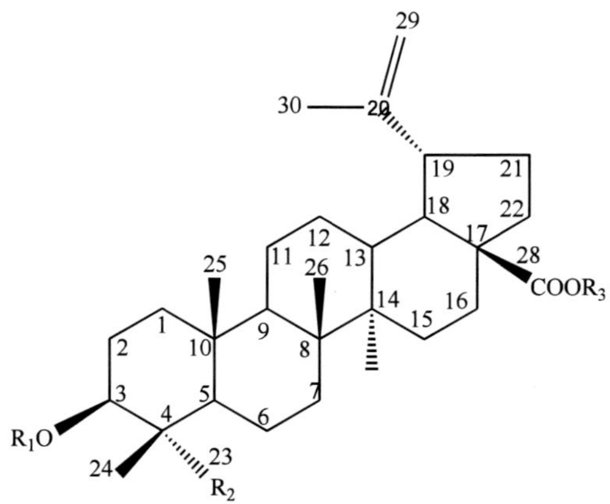

№	Name	Structure	R_1	R_2	R_3	Plant [Ref]
23	betulinic acid	3β-hydroxy-lup-20(29)-en-28-oic acid	H	CH_3	H	*G. struthium* L. [7]
24	gypsophilin	(3β)-3-*O*-(sulfo)lup-20(29)-en-23,28-dioic acid	SO_3H	COOH	H	*G. repens* L. [18]
25	*No common name*	3β-hydroxy-lup-20(29)-en-27-oic acid	H	H	H	*G. struthium* L. [7]

*Aglycone of saponin.

Table 2. Saponins from genus *Gypsophyla*, presented in chronological order

№	Name	Genin*	Sugar moiety**	Species [Ref]
26	gypsoside	3	3-*O*-β-D-gal-(1→4)-*O*-β-D-glc-(1→4)-[α-L-ara-(1→3)]-*O*-β-D-glcA; 28-*O*-β-D-xyl-(1→3)-β-D-fuc-(1→4)-[β-D-xyl-(1→3)-β-D-xyl-(1→2)]-α-L-rha	*G. paniculata* [42]
27	trichoside A	3	3-*O*-β-D-glc-(1→3)-β-D-glcA; 28-*O*-β-D-glc	*G. trichotoma* [46]
28	trichoside B	3	3-*O*-β-D-glc-(1→3)-β-D-glcA; 28-*O*-β-D-glc-(1→4)-β-D-glc	*G. trichotoma* [47]
29	trichoside C	3	3-*O*-β-D-glc-(1→3)-*O*-β-D-glcA; 28-*O*-β-D-gal-(1→4)-*O*-α-L-rha-(1→4)-*O*-β-D-fuc	*G. trichotoma* [48]
30	filoside A	3	3-*O*-β-D-xyl-(1→2)-[β-D-xyl-(1→2)-β-D-gal-(1→3)]-[β-D-gal-(1→4)]-β-D-glcA; 28-*O*-α-L-rha-(1→4)-[α-L-rha-(1→6)]-β-D-glc-(1→2)-β-D-fuc	*G. partinii* [10]
31	filoside B	3	3-*O*-β-D-xyl-(1→2)-[α-L-ara-(1→2)-β-D-xyl-(1→2)-β-D-gal-(1→3)]-[β-D-gal-(1→4)]-β-D-glcA; 28-*O*-α-D-fuc-(1→4)-α-L-ara-(1→2)-α-L-rha	*G. partinii* [11]
32	acutifiloside	3	3-*O*-β-D-gal-(1→4)-[α-L-ara-(1→3)]-β-D-glcA; 28-*O*-β-gal-(1→4)-β-D-glc-(1→4)-[β-D-gal-(1→3)]-[β-D-gal-(1→2)]-β-D-xyl-(1→3)-[β-D-(1→4)]-β-D-fuc	*G. acutifolia* 14]
33	*No common name*	3	3-*O*-glcA	*G. partinii* 36], *G. oldhamiana.* [84]
34	*No common name*	4	3-*O*-β-D-gal-(1→2)-[β-D-xyl-(1→3)]-β-D-glc; 28-*O*-β-D-glc-(1→3)-(β-D-xyl-(1→4)-α-L-rha-(1→2)-β-D-fuc	*G. paniculata* and *G. arostii* [26], *G. oldhamiana* [53]
35	*No common name*	4	3-*O*-β-D-gal-(1→2)-[β-D-xyl-(1→3)]-β-D-glcA; 28-*O*-β-D-ara-(1→4)-β-D-ara-(1→3)-β-D-xyl-(1→4)-α-L-rha-(1→2)-β-D-fuc	*G. paniculata* and *G. arostii* [26]
36	*No common name*	3	3-*O*-β-D-glc-(1→2)-β-D-glcA; 28-*O*-β-D-glc-(1→3)-[β-D-xyl-(1→4)]-α-L-rha-(1→2)-β-D-fuc	*G. paniculata* and *G. arostii* [26]
37	*No common name*	3	3-*O*-β-D-xyl-(1→3)-β-D-gal-(1→2)-β-D-glcA; 28-*O*-β-D-glc-(1→3)-β-D-xyl-(1→4)-α-L-rha-(1→2)-β-D-fuc	*G. paniculata* and *G. arostii* [26] *G. oldhamiana.* [53]
38	*No common name*	4	3-*O*-β-D-gal-(1→2)-[β-D-xyl-(1→3)]-β-D-glcA; methyl ester	*G. oldhamiana* [45]
39	*No common name*	3	3-*O*-β-D-gal-(1→2)-[β-D-xyl-(1→3)]-β-D-glcA; methyl ester	*G. oldhamiana* [45]
40	*No common name*	4	3-*O*-β-D-gal-(1→2)-[β-D-xyl-(1→3)]-β-D-glcA; 28-[*O*-β-D-fuc(1→4)-β-D-glc-(1→3)]-α-L-rha} ester	*G. oldhamiana* [45]
41	*No common name*	6	28-*O*-β-D-glc-(1→6)-β-D-glc	*G. capillaris* [21]
42	*No common name*	4	28-*O*-[β-D-glc(1→2)][β-D-gal(1→6)]-β-D-glc	*G. capillaris* [21]
43	*No common name*	4	28-*O*-β-D-glc-(1→2)-β-D-glc-(1→5)-[β-D-glc-(1→2)]-β-D-glc	*G. capillaris* [22]
44	*No common name*	6	28-*O*-[β-D-glc-(1→3)-β-D-glc(1→2)]-[β-D-gal-(1→6)]-β-D-glc	*G. capillaris* [23]
45	*No common name*	3	28-*O*-(β-glc-(1→2)-β-D-gal-(1→3)]-[β-D-glc-(1→6)]-β-D-gal	*G. capillaris* [23], *G. panicula* [87]
46	*No common name*	6	28-*O*-[β-D-glc-(1→2)-β-D-gal-(1→3)]-[β-D-glc-(1→6)-β-D-gal	*G. capillaris* [23]

Table 2. (Continued)

№	Name	Genin*	Sugar moiety**	Species [Ref]
47	*No common name*	6	28-*O*-(β-glc-(1→2)-β-D-gal-(1→3)]-[β-D-glc-(1→6)]-β-D-gal	*G. capillaris* [23]
48	*No common name*	19	28-[β-D-gal-(6→1)-β-D-glc] ester	*G. capillaris.* [24]
49	*No common name*	3	28-*O*-β-D-glc-(1→2)[β-D-glc-(1→6)]-β-D-glc	*G. bermejoi* [1]
50	*No common name*	8	28-*O*-β-D-glc-(1→2)-[β-D-glc-(1→6)]-β-D-glc	*G. bermejoi* [2]
51	*No common name*	10	28-*O*-β-D-glc-(1→2)-[β-D-glc-(1→6)]-β-D-glc	*G. bermejoi* [2]
52	oldamianoside I	3	3-*O*-β-D-xyl-(1→3)-[β-D-gal-(1→2)]-β-D-glcA	*G. oldhamiana* [68]
53	*No common name*	4	28-{α-L-ara-(1→4)-α-L-ara-(1→3)-β-D-xyl-(1→4)-α-L-rha-(1→2)-β-D-fuc}ester	*G. oldhamiana* [51]
54	*No common name*	14	28-{β-D-glc-(1→3)-[β-D-xyl-(1→4)]-α-L-rha-(1→2)-β-D-fuc}ester	*G. oldhamiana* [51]
55	neogypsoside A	16	3-*O*-[*O*-β-D-gal-(1→2)-[*O*-β-D-xyl-(1→3)]-β-D-glcAp	*G. oldhamiana* [50]
56	neogypsoside B	17	3-*O*-[*O*-β-D-gal-(1→2)-[*O*-β-D-xyl (1→3)]-β-D-glcAp	*G. oldhamiana* [50]
57	*No common name*	3	3-*O*-[β-D-gal-(1→2)-(β-D-xyl-(1→3))-β-D-glcA]; 28-*O*-[3-*O*-arg-β-D-glc-(1→3)-(β-D-xyl-(1→4))-α-L-rha-(1→2)-β-D-fuc]	*G. trichotoma* [31]
58	*No common name*	3	3-*O*-[β-D-gal-(1→2)-(β-L-ara-(1→3))-β-D-glcA]; 28-*O*-[3-*O*-arg-β-D-glc-(1→3)-β-D-xyl-(1→4))-α-L-rha-(1→2)-β-D-fuc]	*G. trichotoma* [31]
59	repensoside A	6	(3β)-3-*O*-(β-D-xyl); 28-{β-D-glc-(1→6)-β-D-gal}ester	*G. repens* [19]
60	repensoside B	6	(3β)-3-*O*-(β-D-xyl); 28-{β-D-xyl-(1→2)-[β-D-glc-(1→6)]-β-D-gal}ester	*G. repens* [19]
61	repensoside C	6	(3β)-3-*O*-(β-D-xyl); 28-{β-D-glc(1→3)-[β-D-glc-(1→6)]-β-D-gal}ester	*G. repens* [19]
62	repensoside D	6	(3β)-3-*O*-{β-D-glc-(1→2)-β-D-gal-(1→2)-[β-D-glc-(1→4)]-β-D-gal	*G. repens* [19]
63	repensoside E	6	(3β)-3-*O*-{β-D-glc-(1→2)-[β-D-xyl-(1→3)]-β-D-glcA}; 28-{α-L-ara-(1→4)-α-L-ara-(1→3)-β-D-xyl-(1→4)-α-L-rha-(1→2)-[β-D-qui-(1→4)]-β-D-fuc}ester	*G. repens* [19]
64	repensoside F	3	(3β)-3-*O*-{β-D-gal-(1→2)-[β-D-xyl-(1→3)]-β-D-glcA}; 28-{α-L-ara-(1→3)-β-D-xyl-(1→4)-α-L-rha-(1→2)-(3-*O*-,4-*O*-diAc-β-D-fuc)}ester	*G. repens* [19]
65	gypsophilinoside	24	28-*O*-β-D-glc ester	*G. repens* [18]
66	*No common name*	4	3-*O*-β-D-gal-(1→2)-[β-D-xyl-(1→3)]-β-D-glcA; 28-*O*-α-L-ara-(1→2)-α-L-ara-(1→3)-β-D-xyl-(1→4)-α-L-rha-(1→2)-β-D-fuc	*G. oldhamiana* [90]
67	*No common name*	3	3-*O*-β-D-gal-(1→2)-[β-D-xyl-(1→3)]-methyl-β-D-glcA;28-*O*-β-D-glc-(1→3)-[β-D-xyl-(1→4)]-α-L-rha-(1→2)-β-D-fuc	*G. oldhamiana* [90]
68	*No common name*	6	23-*O*-β-D-glc; 28-*O*-β-D-glc-(1→3)-[β-D-glc-(1→6)]-β-D-glc	*G. oldhamiana* [90]
69	gypoldoside	4	3-*O*-{β-D-gal-(1→2)-[β-D-xyl-(1→3)]-β-D-glcA; 28-[α-L-ara-(1→2)-α-L-ara-(1→3)-β-D-xyl-(1→4)-α-L-rha-(1→2)-β-D-fuc] ester	*G. oldhamiana* [6]
70	*No common name*	4	3-*O*-β-D-gal-(1→2)-[β-D-gal-(1→3)]-β-D-glcA	*G. odhamiana* [53], *G. paniculata* [85]

№	Name	Genin*	Sugar moiety**	Species [Ref]
71	*No common name*	15	28-[*O*-α-L-ara-(1→4)-α-L-ara-(1→3)-β-D-xyl-(1→4)-α-L-rha-(1→2)-β-D-fuc] ester	*G. oldhamiana* [53]
72	*No common name*	21	28-[*O*-α-L-ara-(1→4)-α-L-ara-(1→3)-β-D-xyl-(1→4)-α-L-rha-(1→2)-β-D-fuc] ester	*G. oldhamiana* [53]
73	*No common name*	3	28-[*O*-α-D-gal-(1→6)-β-D-glc-(1→6)-[β-D-glc-(1→3)]-β-D-glc] ester	*G. oldhamiana* [53], *G. paniculata* [85]
74	*No common name*	3	3-*O*-β-D-gal-(1→2)-β-D-glcA; 28-*O*-β-D-xyl-(1→4)-α-L-rha-(1→2)-β-D-fuc	*G. oldhamiana* [53]
75	*No common name*	3	3-*O*-β-D-gal-(1→2)-[β-D-xyl-(1→3)]-β-D-glcA; 28-*O*-α-L-ara-(1→3)-β-D-xyl-(1→4)-α-L-rha-(1→2)-β-D-fuc	*G. oldhamiana* [53]
76	*No common name*	3	3-*O*-β-D-gal-(1→2)-[β-D-xyl-(1→3)]-β-D-glcA; 28-*O*-(6-*O*-Ac)-β-D-glc-(1→3)-[β-D-xyl-(1→4)]-α-L-rha-(1→2)-β-D-fuc	*G. oldhamiana* [53]
77	*No common name*	3	3-*O*-β-D-gal-(1→2)-[β-D-xyl-(1→3)]-β-D-glcA	*G. paniculata* [85]
78	*No common name*	3	3-*O*-β-D-gal-(1→2)-[β-D-xyl-(1→3)]-β-D-glcA; 28-*O*-β-(Z)-glc-(1→3)-[β-D-xyl-(1→4)]-α-L-rha-(1→2)-β-D-fuc	*G. paniculata* [85], *G. pacifica* [58]
79	*No common name*	11	28-β-glc ester	*G. trichotoma* [44]
80	*No common name*	12	28-β-glc ester	*G. trichotoma* [44]
81	*No common name*	13	28-β-glc ester	*G. trichotoma* [44]
82	*No common name*	3	3-*O*-β-D-gal-(1→2)-[β-D-xyl-(1→3)]-β-D-glcA; 28-*O*-β-D-xyl-(1→4)-α-L-rha-(1→2)-β-D-fuc	*G. pacifica* [58]
83	*No common name*	4	3-*O*-β-D-gal-(1→2)-[β-D-xyl-(1→3)]-β-D-glcA; 28-*O*-β-D-xyl-(1→4)-α-L-rha-(1→2)-β-D-fuc	*G. pacifica* [58]
84	*No common name*	4	3-*O*-β-D-gal-(1→2)-[β-D-xyl-(1→3)]-β-D-glcA; 28-*O*-β-D-glc-(1→3)-[β-D-xyl-(1→4)]-α-L-rha-(1→2)-β-D-fuc	*G. pacifica* [58]
85	*No common name*	4	3-*O*-β-D-gal-(1→2)-[β-D-xyl-(1→3)]-β-D-glcA; 28-*O*-α-L-ara-(1→4)-α-L-ara-(1→3)-β-D-xyl-(1→4)-α-L-rha-(1→2)-β-D-fuc	*G. pacifica* [58]
86	*No common name*	4	3-*O*-β-D-xyl-(1→3)-β-D-glcA	*G. altissima* [13]
87	*No common name*	4	3-*O*-β-D-gal-(1→2)-[β-D-xyl-(1→3)]-β-D-glcA; 28-*O*-(6-*O*-acetyl)-β-D-glc-(1→3)-[β-D-xyl-(1→ 4)]-α-L-rha-(1→2)-β-D-fuc	*G. altissima* [13]
88	*No common name*	4	3-*O*-β-D-gal-(1→2)-6-*O*-Me-β-D-glcA	*G. altissima* [13]
89	*No common name*	3	3-*O*-β-D-gal-(1→2)-[β-D-xyl-(1→3)]-β-D-glcA; 28-O-α-L-ara-(1→4)-α-L-ara-(1→3)-β-D-xyl-(1→4)-α-L-rha-(1→2)-β-D-fuc ester	*G. pacifica* [59]
90	*No common name*	3	3-*O*-β-D-gal-(1→3)-β-D-glcA;28-*O*-β-D-xyl-(1→3)-β-D-xyl-(1→4)-α-L-rha-(1→2)-β-D-fuc ester	*G. pacifica* [59]
91	*No common name*	6	28-*O*-β-D-glc-(1→6)-β-D-glc-(1→6)-[β-D-glc-(1→3)]-β-D-glc ester	*G. pacifica* [59]
92	*No common name*	6	3-*O*-β-D-glc; 28-*O*-α-D-gal-(1→6)-β-D-glc-(1→6)-[β-D-glc-(1→3)]-β-D-glc ester	*G. pacifica* [59]
93	*No common name*	4	3-*O*-β-D-gal-(1→2)-[β-D-xyl-(1→3)]-β-D-glcA; 28-*O*-β-D-glc-(1→3)-[β-D-glc-(1→4)]-α-L-rha-(1→2)-[α-L-ara-(1→4)]-β-D-fuc ester	*G. pacifica* [59]

Table 2. (Continued)

№	Name	Genin*	Sugar moiety**	Species [Ref]
94	*No common name*	4	3-*O*-*β*-D-gal-(1→2)-[*α*-L-ara-(1→3)]-*β*-D-glc; 28-*O*-*α*-L-ara-(1→3)-*β*-D-xyl-(1→4)-[*β*-D-glc-(1→3)]-*α*-L-rha-(1→2)-[*α*-L-rha-(1→4)]-*β*-D-fuc	*G. pacifica* [59]
95	*No common name*	3	3-*O*-*β*-D-gal-(1→2)-[*β*-D-xyl-(1→3)]-*β*-D-glcA; 28-*O*-*β*-D-glc-(1→3)-[*β*-D-xyl-(1→3)-*β*-D-xyl-(1→4)]-*α*-L-rha-(1→2)-*β*-D-fuc	*G. paniculata* [83]
96	*No common name*	4	3-*O*-*β*-D-gal-(1→4)-O-[*β*-D-glc-(1→2)]-*β*-D-glcA	*G. paniculata* [86]
97	*No common name*	4	3-*O*-*β*-D-glc-(1→2)-*O*-[*β*-D-xyl-(1→3)]-*β*-D-glcA	*G. paniculata* [86]
98	*No common name*	22	3-*O*-*β*-D-gal-(1→2)-*O*-[*β*-D-gal-(1→4)]-*β*-D-glcA	*G. paniculata* [86]
99	*No common name*	4	3-*O*-*β*-D-gal-(1→2)-O-[*β*-D-xyl-(1→3)]-*β*-D-glc; methyl ester	*G. paniculata* [86]
100	junceoside C	3	28-*O*-[*β*-D-glc-(1→2)-*β*-D-gal-(1→3)]-[*β*-D-glc-(1→6)]-*β*-D-gal	*G. paniculata* [87]
101	Agro-stemmoside A	1	3-*O*-*β*-D-xyl; 28-*O*-*β*-D-glc-(1→2)-[*β*-D-xyl-(1→6)]-*β*-D-glc-(1→6)-*β*-D-glc	*G. paniculata* [87]
102	*No common name*	3	3-*O*-*α*-L-ara-(1→2)-*O*-[*β*-D-xyl-(1→3)]-*β*-D-glcA; 28-*O*-*β*-D-xyl-(1→3)-*O*-*β*-D-xyl-(1→4)-*O*-*α*-L-rha-(1→2)-4-*O*-[(E)-4-methoxycinnamoyl]-*β*-D-fuc	*G. paniculata* [86]
103	*No common name*	4	3-*O*-*β*-D-xyl-(1→4)-*β*-D-gal-(1→2)-*O*-[*α*-L-ara-(1→3)]-*β*-D-glcA; 28-*O*-*β*-D-xyl-(1→3)-*O*-*β*-D-xyl-(1→4)-*O*-*α*-L-rha-(1→2)-*O*-[*β*-D-qui-(1→4)]-*β*-D-fuc	*G. paniculata* [86]
104	*No common name*	4	3-*O*-*α*-L-ara-(1→3)-*O*-[*β*-D-gal-(1→2)]-*β*-D-glcA; 28-*O*-*β*-D-gal-(1→3)-*O*-*β*-D-xyl-(1→4)-*O*-*α*-L-rha-(1→2)-*β*-D-fuc	*G. paniculata* [86]
105	*No common name*	3	3-*β*-*O*-(*β*-D-gal)-(1→3)-*β*-D-glc; 28-*O*-*β*-D-glc-(1→3)-[*β*-D-xyl-(1→4)]-*α*-L-rha-(1→2)-[*β*-D-fuc-(1→3)]-*α*-L-ara	*G. paniculata* [87]
106	*No common name*	4	3-*O*-*β*-D-gal-(1→2)-*O*-[*β*-D-xyl-(1→3)]-β-D-glcA; 28-*O*-*β*-D-xyl-(1→3)-*O*-*β*-D-xyl-(1→4)-*O*-*α*-L-rha-(1→2)-*O*-[3,4-di-*O*-acetyl-*β*-D-qui -(1→4)]-*β*-D-fuc	*G. paniculata* [87]
107	rubicunoside C	4	3-*O*-*β*-D-gal-(1→2)-[*β*-D-xyl-(1→3)]-*β*-D-glcA; 28-*O*-*β*-D-xyl-(1→4)-*α*-L-rha-(1→4)-[4''-OAc-*β*-D-glc-(1→2)]-*β*-D-fuc	*G. paniculata* [87]
108	*No common name*	4	3-*O*-[*β*-D-gal-(1→2)]-[*β*-D-xyl-(1→3)]-*β*-D-glcA; 28-*O*-[*α*-L-rha-(1→2)]-4-*O*-acetyl-3-*O*-(*E*)-*para*-methoxycinnamoyl-*β*-D-fuc	*G. paniculata* [87]
109	*No common name*	4	3-*O*-[*β*-D-gal-(1→2)]-[*β*-D-xyl-(1→3)]-*β*-D-glcA; 28-*O*-[*α*-L-rha-(1→2)]-4-*O*-acetyl-3-*O*-(*Z*)-*para*-methoxycinnamoyl-*β*-D-fuc	*G. paniculata* [87]

*See Table 1 for the genin structure.

**Abbreviation of sugar moiety: glucose (glc), galactose (gal), xylose (xyl), fucose (fuc), rhamnose (rha), arabinose (ara), glucuronic acid (glcA), glucopyranosiduronic acid (glcAp), quinovose (qui); acetyl (Ac); argirose (arg).

In the 1960s-1970s many Russian scientists isolated many triterpenoid saponins such as: filoside A and filoside B from *G. partinii* Ser. [10-11], acutifiloside from *G. acutifolia* Fisch. [14], trichoside A, B, C and D from *G. trichotoma* Wend. [46-49], gypsoside from *G. capitata* M. Bieb., *G. paniculata* L., *G. pacifica* Kom. [38-39, 43], but some of their structure has not been completely defined, because of the great complexity of the molecule.

During the last years a number of new saponins were isolated from various *Gypsophila* species. Two new 28-nortriterpens and their saponins were obtained from *G. oldhamiana* Miq. [50].

Cevrimli et al. [12] were isolated a new gypsogenin ester from a *G. simonii*. New bidesmosidic saponins were identified in *G. pacifica* [58-59]. New sulfated oleanane type saponins, where the sulfo-group in the aglycone is usually attached to C-3 and C-23, were isolated [2, 44, 52]. A sulfated triterpene and its glucosyl ester with lupane-type skeleton were isolated for the first time from the *Caryophyllaceae*, but also from the plant kingdom [18].

Table 1 and 2 presented triterpene sapogenins and their saponins, isolated from the *Gypsophila* species according to literature up to 2010.

ISOLATION, PURIFICATION AND SEPARATION

Triterpene saponins have a different polarity according to the type of functional group and the sugar chain or chains. That is why there is no one universal way to isolate saponins, but there is a standard extraction procedure that can be followed. The plant material (roots or aerial part) is extracted with different concentrations of MeOH or EtOH. They can vary from 70% to pure MeOH or EtOH. Then, the solvent is evaporated under reduced pressure and thus, crude extract is obtained. One way of purifying is to suspend the extract in MeOH, and precipitate it with Et_2O obtaining crude saponin mixture or to suspend the residue in water and then extract it successively with solvents with increasing polarity $CHCl_3$ or petroleum ether, EtOAC and BuOH [37, 40]. The nonpolar substances, such as aglycones, sterols and others remain in the chloroform extract. The substances with not so long sugar chains that are not so polar remain in the EtOAc extract and the most polar stay in the BuOH extract. Subsequently, the extracts are subjected to purification by chromatographic means. The initial stages of separation of a saponin mixture is a column chromatography (CC) with Silica gel as a stationary phase and different eluents, like $CHCl_3$-MeOH-H_2O mixtures of increasing H_2O content (55:37:5, 55:37:6, 55:37:7) or $CHCl_3$-MeOH-H_2O (100:10:1), $CHCl_3$ content were reduced stepwise until 10:10:1 and finally pure MeOH, $CHCl_3$/MeOH/H_2O 13:7:2, lower phase, $CHCl_3$-MeOH-H_2O (18:11:2) [1-2, 18-19, 22-23, 45-46]. Gel filtration on Sephadex LH-20 with MeOH is used as a preliminary separation of crude saponin fractions as well as chromatography over Diaion HP-20 resin with water/MeOH in different concentrations for water-soluble fractions or CC over D-101 resin with 95% aq. EtOH, or over MCI gel with MeOH/H_2O, 3:7, 5:5, 6:4, 7:3 and 10:0 [58-59].

Nie et al. [57] compared separation characteristics of column packed with MCI-gel, D101 macroporous resin and ODS for the enrichment and separation of oleanane-type triterpenoid saponins with 3,28-*O*-bidesmosides (OTSB) and oleanane-type triterpenoid saponins with 3-*O*-monoglucosides (OTSM) from the *n*-BuOH-soluble portion of *G. pacifica* Kom. The MCI gel showed better separation efficiency, adsorption capacity and faster flow rate than D101 and ODS.

Mostad and Doehl [56] obtained two hydroxylated gypsogenin isomers from *G. arrostii* after acid hydrolysis and separation of aglycones by reversed-phase high-performance liquid chromatography. The compounds were further characterized using direct liquid-inlet liquid chromatography-mass spectrometry.

Medium-pressure Liquid Chromatography (MPLC) or Flash Chromatography with normal (silica gel) or reversed-phase (Rp-8, 56% MeOH, or Rp-8, 41% MeOH) stationary phase, Vacuum liquid chromatography (VLC): RP-18 gel. For better purification results HPLC can be used on a RP-18 with different concentrations of MeCN/H_2O or MeOH/H_2O with or without TFA. For example, one can use 0.1 % TFA [18-19] or 26% MeCN in H_2O containing 0.06% TFA [90]. Nie et al. [59] used HPLC or High Speed Counter Current Chromatography (HSCCC) [62-70% MeOH in H_2O, containing 0.05% trifluoroacetic acid] for purification and separation of saponins.

With the development of separation techniques, high-speed counter-current chromatography (HSCCC) became a new kind of support-free all-liquid partition chromatography. It could bring on higher sample recovery than SLC, and receive larger amounts of sample injection than HPLC; multiform relative pure substances can be obtained at once in large amounts. Furthermore, its separation efficiency exceeds droplet counter-current chromatography (DCCC) and centrifugal partition chromatography (CPC), which are based on the same partition mechanism and have been always applied in separation of saponins [85].

Yao et al. [85] compared acetone precipitation, D101 resin, ODS, and silica gel CC to purify crude extract from the fat soluble components and acquired total saponins of certain purity with HSCCC separation with two-phase solvent system composed of *n*-hexane-*n*-BuOH-MeOH-0.02% TFA (1:9:1:9, v/v) followed by prep. HPLC MeOH-H_2O-0.02% TFA in gradient mode as follows: 5:95 – 100:0 in 50 min and they used it as a superior method for purifying saponins.

Weng et al. [83] described an interesting way to separate saponins from roots of *G. paniculata* L. where the matrix complexity of the raw extract is first reduced by a mild basic hydrolysis (chemical degradation) and the low molecular compounds are removed by extensive dialysis and followed by prep. HPLC.

STRUCTURE ELUCIDATION

Many *Gypsophila* saponins have very complex structure and for their determination is used combination of different chromatographic, chemical and spectral methods. TLC is quick method to identify saponins or sapogenins by comparison with authentic samples in at least three solvent systems [2, 40, 47]. Other chemical methods for structural determination, which were time and sample consuming, were acetylation and methylation [14, 46-49].

Different spectroscopic methods, such as Infrared Spectroscopy (IR), Mass Spectroscopy (MS) and Nuclear Magnetic Resonance (NMR) are usually used for structure elucidation of saponins [15-16, 37, 40]. MS allows one to determine the molecular mass of the compounds, the number of the monosaccharides, and in some cases the sequence of the oligosaccharide chain, using soft ionization methods like Field Desorbtion (FD), Fast Atom Bombardment (FAB) and High Resolution Electrospray Ionization (HR-ESI-MS) [19, 44, 50-53]. Analysis of NMR spectra can provide information about the whole structure of the aglycone and the oligosaccharide moiety. The chemical shifts and coupling constants obtained from the 1D ^{1}H and ^{13}C NMR show the anomeric protons and the methyl groups of the aglycones. The most important information from ^{13}C is if the carbon is glycosylated and the substitute configuration, as well as the linkages between the sugar units [37, 40]. For simple oligosaccharides, use of ^{13}C NMR and MS techniques in combination with some chemical reactions are good enough to establish the structure. However, as in the case of *Gypsophila* saponins where the sugar moiety consists of a large number of sugar residues, the analysis of the structure is very complicated, because of the extensive overlapping of the signals. In these cases the combination with acidic, alkaline and enzymatic hydrolyses can be helpful in receiving data about the linkages in the molecule [1-2, 23, 37, 40, 90].

In recent years new methods used for identification of the new *Gypsophila* saponins have been used; a number of new one dimensional (1D) and two dimensional (2D) NMR techniques such as: 1D Distortionless Enhancement by Polarization Transfer (DEPT), 2D Heteronuclear Multiple Quantum Coherence (HMQC), *Heteronuclear Multiple Bond Correlation* (HMBC), 2D Homonuclear Correlation Spectroscopy (COSY), Double Quantum Filtered COSY (DQF-COSY), Total Correlation Spectroscopy (TOCSY), Homonuclear Hartmann-Hann spectroscopy (HOHAHA), direct ^{1}H-^{13}C 2D Heteronuclear Correlation spectroscopy (HETCOR) and 2D nuclear Overhauser Effect Spectroscopy (NOESY), NOE in rotating frame (ROESY) [15-16, 37, 40]. DEPT helps to distinguish between methane, methylene, methyl and quaternary carbons. COSY and HOHAHA allow the determination of the identity of sugars and the sugar sequence of the sugar moiety. The interactions between each pair of vicinal and geminal protons can be revealed from the COSY and DQF-COSY spectrum. In the TOCSY experiment each network of mutually coupled protons can be detected. NOESY and ROESY provide further information about the anomeric configurations and molecular conformations. To identify the sugar sequence and the inter-glycosidic linkage, homonuclear dipolar coupling (NOE measurements) can be used. HMBC and HMQC provide multi-bond correlation between the anomeric proton and the aglycone carbon and thus help to clarify the connections and also give information about anomeric configurations and the overall conformations [1-2; 31; 37; 40, 50-53]. Frechet et al. [26] were among the first that used a combination of 2D NMR (HOHAHA, COSY) and FAB-MS for structural elucidation when they determined the structure of four new saponins from *G. paniculata* and *G. arostii*. They used a short range HMBC experiment to determine the position of the carboxylic group in the aglycone and of the glucuronic acid, and HOHAHA - for the anomeric proton of the sugars and their direct connectivity.

By combining MS, NMR techniques and hydrolytic experiments two new sulfated saponins isolated from *G. bermejoi* [2] were identified. Assignment of the different resonances to each one of the three residues was achieved through FAB-MS together with acid hydrolysis of the saponins, followed by treatment with $BaCl_2$, which proved the presence of a sulfate group in both molecules [2].

Krasteva et al. [44] used a combination of HR-ESI-MS and different NMR techniques (DEPT, HETCOR, COSY, HMBC, NOESY) to identify three new sulfated saponins. The HMBC showed ester carbon at C-28 and the secondary hydroxyl group at C-16. The place of attachment of the *O*-sulfo unit was determined due the characteristic downfield shift at

δc=87.66 carbon atom. The location of this carbon was established through long-range HMBC correlations with H3-24 (δ=0.83) and H3-23 (δ=1.04) and couplings between C-5 (δc=57.33) and H3-25 (δ=0.97) as well as H3-23 and H3-24, revealing it to be C-3.

Elbandy et al. [18] described a new sulfated lupane triterpene gypsophilin and its glucosyl ester, gypsophilinoside. Again their structure was elucidated with a combination of spectral methods such as 1D and 2D NMR, HR-ESI-MS and FAB-MS. The fragment ion at *m/z* 485 $[M\text{-}H\text{-}80]^-$ showed the presence of a sulfate group $[SO_3]^-$ which was corroborated by the presence of a peak at *m/z* 97 $[OSO_3H]^-$. An extensive 2D NMR analysis of gypsophilin was in favor of a triterpenic lup-20(29)-ene structure which is in good agreement with betulinic acid except for some signals of ring A. The downfield shift observed in the HSQC spectrum at δ 5.41 (dd, *J*=7.9, 2.7 Hz)/δ 83.6 suggested that the aglycone residue was esterified by the SO_3H group at the position C-3.

Two new oleanan type nortriterpen aglycones neogypsogenin A and B and their saponins neogypsoside A and B, obtained from roots of *G. oldhamiana* were identified with the help of new NMR techniques and comparison with the literature data [50]. The chemical shift changes of C(20), C(21), and C(22) were due to the OH group having been removed from C(21). A ROESY experiment showed that that H-C(17) and H-C(18) were not on the same side of the molecular skeleton. Since H-C(17) pointed to the α-side, and H-C(18) to the β-side, the trans D/E ring junction of the aglycone was further confirmed. The differences between neogypsoside A and neogypsoside B concerned the chemical shifts of the C-atoms of rings D and E, including the trisubstituted C=C bond at δ122.1 and 142.1, suggesting the presence of a H-C(17β)-configuration. Later the same research group obtained three new pentacyclic triterpenes [52] in *G. oldhamiana*. The ^{1}H-NMR data of 3α-hydroxyepigypsogenin were very similar to those of gypsogenin, but a signal at δ (H) 3.20 (t, *J*=2.4 Hz) indicated the presence of an α-OH group at C(3). ^{1}H- and ^{13}C-NMR spectra of hederagonic acid showed specific signals of a Me group at δ(H) 1.00 (d, J= 6.5, 3 H) and a ketone C-atom at δ(C) 213.6. In the HMBC spectrum, the correlations indicated C(3) was a carbonyl C-atom, and the Me group giving rise to a doublet was at C(4). The α-configuration of this Me group (Me(23)) was evident from the ROESY spectrum, which showed significant through-space correlation between Me(23) (δ(H) 1.00) and H-C(5) (δ(H) 1.10, Hα), but no correlation between Me(23) and Me(25) (δ(H) 1.12, β-Me)). In the 13C-NMR of hederagenin-3-O-sulfate the chemical shifts of the compound were very similar to those of hederagenin, but the resonance for C(3) was shifted from 70.5 to 79.1 ppm, which revealed that the OH group at C(3) was substituted. However, both ^{1}H- and ^{13}C-NMR spectra did not exhibit any signals due to a sugar moiety or any other substituent. Since HR-ESI-MS and IR data, and acid hydrolysis of the compound suggested the presence of a sulfate group in the molecule, it could be deduced that C(3) was substituted with a sulfate substituent.

Biological Activity

Cytotoxicity and Antitumor Activity

Rao and Sung [63] reported anticarcinogenic properties of *Gypsophila* saponins which include direct cytotoxicity, immunomodulatory effects, bile acid binding and normalization of carcinogen-induced cell proliferation. The mechanisms involve growth of cell membrane permeability in a dose dependent fashion, also alter cell morphology and interact with the cell membrane in different ways. Sung et al. [69] reported that Gypsophila Saponin (GS) and Soybean Saponin (SS) have a significant growth inhibitory effect on colon tumor cells in culture. However, they differ in their mechanism; GS induced a rough and granular cell surface, whereas SS act initially on cytoplasmic material and then cause cell membrane disruption.

Many surveys are conducted on the effects of agrostin and saporin (type I ribosome-inactivating proteins) combined with *Gypsophila* saponins [34, 35, 54, 78, 80-81]. Results of these investigations showed that the variety of bisdesmosidic saponins having an aldehyde group at the position C-23 potentiated the cytotoxicity of agrostin. This group could be a prerequisite for agrostin penetration through the cell membrane [54]. Saponinum album (SA), obtained from *G. paniculata* L., increased the cytotoxicity of the N-glycosidase saporin (up to 100 000-fold) [34] as well as enhancing the toxicity of a chimeric toxin (CT) composed of saporin and human epidermal growth factor up to 385 000-fold [35]. Bachran et al. [3] investigated the therapeutical potential of different saponins and determined that Saponinum album and quillajasaponin enhance the citotoxicity of saporin more than 1,000-fold. In another study of Bachran et al. [4], it was described that CT inhibited the growth of primary oral squamous cell carcinoma cells. They revealed that a combined application of CT with SA reduced the amount of surviving cells.

Weng et al. [79-80] investigated the enhancement of saporin toxicity against U937 cells (ATCC-No, CRL-1593.2) by SA, as well as the indication of apoptosis. They found out that Saponinum album induced a stimulation of the endocytosis of saporin by these cells and the enhancement of cytotoxicity is not based on stimulation of phagocytosis. The combination of saporin with SA increased the cytotoxicity of level of viscumin, a highly toxin type II RIP. Saporin was internalized via clathrin-mediated endocytosis, followed by its release into the endosomal transport system. This effect was not cell line-specific suggesting that saporin exploits a common SA-dependent mechanism to enter cells [78]. To examine this hypothesis the researchers also investigated endocytosis, exocytosis or impaired degradation processes of histidine tagged saporin (^{his}saporin) with or without Saponinum album in ECV-304 cells. They found out that the reason for the higher cytosolic amount of ^{his}saporin in the saponin-treated cells was saponin mediated endosomal escape of saporin [81]. Saponinum album with CT has significant cytotoxic activity on five human cervical carcinoma cell lines (HeLa, CaSki, SiHa, PHCC1 and PHCC2) [5]. In view of potential use of Saponinum album in tumor therapy the authors managed to isolate and characterize a new saponin, which enhanced the cytotoxicity saporin and human epidermal growth factor on HER14 cells [82].

In a study by Weng et al. [83] three isolated saponins from roots of *G. paniculata* L., including one new bisdesmoside saponin, showed toxicity enhancing properties on saporin without causing toxicity by them at 20μg/mL.

The immunologic properties of two new saponins from the roots of *G. oldhamiana* were investigated. The compounds were tested *in vitro* for their lymphocyte proliferation and in T cell activation properties. Saponin 1 showed an immuno-modulatory effect dependent on concentration. It demonstrated a significant enhancement of granulocyte phagocytosis (40-75%) in the concentration range of 10-100 μg/ml [51]. A new saponin, named gypoldoside A, isolated from the same plant was found to be highly active against three different human cancer cell lines, with IC50 values in the low micromolar range. It was tested over human colon (HT29), human gastric (SGC7901), and human hepatoma (PLC/PRF/5) cancer cells. Among the three cell lines tested, saponin acted on PLC/PRF/5 most effectively (IC50μ0.55 mg/ml). Based on these promising results, gypoldoside A and its derivatives could serve as potential antitumor agents for future cancer chemotherapy [6].

Tian et al. [71] conducted experimental studies of the therapeutic effect of *G. oldhamiana* gypsogenin (GOG) on Lewis lung cancer in mice. They concluded that GOG can inhibit the growth and metastasis of Lewis lung cancer, and may also exert its mechanism of tumor control by inhibition of tumor angiogenesis and induction of apoptosis.

Effects on Cell Permeability

Johnson et al. [41] reported that four saponins, including *Gypsophila* saponin inhibited active transport by increasing the general permeability of the enterocytes. They found out that some saponins readily increase the permeability of the small intestinal mucosal cells, thereby inhibiting active nutrient transport, and facilitating the uptake of materials to which the gut would normally be impermeable.

Saponinum album has concentration dependent permeabilization of monolayer cultures of rat hepatocytes. That demonstrated the usefulness of saponin as a tool for investigating the interior of different intracellular compartments [76].

Southon et al. [66] conducted a survey to determine whether there is any indication that dietary *Gypsophila* roots extract from different species saponins reduce mineral utilization in the rat model. Their investigation included diets which were low in Fe or Zn, in addition to a normal mineral-replete diet. The study also demonstrated a hypocholesterolaemic effect of the extract, which was influenced by the Fe content of the diet, or possibly the Fe status of the animal itself. However, the significant reduction in plasma cholesterol observed in rats, given the 'saponin-free' low-Fe diet compared to the other control groups, and the increased potency of the saponin when incorporated into this diet, suggested a saponin-mineral interaction which has not previously been documented. It was found that the addition of *Gypsophila* extract to a semi-synthetic diet had a detrimental effect on Fe status in growing rats, but Zn status as judged by femur Zn was unaffected. Another study demonstrated that the amount of Fe absorbed from a test meal could be reduced in the presence of these saponins, which indicated that the effect on Fe status was probably due to the reduced Fe absorption. Zn absorption was not affected by the saponins, which was in agreement with an earlier finding of no change in femur Zn [67]. Increasing amounts of *Gypsophila* saponin, given in a single meal, progressively reduced the amount of Fe available for absorption but Zn status and absorption were not affected [62].

Gee et al. [28] found out that a range of saponins, commonly present in foods or dietary supplements including Gypsophila saponins reduce the potential difference. Solubility, pH and the chemical form of the saponin were among the factors affecting the nature and magnitude of the de-polarizing effect. The interaction between bile salts and saponins from *Gypsophila* was investigated *in vitro*. There was an evidence of decline in transmural potential difference and an increased rate of mucosal cell proliferation. Serum cholesterol levels were significantly lower [27].

The effects of saponin mixture of *Gypsophila* and glycoalkaloids on the permeability and viability of mammalian intestinal cells have been tested. They showed an increase in gut permeability, which may underline some forms of food allergy and it is assumed to be a local effect, and cells with altered membrane integrity may still remain viable. Sublethal concentrations of saponins and glycoalkaloids may therefore be significant in terms of mediating the occurrence of hypersensitivity to food components [29]. The compounds were also investigated for their effect on the transmucosal passage of β-lactoglobulin across the proximal small intestine of normal and β-lactoglobulin-sensitized rats. An increase in the transmucosal uptake of the milk allergen β-lactoglobulin (βLG) was assessed in non-sensitized and sensitized Brown Norway rats in the presence of Gypsophila saponin. The authors concluded that exposure to food constituents capable of permeabilizing the mucosal epithelium may increase the risk of sensitization to dietary antigens [30].

Wassler et al. [77] investigated the permeabilization of rat hepatocytes by a *Gypsophila* saponin and the effects of dextran. Increasing of the binding of the saponin destabilized the plasma membrane and as a result, ruptured from the colloid osmotic pressure. The lysis that occurred after continuous incubation with the saponin could be inhibited (delayed) by the addition of an osmotically active compound.

Enzyme Inhibitory Activity

Luo et al. [52] studied 12 triterpenoid saponins from the roots of *G. oldhamiana* for α-glucosidase inhibitory activity, such as retarding the uptake of dietary carbohydrates and thus suppressing postprandial hyperglycemia. Four of them exhibited α-glucosidase inhibitory activity and some of them were more potent than acarbose. This is the first example of triterpenoid saponins with α-glucosidase inhibitory activities. Later they isolated another 7 triterpenoid saponins and subjected them to the same research. The results showed that only one of them, which had a methoxycinnamoyl group and gypsogenin, were more active than acarbose. They suggested that the methoxycinnamoyl group played a key role in the enzyme inhibition [86].

Three new and seven known pentacyclic triterpenes were evaluated for their glycogen phosphorylase (GP) inhibitory activity. The results showed that oleanolic acid and hederagenin significantly inhibited GP. Hederagonic acid, gypsogenin, gypsogenic acid, and echinocystic acid exhibited only moderate inhibition.

On the other hand, hederagenin-3-O-sulfate, quillaic acid, and collinsogenin showed no inhibition on GP. Comparing the chemical structure of the active saponins they demonstrated the importance of a C(3)_OH moiety for the activity against GP. The sulfate at C(3)_OH of hederagenin led to the loss of inhibitory activity on GP, which is probably due to the presence of an OH group at C(3) of hederagenin. The 16*a*-OH group had a negative effect on the activity, and the triterpenes with a Me(23) or $HOCH_2$(23) group exhibited more potent activities than those with a CHO(23) or COOH(23) group. More studies are needed to confirm the above proposal [53].

The water-soluble fraction of the roots of *G. oldhamiana* showed potent inhibitory activity against pancreatic lipase dose-dependently with an IC50 value of 0.54 mg/ml. Three gypsosaponins, named gypsosaponin A, B and C, showed inhibitory activity against pancreatic lipase with inhibition of 99.2% and A and C with inhibition of 58.2% and 50.3% in the concentration of 1 mg/ml [90].

The acetylcholinesterase-inhibitory activity of steroidal glycoalkaloids, their aglycones and saponins of *Gypsophila, Quillaja* and *Glycyrrhiza* were investigated. The results of the testing suggested that *Gypsophila* saponins have no acetylcholinesterase-inhibitory activity [64].

Other Biological Activity

Subcutaneous injection of saponins from *G. paniculata*, *Saponaria officinalis*, or *Quillaja saponaria* decreased the ascorbic acid content of the adrenals of hypophysectomized rats [74].

The antagonism between vitamin D and saponins from *Gypsophila*, sugar beet, or lucerne in respect to cartilage formation in certain bones and their mineral content was studied. The saponins counteracted the therapeutic-symptomatic action of vitamin D [9].

Elbary et al. [20] proved that there is a correlation between the haemolytic index and the spermicidal efficacy of some saponins. From the tested saponins, *G. paniculata* saponin was most effective on human sperm. This efficient spermicidal activity was associated with a high hemolytic index and low irritant behavior.

Saponins, isolated from *Panax japonicum*, *G. paniculata*, *Sapindus mukorossi*, *Polygala senega*, *Thea sinensis*, *Bupleurum chinense, Aesculus hippocastanum* and *Styrax japonicus* increased plasma ACTH, corticosterone and glucose. The hemolytic activities of the saponins were correlated with the stimulatory activities of hormone secretion [88].

A protective activity of glucuronogypsogenin (GG) was proven when hepatocytes were treated with it in advance. The authors assumed that GG interacts with the hepatocyte membrane [8].

Gypsophila saponins added to the diet of male Wistar rats, induced enhanced biliary cholesterol secretion, independent of the input of cholesterol from diet [73].

Two triterpene saponins, named saponins A and B from *G. capitata* were responsible for hypocholesteremic effects in rabbits [75]. Ueda [72] reported that the hypocholesterolemic effect of *Gypsophila* saponins was minor as compared with that of protein source or protein content.

Conclusion

This review contains data through 2010 describing triterpenoid saponins, obtained from thirteen *Gypsophila* species. Seventy eight saponins and fifteen triterpens have been isolated from the plants. The recent methods used for their isolation and structure elucidation are discussed. The biological activities of *Gypsophila* saponins are also covered.

References

[1] Acebes, B; Díaz-Lanza, AM; Bernabé, M. A saponin from the roots of *Gypsophila bermejoi*. *Phytochemistry*, 1998, 49, 2077-2079.

[2] Acebes, B; Bernabé, M; Díaz-Lanza, AM; Bartolomé, C. Two new sulfated saponins from the roots of *Gypsophila bermejoi*. *Journal of Natural Products,* 1998, 61, 1557-1559.

[3] Bachran, C; Sutherland, M; Heisler, I; Hebestreit, P; Melzig, MF; Fuchs, H. The saponin-mediated enhanced uptake of targeted saporin-based drugs is strongly dependent on the saponin structure. *Experimental Biology and Medicine*, 2006, 231, 412-420.

[4] Bachran, C; Heisler, I; Bachran, D; Dassler, K; Ervens, J; Matthias, FM; Fuchs, H. Chimeric toxins inhibit the growth of primary oral squamous cell carcinoma cells. *Cancer Biology and Therapy,* 2008, 7, 237-242.

[5] Bachran, D; Schneider, S; Bachran, C; Urban, R; Weng, A; Melzig, MF; Hoffmann, C; Kaufmann, AM; Fuchs, H. Epidermal growth factor receptor expression affects the efficacy of the combined application of saponin and a targeted toxin on human cervical carcinoma cells. *International Journal of Cancer*, 2010, 127, 1453-1461.

[6] Bai, H; Zhong, Y; Xie, YY; Wang, YS; Liu, L. A major triterpenoid saponin from *Gypsophila oldhamiana. Chemistry and Biodiversity*, 2007, 4, 955-960.

[7] Borges Del Castillo, J; Zeitoun, BA; Arriaga, FJ, Vazquez, P. Steryl glucosides of *Gypsophila struthium. Fitoterapia*, 1986, 57, 61-64.

[8] Braut-Boucher, F; Achard-Ellouk, S; Pauthe-Dayde, D; Henry, M; Hoellinger, H. Cytoprotective effects of *Gypsophila* saponins towards isolated rat hepatocytes. *Food Additives and Contaminants*, 1990, 7, 127-130.

[9] Brune, H; Guenther, K. The actions of the saponins as antivitamins. *Zeitschrift für Ernährungswissenschaft*, 1961, 2, 45-64. CA 57:18742.

[10] Bukharov, VG; Karlin, VV; Bukharova, IL; Surkova, LN. Triterpene glycosides of *Gypsophila patrinii* II. The structure of philoside A. *Chemistry of Natural Compounds*, 1974, 10, 607-611.

[11] Bukharov, VG; Karlin, VV; Bukharova, IL; Surkova, LN. Triterpene glycosides of *Gypsophila patrinii* III. The structure of philoside B. *Chemistry of Natural Compounds,* 1974, 10, 612-615.

[12] Cevrimli, BS; Kariptas, E; Yucekutlu, AN. Isolation of saponin from the dried roots of *Gypsophila simonii* Hub. Mor. *Pakistan Journal of Biological Sciences*, 2007, 10, 1944-1946.

[13] Chen, Q; Luo, JG; Kong, LY. Triterpenoid Saponins from *Gypsophila altissima* L. *Chemical and Pharmaceutical Bulletin*, 2010, 58, 412-414.

[14] Chirva, VY; Kintya, PK; Melnikov, VN; Paukov, VN. Structure of the triterpenoid glycoside from *Gypsophila acutifolia. Chemistry of Natural Compounds*, 1974, 10, 336-338.

[15] Connolly, JD; Hill, RA. Triterpenoids. *Natural Product Reports*, 2008, 25, 794-830.

[16] Connolly, JD; Hill, RA. Triterpenoids. *Natural Product Reports,* 2010, 27, 79-132.

[17] Delay, C; Gavin, JA; Aumelas, A; Bonnet, PA; Roumestand, C. Isolation and structure elucidation of a highly haemolytic saponin from the Merck saponin extract using high-field gradient-enhanced NMR techniques. Carbohydrate Research, 1997, 302, 67-78.

[18] Elbandy, M; Miyamoto, T; Lacaille-Dubois, MA. Sulfated lupane triterpene derivatives and a flavone *C*-glycoside from *Gypsophila repens. Chemical and Pharmaceutical Bulletin*, 2007, 55, 808-811.

[19] Elbandy, M; Miyamoto, T; Lacaille-Dubois, MA. New triterpenoidal saponins from *Gypsophila repens*. *Helvetica Chimica Acta*, 2007, 90, 260-270.

[20] Elbary, AA; Nour, SA. Correlation between the spermicidal activity and the haemolytic index of certain plant saponins. *Pharmazie*, 1979, 34, 560-561.

[21] Elgamal, MHA; Soliman, HSM; Karawya, MS; Duddeck, H. Isolation of two triterpene saponins from *Gypsophila capillaris* (Forssk.). *Natural Product Letters,* 1994, 4, 217-222.

[22] Elgamal, MHA; Soliman, HSM; Dueddeck, H; Mikhova, B; Gartmann, M. A novel triterpene saponin from *Gypsophila cappilaris*. *Zeitschrift für Naturforschung B*, 1995, 50, 563-567.

[23] Elgamal, MHA; Soliman, HSM; Karawya, MS; Mikhova, B; Duddeck, H. Isolation of triterpene saponins from *Gypsophila capillaris*. *Phytochemisty*, 1995, 38, 1481-1485.

[24] Elgamal, MHA; Soliman, HSM. Structure of a novel triterpene saponin from *Gypsophila capillaris* Forssk. *Magnetic Resonance in Chemistry*, 1996, 34, 697-702.

[25] Elgar, J. Gypsophila for cut flowers: propagation, production and harvesting. HortFACT. The Horticulture and Food Research Institute of New Zealand Ltd., 1998. Available from: URL: <http: //www.hor tnet. co.nz/publications/hortfacts>.

[26] Frechet, D; Christ, B; du Sorbier, BM; Fischer, H; Vuilhorgne, M. Four triterpenoid saponins from dried roots of *Gypsophila* species. *Phytochemistry*, 1991, 30, 927-931.

[27] Gee, JM; Johnson, IT. Interaction between hemolytic saponins, bile salts and small intestinal mucosa in the rat. *Journal of Nutrition*, 1988, 118, 1391-1139.

[28] Gee, JM; Price, KR; Ridout, CL; Johnson, IT; Fenwick, GR. Effects of some purified saponins on transmural potential difference in mammalian small intestine. *Toxicology in Vitro,* 1989, 3, 85-90.

[29] Gee, JM; Wortley, GM; Johnson, IT; Price, KR; Rutten, AAJJJ; Houbens, GF; Penninks, AH. Effects of saponins and glycoalkaloids on the permeability and viability of mammalian intestinal cells and on the integrity of tissue preparations *in vitro*. *Toxicology in Vitro*. 1996, 10, 117-128.

[30] Gee, JM; Wal, JM; Miller, K; Atkinson, H; Grigoriadou, F; Wijnands, MVW; Penninks, AM; Wortley, G; Johnson, IT. Effect of saponin on the transmucosal passage of β-lactoglobulin across the proximal small intestine of normal and β-lactoglobulin-sensitized rats. *Toxicology*, 1997, 117, 219-228.

[31] Gevrenova, R; Voutquenne-Nazabadioko, L; Harakat, D; Prost, E; Henry, M. Complete 1H- and 13C NMR assignments of saponins from roots of *Gypsophila trichotoma* Wend. *Magnetic Resonance in Chemistry*, 2006, 44, 686-691.

[32] Gevrenova, R; Stancheva, T; Voynikov, Y; Laurain-Mattar, D; Henry, M. Root *in vitro* cultures of six *Gypsophila* species and their saponin contents. *Enzyme and Microbial Technology*, 2010, 47, 97-104.

[33] Hanafy, MS; Lobna, MAS. Saponins production in shoot and callus cultures of *Gypsophila paniculata*. *Journal of Applied Sciences Research*, 2003, 3, 1045-1049.

[34] Hebestreit, P; Weng, A; Bachran, C; Fuchs, H; Melzig, MF. Enhancement of cytotoxicity of lectins by Saponinum album. *Toxicon*, 2006, 47, 330-335.

[35] Heisler, I; Sutherland, M; Bachran, C; Hebestreit, P; Schnitger, A; Melzig, MF; Fuchs, H. Combined application of saponin and chimeric toxins drastically enhances the targeted cytotoxicity on tumor cells. *Journal Control Release*, 2005, 106, 123-137.

[36] Henry, M; Pauthe-Dayde, D; Rochd, M. Extraction and HPLC determination of gypsogenin-3-O-glucoronide. *Journal of Chromatography*, 1989, 477, 413-419.

[37] Hostettmann, K; Marston, A. *Chemistry and Pharmacology of Natural Products: Saponins.* Cambridge, UK: Cambridge University Press; 1995.

[38] Iskenderov, GB; Aliev, RK; Libizov, NI. Saponins from *Gypsophila capitata. Farmatsiya* (Moskow), 1967, 16, 29-34.

[39] Iskenderov, GB. Pharmacochemical study of Azerbaidzhan *Ruscus hyrcanus* and *Gypsophila capitata. Azerbaidzhanskii Meditsinskii Zhurnal*, 1967, 44, 27-30. CA 68:94482.

[40] Jia, Z; Koike, K; Sahu, NP; Nikaido, T. Triterpenoid saponins from *Caryophyllaceae* family. In: Atta-ur-Rahman, editor. *Studies in Natural Products Chemistry*, 2002, 26, 3-61.

[41] Johnson, IT; Gee, JM; Price, K; Curl, C; Fenwick, GR. Influence of saponins on gut permeability and active nutrient transport *in vitro. Journal of Nutrition,* 1986, 116, 2270-2277.

[42] Khorlin, AY; Ovodov, YS; Ovodova, RG. Identity of glycoside and a triterpene saponin from *Gypsophila paniculata* L. *Izvestya Academii Nauk SSSR*, 1963, 8, 1521-1523.

[43] Kochetkov, NK; Khorlin, AJ; Ovodov, JS. The structure of gypsoside – triterpenic saponin from *Gypsophila pacifica* Kom. *Tetrahedron Letters*, 1963, 4, 477-482.

[44] Krasteva, I; Jenet-Siems, K; Kaloga, M; Nikolov, S. 3-O-Sulfo-triterpenoid saponins from *Gypsophila trichotoma* Wend. *Zeitschrift für Naturforschung B*, 2009, 64, 319-322.

[45] Lio, Z; Li, D; Owen, NL; Grant, DM; Cates, RG; Jia, Z. Triterpenoid saponins from *Gypsophila oldhamiana. Journal of Natural Products,* 1995, 58, 1632-1635.

[46] Luchanskaya, VM; Kondarenko, ES; Gorovits, TT; Abubakirov, NK. Triterpenoid glycosides of *Gypsophila trichotoma* III. Structure of trichoside A. *Chemistry of Natural Compounds*, 1971, 7, 142-144.

[47] Luchanskaya, VM; Kondarenko, ES; Abubakirov, NK. Triterpenoid glycosides of *Gypsophila trichotoma* II. Structure of trichoside B. *Chemistry of Natural Compounds*, 1971, 7, 431-434.

[48] Luchanskaya, VM; Kondarenko, ES; Abubakirov, NK. Triterpenoid glycosides of *Gypsophila trichotoma* IV. Structure of trichoside C. *Chemistry of Natural Compounds*, 1971, 7, 586-588.

[49] Luchanskaya, VM; Kondarenko, ES; Abubakirov, NK. Triterpenoid glycosides of *Gypsophila trichotoma* V. Structure of trichoside D. *Chemistry of Natural Compounds*, 1972, 8, 63-65.

[50] Luo, JG; Kong, LY. A Pair of new nortriterpene saponin epimers from the roots of *Gypsophila oldhamiana. Helvetica Chimica Acta*, 2006, 89, 947-953.

[51] Luo, JG; Kong, LY; Takaya, Y; Niwa, M. Two monodesmosidic triterpene saponins from *Gypsophila oldhamiana. Chemical and Pharmaceutical Bulletin*, 2006, 54, 1200-1202.

[52] Luo, JG; Liu, J; Kong, LY. New pentacyclic triterpenes from *Gypsophila oldhamiana* and their biological evaluation as glycogen phosphorylase inhibitors. *Chemistry and Biodiversity*, 2008, 5, 751-757.

[53] Luo, JG; Ma, L; Kong, LY. New triterpenoid saponins with strong *a*-glucosidase inhibitory activity from the roots of *Gypsophila oldhamiana*. *Bioorganic and Medicinal Chemistry*, 2008, 16, 2912-2920.
[54] Melzig, MF; Hebestreit, P; Gaidi, G; Lacaille-Dubois, MA. Structure-activity-relationship of saponins to enhance toxic effects of agrostin. *Planta Medica*, 2005, 71, 1088-1090.
[55] Mossman, S; Evans, L; Baldridge, R; Evans, JT. Immunostimulant compositions comprising aminoalkyl glucosaminide phosphates and saponins. Corixa August 2003: WO 2003/069997.
[56] Mostad, HB; Doehl, J. Separation and characterization of oleanane-type pentacyclic triterpenes from *Gypsophila arrostii* by liquid chromatography-mass spectrometry. *Journal of Chromatography*, 1987, 396, 157-168.
[57] Nie, W; Luo, JG; Wang, XB; Wan, X; Kong, LY. An insight into enrichment and separation of oleanane-type triterpenoid saponins by various chromatographic materials. *Separation and Purification Technology*, 2009, 65, 243-247.
[58] Nie, W; Luo, J; Kong, L. Triterpenoid saponins from roots of *Gypsophila pacifica*. *Chinese Herbal Medicine*, 2010, 2, 145-147.
[59] Nie, W, Luo, J; Kong, L. New triterpenoid saponins from the roots of *Gypsophila pacifica* Kom. *Carbohydrate Research*, 2010, 345, 68-73.
[60] Pasich, B; Terminska, K; Pasich, J. Saponins from *Gypsophila repens* L. Tritepenoids and sterols. *Pharmazie,* 1983, 38, 489.
[61] Pauthe-Dayde, D; Rochd, M; Henry, M. Triterpenoid saponin production in callus and multiple shoot cultures of *Gypsophila* SPP. *Phytochemistry*, 29, 483-487.
[62] Price, KR; Southern, S; Fenwick, GR. The effect of saponins on iron and zinc availability. In: Southgate D, Johnson I and Fenwick GR, editors. Nutrient availability. Royal Society of Chemistry: Thomas Graham House, Cambridge, 1988, pp. 155-157.
[63] Rao, AV; Sung, MK. Saponins as anticarcinogens. *Journal of Nutrition,* 1995, 123, 717-723.
[64] Roddick, JG. The acetylcholinesterase-inhibitory activity of steroidal glycoalkaloids and their aglycones. *Phytochemistry,* 1989, 28, 2631-2634.
[65] Ruzicka, L; Giacomello, G. Polyterpene und Polyterpenoide CVII. Überführung von Gypsogenin (Albsapogenin) in Oleanolsäure. *Helvetica Chimica Acta,* 1936, 19, 1136-1140.
[66] Southon, S; Johnson, IT; Gee, JM; Price, KR. The effect of *Gypsophila* saponins in the diet on mineral status and plasma cholesterol concentration in the rat. *British Journal of Nutrition*, 1988, 59, 49-55.
[67] Southon, S; Wright, GA; Price, KR; Fairwether-Tait, SJ; Fenwick, JR. The effect of three types of saponin on iron and zinc absorbtion from a single meal in the rat. *British Journal of Nutrition*, 1988, 59, 389-396.
[68] Sun, J; Zhong, Y; Yin, J; Liu, L; Wang, B; Zuo, C. Isolation and structure identification of triterpenoids from *Gypsophila oldhamiana*. *Zhongcaoyao*, 2005, 36, 644-646. CA 146:58714.
[69] Sung, MK; Kendall, CW; Koo, MM; Rao, AV. Effect of soybean saponins and gypsophila saponin on growth and viability of colon carcinoma cells in culture. *Nutrition and Cancer*, 1995, 23, 259-270.

[70] Tagiev, SA; Ismailov, AI. Study of sapogenins of *Gypsophila bicolor* root. *Chemistry of Natural Compounds*, 1978, 14, 138-139.

[71] Tian, G; Zhou, L; Zhong, Y; Xu, W; Bai, H; Liu, L; Cui, S. Experimental studies of the therapeutic effect of *Gypsophila oldhamiana* gypsogenin on Lewis lung cancer in mice. *Chinese Journal of Clinical Oncology*, 2008, 5, 206-210.

[72] Ueda, H. Effect of *Gypsophila* saponins on performance and plasma cholesterol concentration in chicks fed diets different in casein content. *Animal Science and Technology*, 1992, 63, 905-911.

[73] Ulloa, N; Nervi, F. Mechanism and kinetic characteristics of the uncoupling by plant steroids of biliary cholesterol from bile salt output. *Biochimica et Biophysica Acta*, 1985, 837, 181-189.

[74] Vacek, L; Kozlik, V. The mechanism of action of saponins on the adrenal cortex. *Arzneimittel-Forschung*, 1961, 11, 325-326. CA 55:101003.

[75] Velieva, MN; Iskenderov, GB; Amiralieva, UA; Gazhieva, GY. Structure and hypocholesteremic properties of saponins from *Gypsophila capitata*. *Azerbaidzhanskii Meditsinskii Zhurnal,* 1988, 65, 40-44. CA 109:70410.

[76] Wassler, M; Jonasson, I; Persson, R; Fries, E. Differential permeabilization of membranes by saponin treatment of isolated rat hepatocytes. *Biochemical Journal,* 1987, 247, 407-415.

[77] Wassler, M; Westman, J; Fries, E. Permeabilization of hepatocytes by a saponin and the effects of dextran. *European Journal of Cell Biology*, 1990, 51, 252-258.

[78] Weng, A; Bachran, C; Fuchs, H; Melzig, MF. Soapwort saponins trigger clathrin-mediated endocytosis of saporin, a type I ribosome-inactivating protein. *Chemico-Biological Interactions*, 2008, 176, 204-211.

[79] Weng, A; Jenett-Siems, K; Görick, C; Melzig, MF. Enhancement of cytotoxicity of ribosome-inactivating-protein type I by saponinum album is not based on stimulation of phagocytosis. *Journal of Pharmacy and Pharmacology*, 2008, 60, 925-930.

[80] Weng, A; Melzig, MF; Bachran, C; Fuchs, H. Enhancement of saporin toxicity against U937 cells by *Gypsophila* saponins. *Journal of Immunotoxicology,* 2008, 5, 287-292.

[81] Weng, A; Bachran, C; Fuchs, H; Krause, E; Stephanowitz, H; Melzig, MF. Enhancement of saporin cytotoxicity of Gypsophia saponins-more than stimulation of endocytosis. *Chemico-Biological Interactions*, 2009, 181, 424-429.

[82] Weng, A; Bachran, D; Görick, C; Bachran, C; Fuchs, H; Melzig, MF. A simple method for isolation of Gypsophila saponins for the combined application of targeted toxins and saponins in tumor therapy. *Planta Medica*, 2009, 75, 1421-1422.

[83] Weng, A; Jenett-Siems, K; Schmieder, P; Bachran, D; Bachran, C; Görick, C; Thakur, M; Fuchs, H; Melzig, MF. A convenient method for saponin isolation in tumor therapy. *Journal of Chromatography B*, 2010, 878, 713-718.

[84] Yang, S; Zhong, Y; Luo, H; Ding, X; Zuo, C. Study on chemical components of *Gypsophila oldhamiana*. *Zhongguo Zhongyao Zazhi,* 2004, 29, 596. CA144:447858.

[85] Yao, S; Luo, J; Huang, X; Kong, L. Application of preparative high-speed counter-current chromatography/preparative high-performance liquid chromatography mode in rapid separation of saponins. *Journal of Chromatography B*, 2008, 824, 69-77.

[86] Yao, S; Ma, L; Luo, JG; Wang, JS; Kong, LY. New triterpenoid saponins from the roots of *Gypsophila paniculata* L. *Helvetica Chimica Acta*, 2010, 93, 361-374.

[87] Yao, S; Ma, L; Luo, JG; Wang, JS; Kong, LY. Triterpenoid saponins from the roots of *Gypsophila paniculata* L. *Chinese Journal of Natural Medicines*, 2010, 8, 28-33.

[88] Yokoyama, H; Hiai, S; Oura, H; Hayashi, T. Effects of total saponins extracted from several crude drugs on rat adrenocortical hormone secretion. *Yakugaku Zasshi*, 1982, 102, 555-559. CA 97:156258.

[89] Yücekutlu, AN; Bildacı, I. Determination of plant saponins and some of *Gypsophila* species: A review of the literature. *Hacettepe Journal of Biology and Chem*istry, 2008, 36, 129-135.

[90] Zheng, Q; Li, W; Han, L; Koike, K. Pancreatic lipase-inhibiting triterpenoid saponins from *Gypsophila oldhamiana. Chemical and Pharmaceutical Bulletin*, 2007, 55, 646-650.

In: Saponins: Properties, Applications and Health Benefits
Editors: Rani Koh and Isaac Tay
ISBN: 978-1-62100-942-9

Chapter 4

POTENTIAL OF TRITERPENOIDS FROM GINSENG (*PANAX QUINQUEFOLIUS* AND *PANAX GINSENG* C.A. MEYER) TO REGULATE CULTURED ADIPOCYTES

Chia-Rou Yeo and David G. Popovich*
Department of Chemistry, National University of Singapore, Singapore

ABSTRACT

The active component of ginseng (*Panax quinquefolius* and *Panax ginseng* C.A. Meyer), is believed to be dammarane type triterpenoids also known as ginsenosides. They can be generally classified into two main groups based on the attached sugar moieties on either position C3 or C6 of the ring structure. There are differences in biological activities attributed to these minor differences in chemical structure. The objective of this review is to focus on the burgeoning interest in the effect of ginseng and ginsenosides on the reduction of risk or risk factors associated to the risk in metabolic abnormalities such as insulin resistance and the metabolic syndrome. For example ginsenosides have been reported to interact with adipocytes and influencing lipid acquisition and increase adiponectin release that can modulate and improve overall metabolic risks.

GINSENG AND METABOLIC SYNDROME

Ginseng species of the *Panax* genus is considered one of the most highly favored traditional medicinal herbs in Asia. There is evidence of ginseng use nearly 5000 years ago, ginseng has been documented in the 'Divine Peasant' as superior non-toxic herbs, served to reinforce vital energy and to invigorate weak bodies [1]. However, to a certain extent, the use

* Corresponding author.
Tel: (65) 6516-4695.
Fax: (65) 6775-7895.
E-mail address: chmpdg@nus.edu.sg.

of ginseng is often based on antidotes or cultural practices, rather than on evidence based science. Ginsengs are slow-growing perennial plants with fleshy roots, not only the roots, but also the leaves, stems, fruits, flowers are now known to display extensive range of effects with multiple plausible mechanisms of action.

Ginseng saponins, termed ginsenosides, are dammarane triterpenoids believed to be the main bioactive components behind its medicinal properties [2, 3]. Ginsenosides are classified based on the position of various water soluble sugar moieties attached to the non-polar aglycone. Polarity of different sugar moieties, including the type, position and number of sugar moieties, gives rise to desirable amphiphilic nature of ginsenosides [4]. The two main classifications of ginsenosides are the protopanaxadiol (PD) and protopanaxatriol (PT) type [5] (**Figure 1**). The PD type has various sugar moieties combinations attached to position C3 of the ring structure and the commonly known ginsenosides are Rb1, Rb2, Rc, Rd, Rg3 and Rh2; while the PT type has two attachment sites at positions C3 and C6 respectively and the commonly represented ginsenosides include Re, Rf, Rg1, Rg2 and Rh1.

The two most popular ginseng species are Asian ginseng (*Panax ginseng* C.A. Meyer) and American ginseng (*Panax quinquefolius*), others may include Japanese ginseng (*Panax japonicus*), Sanchi ginseng (*Panax notoginseng*), and Vietnamese ginseng (*Panax vietnamensis*). Different structure-function relationships are attributed to the different ginsenosides fingerprint profiles generated by respective species.

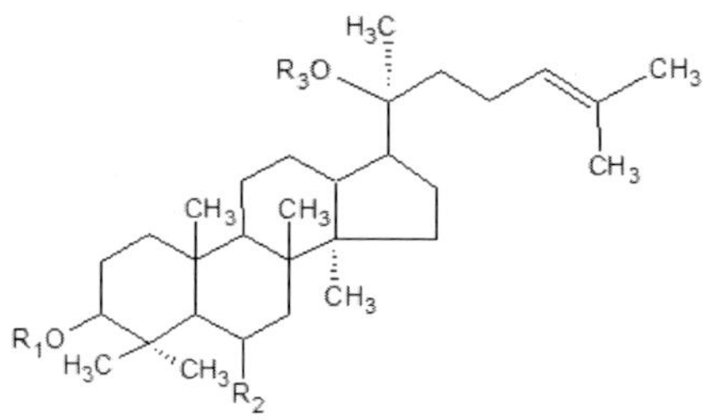

Ginsenosides	R_1	R_2	R_3
20 (S)-protopanaxadiol (PD)			
Rb1	Glc-Glc	H	Glc-Glc
Rb2	Glc-Glc	H	Glc-Ara (p)
Rc	Glc-Glc	H	Glc-Ara (f)
Rd	Glc-Glc	H	Glc
Rg3	Glc-Glc	H	H
Rh2	Glc	H	H
20 (S)-protopanaxatriol (PT)			
Re	H	O-Glc-Rha	Glc
Rf	H	O-Glc-Glc	H
Rg1	H	O-Glc	Glc
Rg2	H	O-Glc-Rha	H
Rh1	H	O-Glc	H

Figure 1. Representative chemical structure of dammarane triterpenoids (ginsenosides) found in ginseng species.

Pharmacological functions of ginseng have been well-explored in diversified areas including anti-cancer[6-9], anti-inflammatory[10-12], anti-arteriosclerosis[13, 14], anti-depressant[15], anti-memory loss research[16, 17]. A recent new area of ginseng research is centered on the potential anti-obesity properties; in a broader perspective, this refers to ginseng and its possible impact on metabolic syndrome and related metabolic consequences. Parallel to the alarming rise in obesity rate around the globe, metabolic syndrome is now under the spotlight and is the focus of much research. Metabolic syndrome (MetS) is a complex disorder with high socioeconomic cost [18]. MetS represents a cluster of cardiometabolic risk factors, including obesity, glucose intolerance and insulin resistance, dyslipidemia, and hypertension [19]. More recently associated with other clinical manifestations including atherosclerosis, polycystic ovarian syndrome (PCOS), pro-inflammatory state, oxidative stress and nonalcoholic fatty liver disease [19].

Obesity-associated metabolic diseases such as type 2 diabetes and cardiovascular diseases have unfortunately prevailed and are now the world's leading causes of mortality, results in estimated 35 million deaths each year [20]. In light of this worldwide epidemic, the use of ginseng saponins to modulate risks of metabolic diseases is of interest. Albeit current literature is insufficient to draw any firm conclusion, a number of research findings have shed light into understanding the metabolic pathways influenced by ginsenosides. Therefore, with the notion that metabolic syndrome, often co-aggregates in obese subjects is particularly a major cause of type 2 diabetes, subsequent sections shall review the health benefits that could be potentiated by ginsenosides in relation to diabetes mellitus and obesity in greater details.

GINSENOSIDES AND DIABETES MELLITUS

According to the World Health Organization (WHO), there is an estimate that over 220 million people worldwide suffering from diabetes. Diabetes mellitus, also known as type 2 diabetes occurs in more than 95% of the diabetic populations [21]. Supported by epidemiological studies and clinical trials, hyperglycemia is known as the principal cause of microvascular (includes retinopathy, neuropathy, nephropathy) and macrovascular complications (includes heart disease, stroke, amputations) [22]. Therefore, effective blood glucose control is crucial in preventing or reversing diabetic complications.

Ginseng saponins have been proposed to act as potential hypoglycemic agents. For example, American ginseng was previously reviewed to be able to improve postprandial glycemia in type 2 diabetic patients by modulating mitochondrial proteins and apoptosis factors and improving pancreatic islet functions [23]. A randomized, placebo-controlled, double-blinded crossover study involving 20 consenting type 2 diabetic subjects, Asian ginseng supplementation was found to have significantly ($P < 0.05$) decreased homeostatic model assessment-insulin resistance (HOMA-IR) by 45%, compared to a 12% decrease in placebo subjects [24].

In-vivo, improved systemic insulin sensitivity and glucose homeostasis was observed utilizing Asian ginseng berry extract in *ob/ob* mice [3]; fasting blood glucose level was lowered and glucose tolerance was significantly improved in KK/Ay mice treated with Sanchi ginseng extract [25, 26]. Ginsenosides Re and Rb1 respectively, were claimed to be the effective constituents behind the pharmacological actions [3, 25]. In recent years, a number of similar studies have been done on diabetic mice or rats incorporating the use of ginsenoside Rh2 [27], ginsenoside Rg3 [28], malonyl ginsenosides [29], Korean red ginseng extract [30], heat-processed American ginseng [31], respectively, to examine potentials of ginseng as anti-hyperglycemic agents. It is noteworthy that the anti-diabetic properties of American ginseng appear to have no direct link to its antioxidant activity [32], suggesting an alternative mechanism of action that is currently unclear. This is in conflict with the findings that ginsenoside Rg3 prevents the progression of renal damage and dysfunction in type 2 diabetic rats by inhibiting oxidative stress and advanced glycation end (AGE) product formation [33] and that ginsenoside Re demonstrated significant antioxidant efficacy against the occurrence of oxidative stress in the eye and kidney in diabetic rats [34].

In-vitro, a handful of mechanistic studies using different target ginsenosides has been performed on 3T3-L1 pre-adipocytes cell model. For instance, ginsenosides compound K and Rg1 were found to enhance glucose uptake in 3T3-L1 adipocytes by up-regulating GLUT4 translocations via activating AMP-activated protein kinase (AMPK) and phosphatidylinositol 3-kinase (PI3K) signaling pathways [35]. Ginsenoside Rb1 as well, promoted GLUT1 and GLUT4 translocations to cell membrane via increasing phosphorylation of insulin receptor substrate-1 (IRS-1) and protein kinase B (PKB), subsequently stimulating PI3K activity [36]. Effects on ginsenosides Rg3 and Re on glucose transport system in mature 3T3-L1 cell were also evaluated. Similarly, glucose uptake and GLUT4 mRNA expression were significantly increased via PI3K pathways involving IRS-1 [37]. With IRS-1 activated by ginsenoside Re, strong suppression of c-Jun NH2-terminal kinase(JNK) and nuclear factor κ-B (NF-κB) then reduce insulin resistance in both 3T3-L1 adipocytes and high-fat diet (HFD) rats [38]. On another note, in rats-isolated pancreatic islets, ginseng extract was found to have significantly enhanced IRS-2 expression, which is the primary and predominate protein delivering insulin/insulin like growth factor (TGF-1) signaling in pancreatic β-cells, resulting in 67% increase in glucose-stimulated insulin secretion [39]. Korean red ginseng (KRG) extract too, stimulated insulin release, however in a glucose-independent manner [40].

In a study comparing insulin-sensitizing thiazolidinedione, rosglitazone to American ginseng extract in male Zucker diabetic fatty (ZDF) rats, while rosglitazone group demonstrated higher decrease in food intake and plasma triglyceride levels ($P < 0.05$), both groups have exhibited marked effects on the genes expression involved in PPAR actions and triglyceride metabolism when compared to controls [41]. When ginsenoside compound K, a major intestinal metabolite of PD type ginsenosides, is used together with metformin (a biguanide used for the treatment of diabetes) in *db/db* mice, the combination of 10 and 150 mg/kg respectively, effectively improved plasma glucose and insulin levels, suggesting synergistic effects [22]. Compound K, used as monotherapy agent, was administered to C57BL/ksJdb/db mice at 25 mg/kg once a day for 6 weeks. Results showed that plasma glucose was lowered by 20.7% and plasma insulin level was increased by 2.2 times, compared to control mice [42]. Altogether, these findings are encouraging as of now further detailed studies are warranted to elucidate the hypoglycemic and anti-diabetic properties of ginsenosides.

Ginsenosides and Obesity

Obesity leads to serious health consequences, posing worldwide health threat [43, 44], with more than 400 million obese and over 1.6 billion overweight adults estimated by WHO [45]. "Metabolically obese" phenotype, which is obese state with adipose tissue centralized in the abdominal area, has increased sharply, even among the lower BMI Asian populations [46]. From a metabolic point of view, abdominal fat tissue produces various adipokines such as TNF-α [47, 48], PAI [49], IL-6 and C-reactive protein [50] at a significantly higher magnitude than subcutaneous adipose tissue.

Therefore, on cellular level, changes in protein signals have garnered much interest among researchers to study the interaction with phytochemicals and anti-obesity mechanisms. One metabolic master protein of interest would be adenosine monophosphate-activated protein kinase (AMPK) that was previously reviewed to play a role in global rise in obesity and diabetes mellitus [51]. AMPK is a key player in regulating pathways that control both energy expenditure and energy intake [52] and the target for anti-diabetic drug metformin [53]. Ginsenoside Rg3 (40 μM) [54] and 20-40 μM of ginsenoside Rh2 [55] effectively activated AMPK expression in 3T3-L1 cells, consequently, adipocyte differentiation was attenuated. On another note, ginsenoside Rh2 at 0.01 to 1 μM was found to have induced adipogenesis via glucocorticoid receptor (GR) activation [56]. When adipocytes were cultured under high cholesterol conditions, ginsenoside Rb2 up-regulated sterol regulatory element binding protein (SREBP), leptin, fatty acid synthase (FAS), glyceraldehyde-3-phosphate dehydrogenase (GPDH) mRNA expressions, and the overall cholesterol and triacylglycerol levels was lowered, suggesting valuable lipid-lowering effects comparable to lovastatin [57]. Peroxisome proliferator-activated receptor (PPARγ), one essential transcription factor well-studied in adipogenesis, was found to be enhanced by PT group ginsenosides [58] and ginsenoside Rb1 [59]; was however inhibited by ginsenoside Rg3 [54]. Inconsistency could be due to structural complexity of steroidal saponins that differ from one another, making specific determinants a challenging task. Glucose-uptake and insulin-sensitizing effects observed in adipocytes thus far were nevertheless in congruence across the reports [35, 58-61].

In recent years, ginsenosides derived from various parts of the plants and species have been utilized in anti-obesity studies in animal models. For example, total chikusetsusaponins, derived from rhizomes of Japanese ginseng were deduced to display anti-obesity effects by inhibiting pancreatic lipase activity and by preventing the increase in body weight and parametrial adipose tissue weight induced by high-fat diet in mice [58]. Pancreatic lipase is a key enzyme for dietary triglycerides digestion, a prerequisite for fat digestion and energy intake; therefore, natural inhibitors of pancreatic lipase are desired players in fighting obesity [62]. Ginsenosides derived from Asian ginseng root [63] as well as ginsenosides isolated from the leaves of American ginseng, particularly PD type ginsenosides, were found effective in inhibiting pancreatic lipase activity dose-dependently [64]. Likewise, PD-type saponins rather than the PT-type were reported to be the major contributing components, inhibiting energy gain, normalizing hypothalamic neuropeptides and serum biochemicals related to weight gain [65].

In *ob/ob* mice, concurrent with decrease in fasting blood glucose levels, American ginseng berry juice also significantly ($P<0.05$) reduced body weight after 10 days of administration [66]. Noteworthy, a comparison study in *ob/ob* mice, pointed out that American ginseng berry extract only showed profound anti-obesity effect when administered intraperitoneally but not orally [67]. This suggested that route of entry and bioavailabilities have to be taken into careful considerations for accurate determination of activity. Other studies suggesting intensified anti-obesity effects have been demonstrated on wild ginseng extract [68], crude saponins of Korean Red Ginseng [69], Korean white ginseng extract [70], saponins from steams and leaves of American ginseng [71], and vinegar-processed form of ginsenosides from Asian ginseng [72] in *ob/ob* mice.

Our research group has recently presented baseline reports with ginsenosides derived from American ginseng [73] and Asian ginseng [74] respectively on 3T3-L1 cell line. Dose-dependent cytotoxic effects were observed in both extracts on 3T3-L1 preadipocytes. American ginseng extract had a LC50 value of 40.3 ± 5 μgmL^{-1} while LC50 for Asian ginseng extract was 18.2 ± 5 μgmL^{-1}. Modest changes were found in cell cycle analysis. Upon the induction of adipogenesis, western blot analysis showed significantly up-regulated adiponectin expression in both extracts. However, different effective concentrations were noted, 20.2 μgmL^{-1} was needed for American ginseng while 10 μgmL^{-1} was sufficient for significant changes with Asian ginseng. Adiponectin functions as insulin sensitizer [75-78] and hypoadiponectinemia in human subjects have been exhibited in a wide range of metabolic diseases, including diabetes mellitus, hypertension, coronary artery disease, lipodystrophy, non-alcoholic hepatic steatosis, and obesity [79]. Anti-obesity effects of ginsenosides, whether in a cocktail or as individual ginsenosides, require future mechanistic studies to provide additional evidence with regards to interactions between ginsenosides and adipokines signaling.

REFERENCES

[1] Yun, T. K. Brief introduction of Panax ginseng C.A. Meyer. *Journal of Korean Medical Science* (2001), *16 Suppl*, S3-S5.

[2] Attele, A. S.; Wu, J. A.; Yuan, C. S. Ginseng pharmacology: multiple constituents and multiple actions. *Biochemical Pharmacology* (1999), *58*, 1685-1693.

[3. Attele, A. S.; Zhou, Y. P.; Xie, J. T.; Wu, J. A.; Zhang, L.; Dey, L.; Pugh, W.; Rue, P. A.; Polonsky, K. S.; Yuan, C. S. Antidiabetic effects of Panax ginseng berry extract and the identification of an effective component. *Diabetes* (2002), *51*, 1851-1858.

[4] Popovich, D. G.; Kitts, D. D. Structure-function relationship exists for ginsenosides in reducing cell proliferation and inducing apoptosis in the human leukemia (THP-1) cell line. *Archives of Biochemistry and Biophysics* (2002), *406*, 1-8.

[5] Gillis, C. N. Panax ginseng pharmacology: A nitric oxide link? *Biochemical Pharmacology* (1997), *54*, 1-8.

[6] Qi, L. W.; Wang, C. Z.; Yuan, C. S. American ginseng: potential structure-function relationship in cancer chemoprevention. *Biochemical Pharmacology* (2010), *80*, 947-954.

[7] Shin, H. R.; Kim, J. Y.; Yun, T. K.; Morgan, G.; Vainio, H. The cancer-preventive potential of Panax ginseng: a review of human and experimental evidence. *Cancer Causes & Control: CCC* (2000), *11*, 565-576.

[8] Shibata, S. Chemistry and cancer preventing activities of ginseng saponins and some related triterpenoid compounds. *Journal of Korean Medical Science* (2001), *16 Suppl*, S28-S37.

[9] Xie, J. T.; Wang, C. Z.; Zhang, B.; Mehendale, S. R.; Li, X. L.; Sun, S.; Han, A. H.; Du, W.; He, T. C.; Yuan, C. S. In vitro and in vivo anticancer effects of american ginseng berry: exploring representative compounds. *Biological & Pharmaceutical Bulletin* (2009), *32*, 1552-1558.

[10] Park, J. S.; Park, E. M.; Kim, D. H.; Jung, K.; Jung, J. S.; Lee, E. J.; Hyun, J. W.; Kang, J. L.; Kim, H. S. Anti-inflammatory mechanism of ginseng saponins in activated microglia. *Journal of Neuroimmunology* (2009), *209*, 40-49.

[11] Yim, H. W.; Jong, H. S.; Kim, T. Y.; Choi, H. H.; Kim, S. G.; Song, S. H.; Kim, J.; Ko, S. G.; Lee, J. W.; Kim, T. Y.; Bang, Y. J. Cyclooxygenase-2 inhibits novel ginseng metabolite-mediated apoptosis. *Cancer Research* (2005), *65*, 1952-1960.

[12] Lee, J. S.; Choi, H. S.; Kang, S. W.; Chung, J. H.; Park, H. K.; Ban, J. Y.; Kwon, O. Y.; Hong, H. P.; Ko, Y. G. Therapeutic effect of Korean red ginseng on inflammatory cytokines in rats with focal cerebral ischemia/reperfusion injury. *The American Journal of Chinese Medicine* (2011), *39*, 83-94.

[13] Guo, J.; Gan, X. T.; Haist, J. V.; Rajapurohitam, V.; Zeidan, A.; Faruq, N. S.; Karmazyn, M. Ginseng inhibits cardiomyocyte hypertrophy and heart failure via NHE-1 inhibition and attenuation of calcineurin activation. *Circulation Heart Failure* (2011), *4*, 79-88.

[14] Zhou, H.; Hou, S. Z.; Luo, P.; Zeng, B.; Wang, J. R.; Wong, Y. F.; Jiang, Z. H.; Liu, L. Ginseng protects rodent hearts from acute myocardial ischemia-reperfusion injury through GR/ER-activated RISK pathway in an endothelial NOS-dependent mechanism. *Journal of Ethnopharmacology* (2011), *135*, 287-298.

[15] Xu, C.; Teng, J.; Chen, W.; Ge, Q.; Yang, Z.; Yu, C.; Yang, Z.; Jia, W. 20(S)-protopanaxadiol, an active ginseng metabolite, exhibits strong antidepressant-like effects in animal tests. *Progress in Neuro-Psychopharmacology & Biological Psychiatry* (2010), *34*, 1402-1411.

[16] Chuang, C. M.; Hsieh, C. L.; Lin, H. Y.; Lin, J. G. Panax Notoginseng Burk attenuates impairment of learning and memory functions and increases ED1, BDNF and beta-secretase immunoreactive cells in chronic stage ischemia-reperfusion injured rats. *The American Journal of Chinese Medicine* (2008), *36*, 685-693.

[17] Nishijo, H.; Uwano, T.; Zhong, Y. M.; Ono, T. Proof of the mysterious efficacy of ginseng: basic and clinical trials: effects of red ginseng on learning and memory deficits in an animal model of amnesia. *Journal of Pharmalogical Sciences* (2004), *95*, 145-152.

[18] Kassi, E.; Pervanidou, P.; Kaltsas, G.; Chrousos, G. Metabolic syndrome: definitions and controversies. *BMC Medicine* (2011), *9*, 48.

[19] Bruce, K. D.; Cagampang, F. R. Epigenetic priming of the metabolic syndrome. *Toxicology Mechanisms and Methods* (2011), *21*, 353-361.

[20] Simmons, R. K.; Alberti, K. G.; Gale, E. A.; Colagiuri, S.; Tuomilehto, J.; Qiao, Q.; Ramachandran, A.; Tajima, N.; Brajkovich, M., I; Ben-Nakhi, A.; Reaven, G.; Hama, S. B.; Mendis, S.; Roglic, G. The metabolic syndrome: useful concept or clinical tool? Report of a WHO Expert Consultation. *Diabetologia* (2010), *53*, 600-605.

[21] Xie, W.; Zhao, Y.; Zhang, Y. Traditional chinese medicines in treatment of patients with type 2 diabetes mellitus. *Evidence-Based Complementary and Alternative Medicine: ECAM* (2011), *2011*, 726723.

[22] Yoon, S. H.; Han, E. J.; Sung, J. H.; Chung, S. H. Anti-diabetic effects of compound K versus metformin versus compound K-metformin combination therapy in diabetic db/db mice. *Biological & Pharmaceutical Bulletin* (2007), *30*, 2196-2200.

[23] Wu, Z.; Luo, J. Z.; Luo, L. American ginseng modulates pancreatic beta cell activities. *Chinese Medicine* (2007), *2*, 11.

[24] Ma, S. W.; Benzie, I. F.; Chu, T. T.; Fok, B. S.; Tomlinson, B.; Critchley, L. A. Effect of Panax ginseng supplementation on biomarkers of glucose tolerance, antioxidant status and oxidative stress in type 2 diabetic subjects: results of a placebo-controlled human intervention trial. *Diabetes, Obesity & Metabolism* (2008), *10*, 1125-1127.

[25] Yang, C. Y.; Wang, J.; Zhao, Y.; Shen, L.; Jiang, X.; Xie, Z. G.; Liang, N.; Zhang, L.; Chen, Z. H. Anti-diabetic effects of Panax notoginseng saponins and its major anti-hyperglycemic components. *Journal of Ethnopharmacology* (2010), *130*, 231-236.

[26] Chen, Z. H.; Li, J.; Liu, J.; Zhao, Y.; Zhang, P.; Zhang, M. X.; Zhang, L. Saponins isolated from the root of Panax notoginseng showed significant anti-diabetic effects in KK-Ay mice. *The American Journal of Chinese Medicine* (2008), *36*, 939-951.

[27] Lee, W. K.; Kao, S. T.; Liu, I. M.; Cheng, J. T. Ginsenoside Rh2 is one of the active principles of Panax ginseng root to improve insulin sensitivity in fructose-rich chow-fed rats. *Hormone and Metabolic Research* (2007), *39*, 347-354.

[28] Kang, K. S.; Yamabe, N.; Kim, H. Y.; Park, J. H.; Yokozawa, T. Therapeutic potential of 20(S)-ginsenoside Rg(3) against streptozotocin-induced diabetic renal damage in rats. *European Journal of Pharmacology* (2008), *591*, 266-272.

[29] Liu, Z.; Wang, L. J.; Li, X.; Hu, J. N.; Chen, Y.; Ruan, C. C.; Sun, G. Z. Hypoglycemic effects of malonyl-ginsenosides extracted from roots of Panax ginseng on streptozotocin-induced diabetic mice. *Phytotherapy Research* (2009), *23*, 1426-1430.

[30] Lee, H. J.; Lee, Y. H.; Park, S. K.; Kang, E. S.; Kim, H. J.; Lee, Y. C.; Choi, C. S.; Park, S. E.; Ahn, C. W.; Cha, B. S.; Lee, K. W.; Kim, K. S.; Lim, S. K.; Lee, H. C. Korean red ginseng (Panax ginseng) improves insulin sensitivity and attenuates the development of diabetes in Otsuka Long-Evans Tokushima fatty rats. *Metabolism: Clinical and Experimental* (2009), *58*, 1170-1177.

[31] Kim, H. Y.; Kang, K. S.; Yamabe, N.; Nagai, R.; Yokozawa, T. Protective effect of heat-processed American ginseng against diabetic renal damage in rats. *Journal of Agricultural and Food Chemistry* (2007), *55*, 8491-8497.

[32] Xie, J. T.; Wang, C. Z.; Li, X. L.; Ni, M.; Fishbein, A.; Yuan, C. S. Anti-diabetic effect of American ginseng may not be linked to antioxidant activity: comparison between American ginseng and Scutellaria baicalensis using an ob/ob mice model. *Fitoterapia* (2009), *80*, 306-311.

[33] Kang, K. S.; Yamabe, N.; Kim, H. Y.; Park, J. H.; Yokozawa, T. Effects of heat-processed ginseng and its active component ginsenoside 20(S)-Rg3 on the progression of renal damage and dysfunction in type 2 diabetic Otsuka Long-Evans Tokushima Fatty rats. *Biological & Pharmaceutical Bulletin* (2010), *33*, 1077-1081.

[34] Cho, W. C.; Chung, W. S.; Lee, S. K.; Leung, A. W.; Cheng, C. H.; Yue, K. K. Ginsenoside Re of Panax ginseng possesses significant antioxidant and

antihyperlipidemic efficacies in streptozotocin-induced diabetic rats. *European Journal of Pharmacology* (2006), *550*, 173-179.

[35] Huang, Y. C.; Lin, C. Y.; Huang, S. F.; Lin, H. C.; Chang, W. L.; Chang, T. C. Effect and Mechanism of Ginsenosides CK and Rg1 on Stimulation of Glucose Uptake in 3T3-L1 Adipocytes. *Journal of Agricultural and Food Chemistry* (2010).

[36] Shang, W.; Yang, Y.; Zhou, L.; Jiang, B.; Jin, H.; Chen, M. Ginsenoside Rb1 stimulates glucose uptake through insulin like signaling pathway in 3T3-L1 adipocytes. *The Journal of Endocrinology* (2008), *198*, 561-569.

[37] Lee, O. H.; Lee, H. H.; Kim, J. H.; Lee, B. Y. Effect of ginsenosides Rg3 and Re on glucose transport in mature 3T3-L1 adipocytes. *Phytotherapy Research* (2011), *25*, 768-773.

[38] Zhang, Z.; Li, X.; Lv, W.; Yang, Y.; Gao, H.; Yang, J.; Shen, Y.; Ning, G. Ginsenoside Re reduces insulin resistance through inhibition of c-Jun NH2-terminal kinase and nuclear factor-kappaB. *Molecular Endocrinology* (2008), *22*, 186-195.

[39] Park, S. M.; Hong, S. M.; Sung, S. R.; Lee, J. E.; Kwon, D. Y. Extracts of Rehmanniae radix, Ginseng radix and Scutellariae radix improve glucose-stimulated insulin secretion and beta-cell proliferation through IRS2 induction. *Genes & Nutrition* (2008), *2*, 347-351.

[40] Kim, K.; Kim, H. Y. Korean red ginseng stimulates insulin release from isolated rat pancreatic islets. *Journal of Ethnopharmacology* (2008), *120*, 190-195.

[41] Banz, W. J.; Iqbal, M. J.; Bollaert, M.; Chickris, N.; James, B.; Higginbotham, D. A.; Peterson, R.; Murphy, L. Ginseng modifies the diabetic phenotype and genes associated with diabetes in the male ZDF rat. *Phytomedicine: International Journal of Phytotherapy and Phytopharmacology* (2007), *14*, 681-689.

[42] Yuan, H. D.; Kim, S. J.; Chung, S. H. Beneficial effects of IH-901 on glucose and lipid metabolisms via activating adenosine monophosphate-activated protein kinase and phosphatidylinositol-3 kinase pathways. *Metabolism: Clinical and Experimental* (2011), *60*, 43-51.

[43] Flegal, K. M.; Carroll, M. D.; Ogden, C. L.; Curtin, L. R. Prevalence and trends in obesity among US adults, 1999-2008. *JAMA: the Journal of the American Medical Association* (2010), *303*, 235-241.

[44] Low, S.; Chin, M. C.; urenberg-Yap, M. Review on epidemic of obesity. *Annals of the Academy of Medicine, Singapore* (2009), *38*, 57-59.

[45] Drew, B. S.; Dixon, A. F.; Dixon, J. B. Obesity management: update on orlistat. *Vascular Health and Risk Management* (2007), *3*, 817-821.

[46] Chan, J. C.; Malik, V.; Jia, W.; Kadowaki, T.; Yajnik, C. S.; Yoon, K. H.; Hu, F. B. Diabetes in Asia: epidemiology, risk factors, and pathophysiology. *JAMA: the Journal of the American Medical Association* (2009), *301*, 2129-2140.

[47] van, H., V; Dicker, A.; Ryden, M.; Hauner, H.; Lonnqvist, F.; Naslund, E.; Arner, P. Increased lipolysis and decreased leptin production by human omental as compared with subcutaneous preadipocytes. *Diabetes* (2002), *51*, 2029-2036.

[48] Bertin, E.; Nguyen, P.; Guenounou, M.; Durlach, V.; Potron, G.; Leutenegger, M. Plasma levels of tumor necrosis factor-alpha (TNF-alpha) are essentially dependent on visceral fat amount in type 2 diabetic patients. *Diabetes & Metabolism* (2000), *26*, 178-182.

[49] Alessi, M. C.; Peiretti, F.; Morange, P.; Henry, M.; Nalbone, G.; Juhan-Vague, I. Production of plasminogen activator inhibitor 1 by human adipose tissue: possible link between visceral fat accumulation and vascular disease. *Diabetes* (1997), *46*, 860-867.

[50] You, T.; Nicklas, B. J.; Ding, J.; Penninx, B. W.; Goodpaster, B. H.; Bauer, D. C.; Tylavsky, F. A.; Harris, T. B.; Kritchevsky, S. B. The metabolic syndrome is associated with circulating adipokines in older adults across a wide range of adiposity. *The Journals of Gerontology. Series A, Biological Sciences and Medical Sciences* (2008), *63*, 414-419.

[51] Hardie, D. G.; Hawley, S. A.; Scott, J. W. AMP-activated protein kinase--development of the energy sensor concept. *The Journal of Physiology* (2006), *574*, 7-15.

[52] Carling, D. AMP-activated protein kinase: balancing the scales. *Biochimie* (2005), *87*, 87-91.

[53] Towler, M. C.; Hardie, D. G. AMP-activated protein kinase in metabolic control and insulin signaling. *Circulation Research* (2007), *100*, 328-341.

[54] Hwang, J. T.; Lee, M. S.; Kim, H. J.; Sung, M. J.; Kim, H. Y.; Kim, M. S.; Kwon, D. Y. Antiobesity effect of ginsenoside Rg3 involves the AMPK and PPAR-gamma signal pathways. *Phytotherapy Research* (2009), *23*, 262-266.

[55] Hwang, J. T.; Kim, S. H.; Lee, M. S.; Kim, S. H.; Yang, H. J.; Kim, M. J.; Kim, H. S.; Ha, J.; Kim, M. S.; Kwon, D. Y. Anti-obesity effects of ginsenoside Rh2 are associated with the activation of AMPK signaling pathway in 3T3-L1 adipocyte. *Biochemical and Biophysical Research Communications* (2007), *364*, 1002-1008.

[56] Niu, C. S.; Yeh, C. H.; Yeh, M. F.; Cheng, J. T. Increase of adipogenesis by ginsenoside (Rh2) in 3T3-L1 cell via an activation of glucocorticoid receptor. *Hormone and Metabolic Research* (2009), *41*, 271-276.

[57] Kim, E. J.; Lee, H. I.; Chung, K. J.; Noh, Y. H.; Ro, Y.; Koo, J. H. The ginsenoside-Rb2 lowers cholesterol and triacylglycerol levels in 3T3-L1 adipocytes cultured under high cholesterol or fatty acids conditions. *BMB Reports* (2009), *42*, 194-199.

[58] Han, K. L.; Jung, M. H.; Sohn, J. H.; Hwang, J. K. Ginsenoside 20S-protopanaxatriol (PPT) activates peroxisome proliferator-activated receptor gamma (PPARgamma) in 3T3-L1 adipocytes. *Biological & Pharmaceutical Bulletin* (2006), *29*, 110-113.

[59] Shang, W.; Yang, Y.; Jiang, B.; Jin, H.; Zhou, L.; Liu, S.; Chen, M. Ginsenoside Rb1 promotes adipogenesis in 3T3-L1 cells by enhancing PPARgamma2 and C/EBPalpha gene expression. *Life Sciences* (2007), *80*, 618-625.

[60] Kim, J. J.; Xiao, H.; Tan, Y.; Wang, Z. Z.; Paul, S. J.; Qu, X. The effects and mechanism of saponins of Panax notoginseng on glucose metabolism in 3T3-L1 cells. *The American Journal of Chinese Medicine* (2009), *37*, 1179-1189.

[61] Park, S.; Ahn, I. S.; Kwon, D. Y.; Ko, B. S.; Jun, W. K. Ginsenosides Rb1 and Rg1 suppress triglyceride accumulation in 3T3-L1 adipocytes and enhance beta-cell insulin secretion and viability in Min6 cells via PKA-dependent pathways. *Bioscience, Biotechnology, and Biochemistry* (2008), *72*, 2815-2823.

[62] de la Garza, A. L.; Milagro, F. I.; Boque, N.; Campion, J.; Martinez, J. A. Natural inhibitors of pancreatic lipase as new players in obesity treatment. *Planta Medica* (2011), *77*, 773-785.

[63] Karu, N.; Reifen, R.; Kerem, Z. Weight gain reduction in mice fed Panax ginseng saponin, a pancreatic lipase inhibitor. *Journal of Agricultural and Food Chemistry* (2007), *55*, 2824-2828.

[64] Liu, R.; Zhang, J.; Liu, W.; Kimura, Y.; Zheng, Y. Anti-Obesity effects of protopanaxdiol types of Ginsenosides isolated from the leaves of American ginseng (Panax quinquefolius L.) in mice fed with a high-fat diet. *Fitoterapia* (2010).

[65] Kim, J. H.; Kang, S. A.; Han, S. M.; Shim, I. Comparison of the antiobesity effects of the protopanaxadiol- and protopanaxatriol-type saponins of red ginseng. *Phytotherapy Research* (2009), *23*, 78-85.

[66] Xie, J. T.; Wang, C. Z.; Ni, M.; Wu, J. A.; Mehendale, S. R.; Aung, H. H.; Foo, A.; Yuan, C. S. American ginseng berry juice intake reduces blood glucose and body weight in ob/ob mice. *Journal of Food Science* (2007), *72*, S590-S594.

[67] Dey, L.; Zhang, L.; Yuan, C. S. Anti-diabetic and anti-obese effects of ginseng berry extract: comparison between intraperitoneal and oral administrations. *The American Journal of Chinese Medicine* (2002), *30*, 645-647.

[68] Mollah, M. L.; Kim, G. S.; Moon, H. K.; Chung, S. K.; Cheon, Y. P.; Kim, J. K.; Kim, K. S. Antiobesity effects of wild ginseng (Panax ginseng C.A. Meyer) mediated by PPAR-gamma, GLUT4 and LPL in ob/ob mice. *Phytotherapy Research* (2009), *23*, 220-225.

[69] Kim, J. H.; Hahm, D. H.; Yang, D. C.; Kim, J. H.; Lee, H. J.; Shim, I. Effect of crude saponin of Korean red ginseng on high-fat diet-induced obesity in the rat. *Journal of Pharmacological Sciences* (2005), *97*, 124-131.

[70] Lee, Y. S.; Cha, B. Y.; Yamaguchi, K.; Choi, S. S.; Yonezawa, T.; Teruya, T.; Nagai, K.; Woo, J. T. Effects of Korean white ginseng extracts on obesity in high-fat diet-induced obese mice. *Cytotechnology* (2010).

[71] Liu, W.; Zheng, Y.; Han, L.; Wang, H.; Saito, M.; Ling, M.; Kimura, Y.; Feng, Y. Saponins (Ginsenosides) from stems and leaves of Panax quinquefolium prevented high-fat diet-induced obesity in mice. *Phytomedicine: International Journal of Phytotherapy and Phytopharmacology* (2008), *15*, 1140-1145.

[72] Yun, S. N.; Ko, S. K.; Lee, K. H.; Chung, S. H. Vinegar-processed ginseng radix improves metabolic syndrome induced by a high fat diet in ICR mice. *Archives of Pharmacal Research* (2007), *30*, 587-595.

[73] Yeo, C. R.; Lee, S. M.; Popovich, D. G. Ginseng (*Panax quinquefolius*) Reduces Cell Growth, Lipid Acquisition and Increases Adiponectin Expression in 3T3-L1 Cells. *Evidence-Based Complementary and Alternative Medicine* (2010), *doi:10.1093/ecam/neq051*.

[74] Yeo, C. R.; Yang, C.; Wong, T. Y.; Popovich, D. G. A quantified ginseng (Panax ginseng C.A. Meyer) extract influences lipid acquisition and increases adiponectin expression in 3T3-L1 cells. *Molecules.* (2011), *16*, 477-492.

[75] Gil-Campos, M.; Canete, R. R.; Gil, A. Adiponectin, the missing link in insulin resistance and obesity. *Clinical Nutrition* (2004), *23*, 963-974.

[76] Whitehead, J. P.; Richards, A. A.; Hickman, I. J.; Macdonald, G. A.; Prins, J. B. Adiponectin--a key adipokine in the metabolic syndrome. *Diabetes, Obesity & Metabolism* (2006), *8*, 264-280.

[77] Whitehead, J. P.; Richards, A. A.; Hickman, I. J.; Macdonald, G. A.; Prins, J. B.; Weyer, C.; Funahashi, T.; Tanaka, S.; Hotta, K.; Matsuzawa, Y.; Pratley, R. E.; Tataranni, P. A. Adiponectin--a key adipokine in the metabolic syndrome Hypoadiponectinemia in obesity and type 2 diabetes: close association with insulin resistance and hyperinsulinemia. *Diabetes, Obesity & Metabolism* (2006), *8*, 264-280.

[78] Dridi, S.; Taouis, M. Adiponectin and energy homeostasis: consensus and controversy. *The Journal of Nutritional Biochemistry* (2009), *20*, 831-839.

[79] Deng, Y.; Scherer, P. E. Adipokines as novel biomarkers and regulators of the metabolic syndrome. *Annals of the New York Academy of Sciences* (2010), *1212*, E1-E19.

In: Saponins: Properties, Applications and Health Benefits ISBN: 978-1-62100-942-9
Editors: Rani Koh and Isaac Tay

Chapter 5

SAPONIN USE AS ANTIMICROBIAL IN FIBROUS AND CONSUMER PRODUCTS

Vivechana Dixit and S. Kay Obendorf
Fiber Science, Cornell University, Ithaca, NY, US

ABSTRACT

Natural antimicrobials recently have been used to replace synthesized compounds in materials and consumer products offering the opportunity to reduce hazardous effects on health and environment. Research results show that saponin, a natural bio-degradable and non-toxic biopolysaccharide derived from plants, has potential to be used as a natural antimicrobial compound. Saponin has exhibited high antimicrobial activity against a wide variety of pathogenic and microorganisms, including fungi and bacteria. The antimicrobial action is influenced by intrinsic factors such as the type of saponin, the degree of saponin polymerization and extrinsic factors such as the microbial organism, the environmental conditions and presence of the other components. In this article we described properties, a number of applications and health related benefits of saponin when used as biodegradable antimicrobials in fibrous materials and consumer products. Chemical and biochemical antimicrobial saponins derived from natural sources and activities against a range of microorganisms are also outlined.

1. INTRODUCTION

Natural products have proven to be rich sources of compounds with surfactant properties. Saponins are natural surfactants produced by the soapwort plant, *Quillaja saponaria* (Sparg et al. 2004, Magota et al. 1991). They are a major family of secondary metabolites that have strong biologic activities, such as growth-promoting, antimicrobial, and insecticidal effects (Avato et al. 2006, De Lucca et al. 2006, Yang et al. 2006, Barile et al. 2007). Because of their well-known functional activities, they have been used as surfactants (Roy et al. 1997, Andreuccetti et al. 2010), anti-inflammatory and anti-arthritic agents (Cheeke et al. 2006), fungicides (Zhang et al. 2005), insecticides (San Martín and Briones 1999), anticancer agents

(Lacaille-Dubois 2005, Raghupathi et al. 2011), cosmetics (Murakami 1986), food preservatives (San Martín and Briones 1999), and wound healing (Kanzaki et al. 1998). Some types of saponins are biocompatible, nontoxic, and biofunctional, thus they can be used as a food additives. Saponin also has been documented for use as films or coating as lysing agent (Umlas and Fallon 1971, Gleeson 1997).

Increased use of antibacterial and antifungal agents has resulted in the development of natural antimicrobial materials. Saponin coating improves antifungal properties of textile surfaces making them safe against different types of fungi (Dixit et al. 2010). Research has shown that the antifungal activity of saponins is associated with their individual aglycone moieties as well as the number and structure of monosaccharide units in the sugar chains. The sugar chain in each saponin plays a key role in its antifungal activity by forming complexes with cell membrane sterols (De Lucca et al. 2006, Yang et al. 2006). In this chapter, we summarized properties and application of saponins as antimicrobial agents in fibrous and consumer products.

2. General Properties

Saponins are high molecular weight glycosides. Based upon structure, saponins can be divided into two main classes: triterpenoid and steroid saponins. Both are derived from the 30 carbon atoms containing precursor oxidosqualene. The steroid saponins have three methyl groups removed, *i.e.* they are molecules with 27 C-atoms, whereas in the triterpenoid saponins all 30 C-atoms are retained. With a single sugar chain, saponins are known as monodesmosidic saponins, while with two sugar chains they are known as bidesmosidic saponins. In monodesmosidic saponins, the sugar chain is typically attached by a glycosidic ether linkage at the C-3 of the aglycone. In addition to the C-3 linked sugar chain, bidesmosidic saponins have a second sugar chain bound at C-28 (triterpene saponins) or at C-26 (steroid saponins) by an ester linkage (Sun et al. 2009). Saponins are non-ionic biosurfactants with some acidic and ionizable functional groups. Therefore, they exhibit different solubility properties compared to synthetic non-ionic surfactants and anionic rhamnoplid biosurfactants (Zhou et al. 2011).

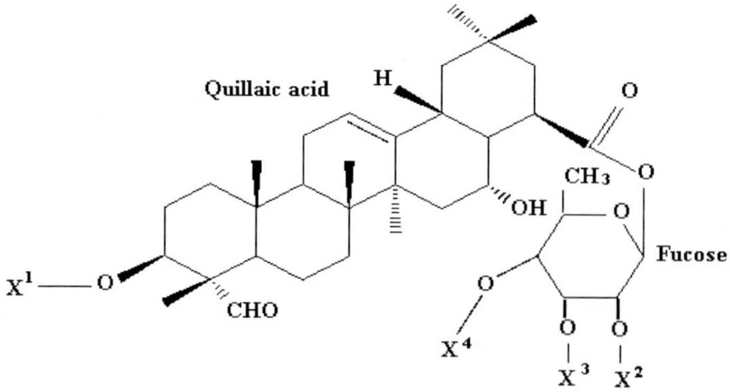

Recchiae et al. 1995.

Figure 1. Common chemical structure of *Quillaja* saponin.

Quillaja saponin is a bidesmosidic saponin. It is a mixture of approximately 20 structurally related triterpenoid glycosides with minimal differences between them (Higuchi and Komori 1987, De Lucca et al. 2006). Figure 1 shows the general chemical structure of *Quillaja* saponin, where X^1 at C-3 is a disaccharide or trisaccharide and C-28 is an oligosaccharide with X^2-, X^3-, and X^4- substituted fucose (Bankefors et al. 2008). Important structural features that distinguish *Q. saponaria* saponins from those of other plant species are the presence of a fatty acid domain and a triterpene aldehyde group at position C-4 (San Martín and Briones 1999).

3. Antifungal Activity

Saponins exhibit a wide range of biological activities. A number of researchers have focused on the antifungal action modes of saponins as reviewed by Morrissey and Osbourn (1999). The major advantage of using saponins as an antifungal agent is that they are plant derived natural product that are biodegradable and biocompatible. Keukens et al. (1995) developed a model for sterol-mediated glycoalkaloid induced membrane disruption. According to their results, the sugar chain in each saponin is necessary and plays a key role for its antifungal activity. The formation of stable saponin-sterol complexes may be mediated by interactions between the sugar residues of the saponin molecules. The sugar chain attached to C-3 is usually critical for both the membrane-permeabilizing and antifungal properties of saponins. The removal of these sugar residues often results in loss of biological activity (De Lucca et al. 2006, Yang et al. 2006, Keukans et al. 1995, Morrissey and Osbourn 1999, Fujita and Kubo 2005). Other important parameters affecting antifungal activity of saponins are molecular weight, concentration of saponins, and type of challenge microorganism.

In summary, two major suggested antimicrobial mechanisms are: 1) membrane insertion of the saponins and binding to sterols and 2) formation of a stable irreversible glycoalkoid/sterol complexes and loss of membrane integrity.

4. Applications

The possibilities of developing saponin as a natural antimicrobial have increased over time. Saponins are applied to extend the storage life of different categories of food materials such as rice and beans, pickled vegetables, processed fish meat, and fermented seasonings. Miyakoshi et al. (2000) showed that saponin can be used as anti-deteriorating agents in food. Matsuura (2001) suggested the application of saponin as a cholesterol-lowering agent. Saponin micelles form insoluble aggregates with cholesterol that can be removed by filtration. Tiwari et al. (2008) demonstrated the use of saponin as a contraceptive. San Martin and Briones (1999) and Güçlü-Ustündağ and Mazza (2007) reported different industrial uses and properties of saponins. For example, saponins can be uses as foaming agent and emulsifier in food and beverages, additives for animal feed, wetting agents in agriculture, biopesticides, and seed germination and plant growth stimulants. For cosmetics application, saponins are used in shampoos, hair tonic, and hand creams.

Fungi can be harmful pathogenic agents, and saponins have been used for decades as effective fungicides (Barlie et al. 2007, Sautour et al. 2005). Materials used in filtration can be treated to improve the surface activity against fungal growth or biofouling. Antifungal agents need to be effective against a broad spectrum of fungal species; support high hygiene standards; have low toxicity to humans, durability, and no negative effect on the substrate; and be cost effective and environment friendly (Gao and Cranston 2008). This can be accomplished by using an eco-friendly approach such as using plant derived natural antimicrobial products as an additive for functional modification of coating or finishing agents on fabric surfaces or for inclusion in manufactured fibers. Chitosan and triclosan have been used as antimicrobial agents (Lim and Hudson 2004, Kim et al. 1998, Park et al. 1986, Kalyon and Olgun 2001). Similarly, alternative materials can be explored using saponin as the antifungal coating. Due to the advanced coating technology and ability to produce designed materials for implants, adhesives, coatings, packaging, and drug delivery systems, use of natural antifungal agents is an important innovation for numerous applications.

Saponins utilization as a modifier in film formation has been reported by Umlas and Fallon (1971), Gleeson (1997), and Andreuccett et al. (2010). Gleeson (1997) used saponin as a lysing agent for preparation of thick film. They showed that the modified saponin allows clearer identification of gametocytes without affecting parasite morphology. Amphiphilic surfactant molecules soluble in water can bind to protein molecules by electrostatic interactions in the case of ionic surfactants, and also by hydrophobic interactions (Pugnaloni et al. 2004). A similar approach was used by Andreuccett et al. (2010) to incorporate saponin as an emulsifier in the production of biodegradable film. They suggested that incorporation of hydrophobic plasticizer-acetyltriethyl citrate and reduction in film drying time were possible due the use of yucca (saponin) in the formulation. In the case of yucca, non-ionic saponin containing sugars, hydrophobic interactions with the protein and the hydrophobic plasticizer and associations via hydrogen bonds with polar groups of the protein may be favored. The same kind of interaction was observed for films containing amphiphilic surfactants and modified starches or hydroxypropyl methyl cellulose (Villalobos et al. 2006, Chen et al. 2009).

Saponin adhesion on or within fibers could be extremely attractive for development of materials to improve the indoor air quality. As the external uses of saponins, *e.g.* washing soap, have had no toxic effects on human skin and eyes (Roy et al. 1997), use in consumer or household products are possible. Saponin/cellulose nanocomposites could be a valid option for such purposes because of the large nanofiber /polymer interface area that ensures high reactivity and the formation of a microporous membrane. Therefore, these nanofibrous materials are prime candidates for many applications such as reinforced nanocomposites, tissue engineering scaffolds, cosmetics, biosensor/chemosensors, drug delivery, protective clothing, and filtration media. A large number of synthesis and fabrication methods for producing these nanofibers have already been reported (Doshi and Reneker 1995, Rambo et al. 2008). In particular, electrospinning has been the subject of much attention over the past decade. Cellulose, a sustainable organic substance and a primary structural component of the cell walls of plants, is important as a renewable resource and biodegradable polymeric material. Cellulose whiskers and fibrils have great potential for use as reinforcement in nanocomposites. Cellulose based nanofibrous materials are used in a broad range of applications due to good thermal stability, chemical resistance, and abundance (Siro and Plackett 2010).

Recent work has been reported on the study and development of saponin/cellulose based nanofibrous materials with antifungal properties (Dixit et al. 2010). Use of *Quillaja* saponin was explored as an antifungal agent in the form of an additive with cellulose acetate to fabricate antifungal nanofibrous membrane. We used an approach to design surfaces that inhibit growth and proliferation of fungal cells. Antifungal agents can be incorporated within and on the surfaces of nanofibrous material and the presence and/or release of the antimicrobial agent in the material can reduce the number of live cells on or near a surface. In our study, we developed a materials-based approach to inhibit fungal growth by incorporating saponin as an additive in a cellulose acetate nanofibrous membrane. However, the poor solubility of cellulose acetate in common solvents and low melting temperature significantly limit its practical applications (Berglund 2005, Samir et al. 2005, Abe et al. 2007). To obtain regenerated cellulose (RC) nanofiber, first cellulose acetate (CA) nanofibers were prepared and then these were treated in alkaline solution to completely remove the acetyl groups to form cellulose.

The treatment to mix saponin with cellulose involved: 1) the preparation of saponin powder solution in water and then adding acetone /DMF (*N N*- dimethylformamide) and 2) the preparation of cellulose acetate solution in acetone/DMF/water. After combining these two and continuous magnetic stirring overnight, a homogeneous spinning solution was formed for electrospinning. After electrospun fiber formation, chemical and physical properties of the nanofibrous membrane were characterized using scanning electron microscopy (SEM), attenuated total reflectance-Fourier transform infrared spectroscopy (ATR–FTIR), differential scanning calorimetry (DSC), and tensile properties.

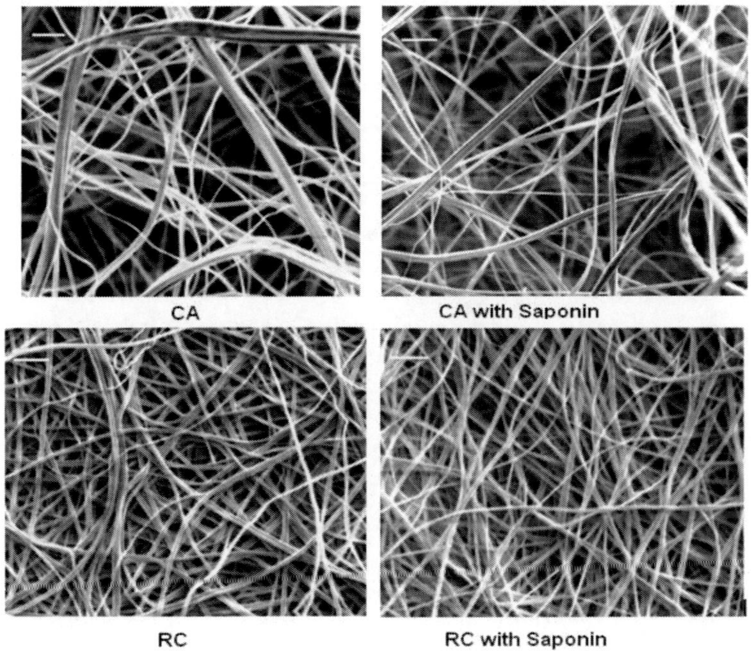

Dixit et al. 2010.

Figure 2. SEM images for electrospun nanofibrous membranes of cellulose acetate (CA) and regenerated cellulose (RC) with and without loading with *Quillaja* saponin. Scale bar is 5 μm.

The fibrous structure of the saponin loaded fibrous was maintained during the deacetylation (Figure 2). Conversion of cellulose acetate (CA) into cellulose (RC) was confirmed by FTIR by monitoring the disappearance of carbonyl absorption peak at 1742 ~ 1744 cm^{-1}(C=O), 1365~ 1370 cm^{-1} ($C-CH_3$). The increase in hydroxyl groups in the regenerated cellulose was seen in the spectrum by the increase in the absorption peak at around 3400-3500 cm^{-1} (Figure 3). The anti-fungal properties of saponin loaded fibrous membrane were demonstrated by comparing the spore counts after 0 and 24 h time against two household fungi, *Penicillium roguefortii and Aspergillus ochraceus* with control sample (Table 1). The saponin-loaded membrane had reductions of 80.4 % and 53.6 % for *Penicillium roguefortii* and *Aspergillus ochraceus*, respectively. Fibers containing *Quillaja* saponin have potential for both household and medical applications.

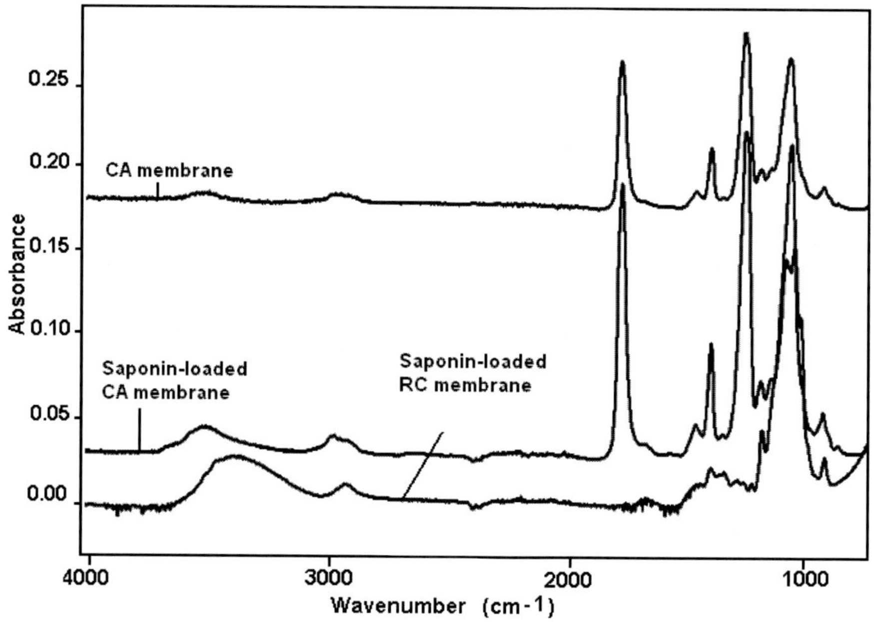

Dixit et al. 2010.

Figure 3. FTIR spectra of (A) *Quillaja* saponin and (B) electrospun CA membrane, CA membrane loaded with saponin, and RC membrane loaded with saponin.

Table 1. Spore counts ($x10^9$/mL) at 0 and 24 hours with regenerated cellulose (RC) control and RC loaded with *Quillaja* saponin

Fungus	0 h		24 h		Reduction (%)
	Control RC	Saponin loaded RC	Control RC	Saponin loaded RC	
Penicillium roguefortii	11.1±3.05	9.5±2.08	24.8±3.5	1.9±4.9	80.4
Aspergillus ochraceus	3.7±2.5	2.8±2.6	9.6±5.9	1.3±2.0	53.6

Dixit et al. 2010.

CONCLUSION

In conclusion, natural compounds can be loaded within and on cellulose based nanofibers. These nanofibers are good candidates for the development of biofunctional materials for use in medical textiles and personal protective equipment. The saponin added cellulose nanofibrous membranes are extremely attractive materials as they possess antifungal properties. Preliminary investigations of saponin -based systems provided useful indications about the possibility of extending the preparation approach to analogous nanocomposites possessing different biological properties. Finally, nanofibers can be used in a number of industrial applications, and their use is increasing each year. The application of these developed nanofibrous material can be envisaged in the preparation of antibacterial paints/coatings to be used in households, medical textile, biomedical/ hospital, food-packaging field, and aerospace industries, and their use may be ubiquitous in coming years especially for medical textiles and applications in personal protection.

REFERENCES

Abe K, Iwamoto S and Yano H (2007) Obtaining cellulose nanofibers with a uniform width of 15 nm from wood, *Biomacromolecules*, *8*(10): 3276–3278.

Andreuccetti C, Carvalho R A, and Grosso CRF (2010) Gelatin-based films containing hydrophobic plasticizers and saponin from *Yucca schidigera* as the surfactant, *Food Res Int* 43:1710–1718.

Avato P, Bucci R, Tava A, Vitali C, Rosato A, Bialy Z, and Jurzysta M (2006) Antimicrobial activity of saponins from *Medicago* sp.: structure-activity relationship, *Phytother Res* 20:454–457.

Bankefors J, Nord LI, and Kenne L (2008) Structural classification of *Quillaja* saponins by electrospray ionization ion trap multiple-stage mass spectrometry in combination with multivariate analysis, proof of concept, *Chemometr Intell Lab* 90:178–187.

Barile E, Bonanomi G, Antignani V, Zolfaghari B, Sajjadi SE, Scala F, and Lanzotti V (2007) Saponins from *Allium minutiflorum* with antifungal activity, *Phytochemistry* 68:596–603.

Berglund LA. (2005) In *Natural Fibers, Biopolymers and Their Biocomposites*; Eds. Mohanty AK, Misra M, and Drzal LT, CRC Press: Boca Raton, FL, pp. 807−832.

Cheeke PR, Piacente S, and Oleszek W (2006) Anti-inflammatory and anti-arthritic effects of *Yucca schidigera*: a review, *J Inflamm* 29(3):6-13.

Chen C-H, Kuo W-S, and Lai L-S (2009) Effect of surfactants on water barrier and physical properties of tapioca starch/decolorized hsian-tsao leaf gum films, *Food Hydrocolloid*, 23:714–721.

De Lucca AJ, Boue S, Palmgren MS, Maskos K, and Cleveland TE (2006) Fungicidal properties of two saponin Capsicum frutescens and the relationship structure and fungicidal activity, *Can J Microbiol* 52:336–342.

Doshi J and Reneker D H (1995), Electrospinning process and applications of electrospun fibers, *J Electrostat*, 35:151-160.

Dixit V, Tewari J, and Obendorf SK (2010) Fungal growth inhibition of regenerated cellulose nanofibrous membranes containing *Quillaja* saponin, *Arch Environ Contam Toxicol* 59:417–423.

Fujita K-I and Kubo I (2005) Multifunctional action of antifungal polygodial against Saccharomyces cerevisiae: Involvement of pyrrole formation on cell surface in antifungal action, *Bioorg Med Chem* 13:6742–6747.

Gao Y and, Cranston R (2008) Recent advances in antimicrobial treatments of textiles, *Text Res J* 78: 60-72.

Gleeson RM (1997) An improved method for thick film preparation using saponin as a lysing agent, *Clin Lab Haem* 19(4): 249–251.

Güçlü-Ustündağ O and Mazza G (2007) Saponins: properties, applications and processing, *Crit Rev Food Sci Nutr.* 47(3):231-58.

Higuchi R and Komori T (1987) Structures of compounds derived from the acyl moieties of Quillajasaponin, *Phytochemistry* 26:2357-2360.

Kalyon BD and, Olgun U (2001) Antibacterial efficacy of triclosan-incorporated polymers, *Am J Infect Contr* 29:124-125.

Kanzaki T, Morisaki N, Shiina R, and Saito Y (1998) Role of transforming growth factor-β pathway in the mechanism of wound healing by saponin from *Ginseng radix* rubra, *Brit J Pharmacol* (1998) 125:255-262.

Keukens EAJ, de Vrije T, van den Boom C, de Waard P, Plasman HH, Thiel F, Chupin V, Jongen WMF, and de Kruijff B (1995) Molecular basis of glycoalkaloid induced membrane disruption, *Biochim Biophys Acta* 1240:216-228

Kim YH, Choi H-M, and Yoon JH (1998) Synthesis of a quaternary ammonium derivative of chitosan and its application to a cotton antimicrobial finish. *Text Res J* 68:428–434.

Lacaille-Dubois MA (2005) Bioactive saponins with cancer related and immunomodulatory activity: recent developments, *Stud Nat Prod Chem* 32(12):209–246.

Lim SH and, Hudson SM (2004) Application of a fiber-reactive chitosan derivative to cotton fabric as an antimicrobial textile finish. *Carbohyd Polym* 56: 227–234.

Magota H, Okubo K, Shimoyamada M, Suzuki M, and Maruyama M (March 1, 1991) Isolation of steroidal saponin as antifungal agent, *Japanese Patent JP* 3048694.

Matsuura H (2001) Saponins in garlic as modifiers of the risk *J Nutr* 131(3S):1000S-1005S

Miyakoshi M, Tamura Y, Masuda H, Mizutani K, Tanaka O, Ikeda T, Ohtani K, Kasai R, and Yamasaki K (2000) Anti-yeast steroidal saponins from *Yucca schidigera* (Mohave Yucca), a new anti-food-deteriorating agent, *J Nat Prod* 63:332-338.

Morrissey JP and Osbourn AE (1999) Fungal resistance to plant antibiotics as a mechanism of pathogenesis, *Microbiol Mol Biol* Rev 63:708–724.

Murakami F (1986) Water-soluble perfumes containing essential oils solubilized by saponins, Japanese Patent JP 61266496.

Park WH, Lee KY, Choi JH, Ha WS, and Chang BH (1996) Characterization of chitosan-treated wool fabric. I. Antimicrobial and deodorant activities. *J Korean Fiber Soc* 33: 855–860.

Pugnaloni LA, Dickinson E, Ettelaie R, Mackie AR, and Wilde PJ (2004). Competitive adsorption of proteins and low-molecular-weight surfactants: Computer simulation and microscopic imaging, *Adv Colloid Interfac* 107:27–49.

Ragupathi G, Gardner JR, Livingston PO, and Gin DY (2011) Natural and synthetic saponin adjuvant QS-21 for vaccines against cancer, *Expert Rev Vaccines* 10(4):463-47.

Rambo CR, Recouvreux DOS, Carminatti CA, Pitlovanciv AK, Antônio RV and Porto LM, (2008) Template assisted synthesis of porous nanofibrous cellulose membranes for tissue engineering, *Mater Sci Eng* C 28:549–554.

Recchia J, Lurantos MHA, Amsden JA, Storey J, and Kensil CR (1995) A semisynthetic *Quillaja* saponin as a drug delivery agent for aminoglycoside antibiotics, *Pharmaceut Res* 12:1917-1923.

Roy D, Kommalapati RR, Mandava SS, Valsaraj KT, and Constant WD (1997) Soil washing potential of a natural surfactant, *Environ Sci Technol* 31:670-675.

Samir MASA, Alloin F, and Dufresne A (2005) Review of recent research into cellulosic whiskers, their properties and their application in nanocomposite field, *Biomacromolecules* 6:612–626.

San Martín RS and Briones R (1999) Industrial uses and sustainable supply of *Quillaja saponaria* (Rosaceae) saponins, *Econ Bot* 53(3):302-311.

Sautour M, Miyamoto T, and Lacaille-Dubois M-A (2005) Steroidal saponins from *Smilax medica* and their antifungal activity, *J Nat Prod* 68:1489-93.

Siro I and Plackett D (2010) Microfibrillated cellulose and new nanocomposite materials: a review, *Cellulose* 17(3): 459-494.

Sparg SG, Light ME, and van Staden J (2004) Biological activities and distribution of plant saponins, *J Ethnopharmacol* 94:219–43.

Sun H X, Xie Y, and Ye YP (2009) Advances in saponin-based adjuvant, *Vaccine* 27(12):1787-1796.

Tiwari P, Singh D, and Singh MM (2008) Anti-*Trichomonas* activity of *Sapindus* saponins, a candidate for development as microbicidal contraceptive, *J Antimicrob Chemother* 62(3):526-534.

Umlas J and Fallon JN (1971) New thick-film technique for malaria diagnosis - use of saponin stromatolytic solution for lysis, *Am J Trop Med Hyg* 20(4):527-529

Villalobos R, Hernández-Muñoz P, and Chiralt A (2006) Effect of surfactants on water sorption and barrier properties of hydroxypropyl methylcellulose films, *Food Hydrocolloid* 20:502–509

Yang C-R, Zhang Y, Jacob MR, Khan SI, Zhang Y-J, and Li X-C (2006) Antifungal activity of C-27 steroidal saponins, *Antimicrob Agents Chemother* 50:1710–1714

Zhang J-D, Cao Y-B, Xu Z, Sun H-H, An M-M, Yan L, Chen H-S, Gao P-H, Wang Y, Jia X-M, and Jiang Y-Y (2005) *In vitro* and *in vivo* antifungal activities of the eight steroid saponins from *Tribulus terrestris* L. with potent activity against fluconazole-resistant fungal pathogens, *Biol Pharm Bull* 28(12):2211-2215.

Zhou W, Yang J, Lou L, and Zhu L (2011) Solubilization properties of polycyclic aromatic hydrocarbons by saponin, a plant-derived biosurfactant, *Environ Pollut* 159:1198-1204.

In: Saponins: Properties, Applications and Health Benefits ISBN: 978-1-62100-942-9
Editors: Rani Koh and Isaac Tay

Chapter 6

EVIDENCE OF BIOACTIVITY FROM *GANODERMA LUCIDUM* TRITERPENOIDS IN CULTURED CELL MODELS

Weimei Ruan and David G. Popovich*

Department of Chemistry, National University of Singapore, Singapore

ABSTRACT

Triterpenoids are a structurally diverse class of potential bioactive molecules found in a variety of plants. This review will focus on a medicinal mushroom *Ganoderma lucidum* which is also known as either lingzhi or reishi mushroom. This mushroom has a long history of use in traditional Chinese medicine. Triterpenoids either isolated or present in extracts of *Ganoderma lucidum* have multiple reported bioactive effects which include chemoprevention by inducing multiple types of programmed cell death. *Ganoderma lucidum* can also influence other metabolic states such as reducing inflammatory markers and possess anti-diabetic properties among others and these may have an influence on improving metabolic control.

Ganoderma lucidum is a medicinal mushroom (also known as Ling zhi in Chinese and Reshi in Japanese), is a well-known Chinese traditional medicine that has been used to promote longevity and treat weakness for centuries. Research has centered on *Ganoderma lucidum* recently due to its multiple pharmacological activities, including anti-inflammatory [1], anti-tumorigenic [2], anti-herpetic[3], anti-virus [4], anti-ulcerogenic [5], anti-allergic [6], anti-angiogenic [7], anti-diabetic [8], hypoglycimic activity [9], and osteoclastogenesis-regulated effects [10]. Triterpenoids are one of the major classes of potential bioactive compounds in *Ganoderma lucidum*. Hundreds of triterpenoids from *Ganoderma lucidum* have been isolated and identified and these triterpenoids are exclusively found in genus Ganoderma [11].

* Corresponding author.
Tel: (65) 6516-4695.
Fax: (65) 6775-7895.
E-mail address: chmpdg@nus.edu.sg.

TRITERPENOIDS FROM *GANODERMA LUCIDUM*

Triterpenoids derived from *Ganoderma lucidum* are oxygenated tetracyclic triterpenoids. The majority of these triterpenoids are ganoderic acids (C30) and licidenic acid (C27). In addition to the two major triterpenoids, ganolucidic acids, ganoderenic acids, ganoderiols, ganodermadiol, ganodermatriol, ganodermanondiol, ganodermanontriol, lucidumols, ganoderic aldehydes and lucialdehydes are also found in *Ganoderma lucidum*. New triterpenoids are continuously discovered by different research groups. For example, 7-O-ethyl ganoderic acid O (GA-O) was recently found from fermented mycelia of *Ganoderma lucidum* by silica gel chromatography [12]. A novel ganoderic acid, ganoderic acid FWI was found in a methanolic extract [13]. Additionally, new triterpenoid derivatives such as ganofuran B, butyl ganoderate and butyl lucidenate were discovered [14, 15]. Nevertheless, many more triterpenoids from *Ganoderma lucidum* likely remain undiscovered and worthwhile to explore. Chemical structures of representative triterpenoids identified from *Ganoderma lucidum* are shown in Figure 1.

ANTI-INFLAMMATORY, ADIPOGENESIS AND OSTEOCLAST DIFFERENTIATION EFFECT IN CULTURED CELLS

Triterpenoids from *Ganoderma lucidum* have been reported to exhibit diverse bioactivity in variety of cell culture models. Extracts of triterpenoids from *Ganoderma lucidum* possessed anti-inflammatory effects on lipopolysaccharide (LPS)-stimulated macrophages by suppressing secretion of potentially harmful cytokines tumor necrosis factor-α (TNF-α) and interleukin-6 (IL-6) [1].

Butyl ganoderate A and butyl lucidenate N isolated from *Ganoderma lucidum* were demonstrated to inhibit adipogenesis in 3T3-L1 cells by down-regulation of the adipogenic transcription factor sterol regulatory element-binding protein (SREBP)-1c and its target genes, such as fatty acid synthase (FAS)and acetyl-CoA carboxylase (ACC) [16]. Another triterpenoid T-butyl lucidenate B was also shown to exert adipogenesis inhibitory effect by reduction of triglyceride accumulation and suppression of glycerol-3-phosphate dehydrogenase (GPDH) activity and gene expressions of peroxisome proliferator-activated receptor (PPAR)γ, CCAAT/enhancer-binding proteins(C/EBP)α, and SREBP-1c [17]. Recently, a *Ganoderma lucidum* extract containing approximately 10% of ganoderic acid A was reported to promote adipocyte differentiation and adiponectin production by activating PPARγ and PPARα [18]. Production of adiponectin is associated with an improvement in metabolic control.

Triterpenoids from *Ganoderma Lucidum* could be beneficial in osteoclastogenesis therapeutics. Inhibition of osteoclast differentiation helps in preventing excessive osteoclastic bone resorption which is believed to be responsible for osteopenic diseases such as osteoporosis and rheumatoid arthritis. Ganoderic acid DM and ganoderic acid F were found to exhibit cytotoxicities and inhibit osteoclast differentiation in RAW264 mouse leukaemic monocyte-macrophage cells. These effects were mediated by suppression of c-Fos and the nuclear factor of activated T cells c1 (NFATc1) which subsequently suppressed expression of dendritic cell−specific transmembrane protein (DC-STAMP) and reduced osteoclast fusion [19]. Additionally, a structure-activity relationship was related to the inhibitory activity [10].

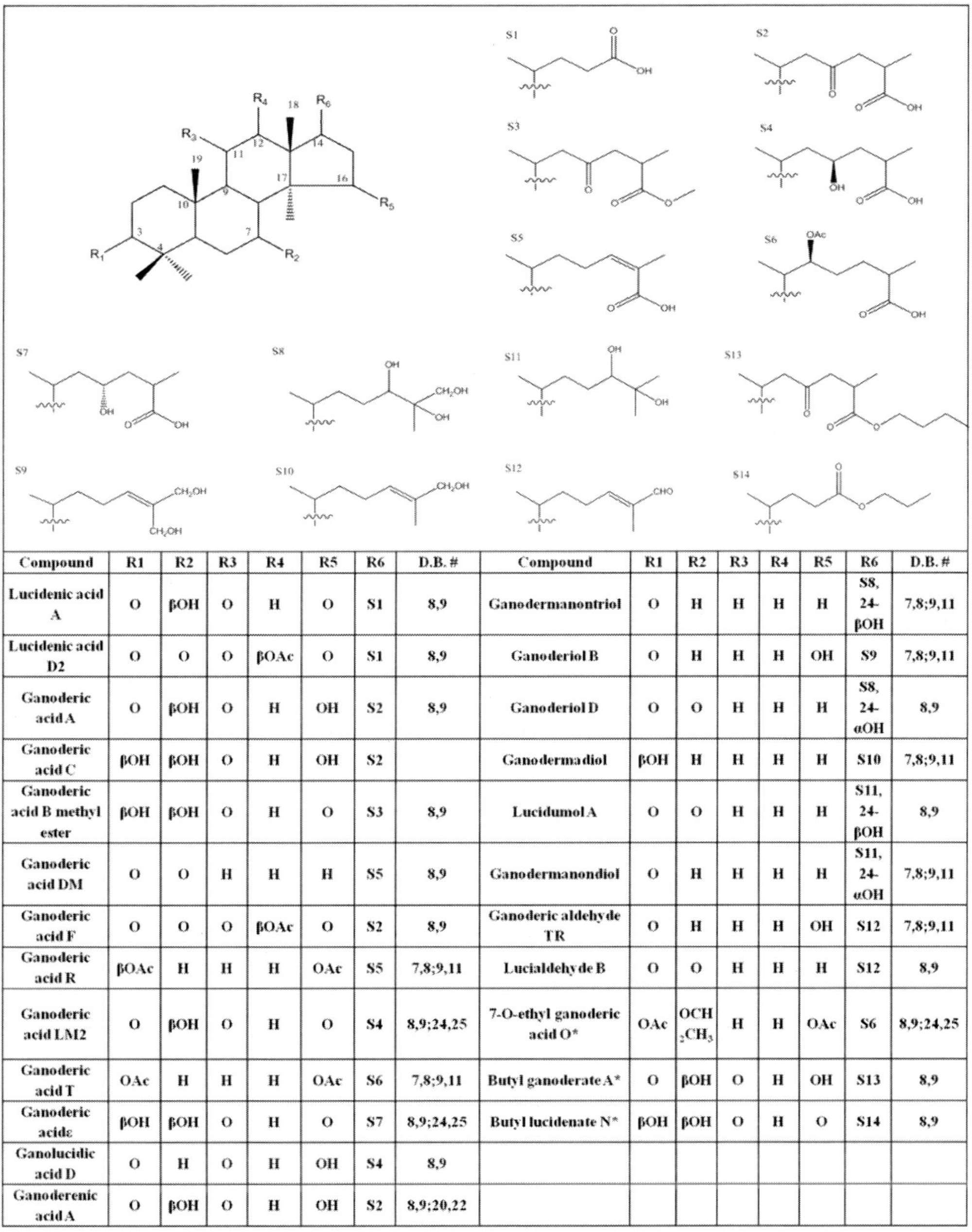

Compound	R1	R2	R3	R4	R5	R6	D.B. #	Compound	R1	R2	R3	R4	R5	R6	D.B. #
Lucidenic acid A	O	βOH	O	H	O	S1	8,9	Ganodermanontriol	O	H	H	H	H	S8, 24-βOH	7,8;9,11
Lucidenic acid D2	O	O	O	βOAc	O	S1	8,9	Ganoderiol B	O	H	H	H	OH	S9	7,8;9,11
Ganoderic acid A	O	βOH	O	H	OH	S2	8,9	Ganoderiol D	O	O	H	H	H	S8, 24-αOH	8,9
Ganoderic acid C	βOH	βOH	O	H	OH	S2		Ganodermadiol	βOH	H	H	H	H	S10	7,8;9,11
Ganoderic acid B methyl ester	βOH	βOH	O	H	O	S3	8,9	Lucidumol A	O	O	H	H	H	S11, 24-βOH	8,9
Ganoderic acid DM	O	O	H	H	H	S5	8,9	Ganodermanondiol	O	H	H	H	H	S11, 24-αOH	7,8;9,11
Ganoderic acid F	O	O	O	βOAc	O	S2	8,9	Ganoderic aldehyde TR	O	H	H	H	OH	S12	7,8;9,11
Ganoderic acid R	βOAc	H	H	H	OAc	S5	7,8;9,11	Lucialdehyde B	O	O	H	H	H	S12	8,9
Ganoderic acid LM2	O	βOH	O	H	O	S4	8,9;24,25	7-O-ethyl ganoderic acid O*	OAc	OCH_2CH_3	H	H	OAc	S6	8,9;24,25
Ganoderic acid T	OAc	H	H	H	OAc	S6	7,8;9,11	Butyl ganoderate A*	O	βOH	O	H	OH	S13	8,9
Ganoderic acidε	βOH	βOH	O	H	O	S7	8,9;24,25	Butyl lucidenate N*	βOH	βOH	O	H	O	S14	8,9
Ganolucidic acid D	O	H	O	H	OH	S4	8,9								
Ganoderenic acid A	O	βOH	O	H	OH	S2	8,9;20,22								

Figure 1. Chemical structures of triterpenoids from *Ganoderma lucidum* # refers to double bonds, * represents newly discovered triterpenoids.

Table 1. Summary of the type of cell death in specific cell lines using triterpenoids from *Ganoderma lucidum*

Components	Responsive cell lines	Type of cell death	Molecular mechanisms involved	Reference
Methanol extracts	transplantable B16 murine melanoma cells, mouse fibrosarcoma L929 cells ,rat astrocytoma C6 cells	Apoptosis and necrosis	Upregulation of 1. p53 2. caspase-3 Downregulation of 1. Bcl-2	[22]
Methanol extracts	interleukin 3-dependent lymphoma (DA-1)	Apoptosis	Downregulation of 1. NFkB-p65 2. Inactive caspase 3	[23]
Methanol extract with possible triteropenoids	NB4 human leukemia cells.	Apoptosis	Downregulation of 1. p53 2. Akt 3. Erk 4. Bcl2/Bax ratio.	[24]
Triterpenoid-rich ethanol extract	platelet-derived growth factor (PDGF-BB)-activated rat hepatic stellate cells (HSC-T6)	Apoptosis	Upregulation of 1. JNK Downregulation of 1. cyclins D1 and D2 2. PDGFβR 3. Akt 4. α-SMA.	[25]
Ethanol extracts of triterpenoids	human hepatomaHep 3B and HepG2 cells, breast cancer cells (MCF-7 and MDA-MB-231) and myeloid leukemia cells (HL-60)	Apoptosis	Not Detected	[26, 27]
Ethanol extract	AGS human gastric carcinoma cells	Apoptosis	Upregulation of 1. death receptor 5 2. TRAIL 3. caspase-3,8 and 9 Downregualtion of 1. Akt 2. Bcl-2 3. Bid 4. XIAP 5. survivin Degradation of poly (ADP-ribose) polymerase	[28]

Components	Responsive cell lines	Type of cell death	Molecular mechanisms involved	Reference
Triterpene-enriched extract	SW620 human colorectal carcinoma cells	Apoptosis	Upregulation of 1. p53 2. caspase 3 Downreguation of 1. Bcl-2/Bax ratio	[29]
Ganoderic acid Me	HCT-116 human colon carcinoma cells	Apoptosis	Upregulation of 3. p53 4. caspase 3 Downreguation of 1. Bcl-2/Bax ratio 2. Mitochondria membrane potential Release of cytochrome c	[30]
Ganoderic acid Mf and ganoderic acid S	human cervical carcinoma HeLa cells	Apoptosis	Downregulation of 1. Bcl-2/Bax ratio 2. caspase-3and 9 3. mitochondria membrane potential Release of cytochrome c	[31]
Triterpenoids from *Ganoderma lucidum*	HT-29 human colon cancer cells	Autophagy	Upregulation of 1. Beclin-1 2. LC-3 Downregulation of 1. p38 MAPK Formation of autophagic vacuoles	[32]
Ganoderiol F	HepG2 cells.	Senescence	Upregulation of 1. EKR 2. p16 Inhibition of 1. DNA synthesis 2. topoisomerases activity	[33]
Ganoderic acid A and ganoderic acid H	MDA-MB-231 breast cancer cells	Antimetastasis	Downregulation of 1. AP-1 2. NF-κB 3. Cdk4 4. secretion of uPA	[34]
Ganoderic acid T	95-D human highly metastatic lung tumor cells	Antimetastasis	Downregulation of 1. MMP-2 and MMP-9 2. NF-κB.	[35]

Table 1. (Continued)

Components	Responsive cell lines	Type of cell death	Molecular mechanisms involved	Reference
Lucidenic acids A, B, C and N	phorbol-12-myristate-13-acetate (PMA)-induced HepG2 cells	Antimetastasis	Downregulation of 1. MMP-9 2. ERK1/2 3. AP-1 4. NF-kB	[36]

CHEMOPREVENTION

The most extensively studied of *Ganoderma lucidum* triterpenoids bioactivity is their anti-tumor or chemo-preventative effects. Both triterpenoid extracts from *Ganoderma lucidum* and individual isolated triterpenoids have been reported to inhibit cell growth and in various carcinoma cells. Preliminary research has focused on the cytotoxic properties of triterpenoids from *Ganoderma lucidum* on tumor cells. For instance, ethanol extracts from *Ganoderma lucidum* have been studied using human cervical carcinoma HeLa cells [20]. Additionally, individual triterpenoids including lucidenic acid N, lucidenic acid A, and ganoderic acid E have been showed significant cytotoxicity in hepatic carcinoma cells Hep-G2 and murine P-388 lymphocytic leukemia cells [21]. The molecular mechanism involved includes multiple programmed cell death such as apoptosis, autophagy, senescence and also may reduce or prevent cellular metastasis. The chemo-preventative properties from *Ganoderma lucidum* triterpenoids are summarized in Table 1.

PROGRAMMED CELL DEATH

Apoptosis

One of the most commonly studied bioactive properties of natural produce is the ability to induce apoptosis in cancer cell lines. Methanol extracts containing ganoderic acids and triterpenoid derivatives were found to induce apoptosis and necrosis in transplantable B16 murine melanoma cells, mouse fibrosarcoma L929 cells and rat astrocytoma C6 cells. The apoptotic cell death involved was caspase-dependent and mediated by up-regulation of tumor suppressor protein p53 and suppression of anti-apoptotic protein B-cell lymphoma (Bcl)-2 expression [22]. Another methanol extract possibly containing triterpenoids was also indicated to cause apoptosis in interleukin 3-dependent lymphoma cells (DA-1) with reduction of expression of nuclear factor kappa B (NFkB)-p65 factor and inactivated caspase-3 [23]. Additionally, induction of apoptosis in NB4 human leukemia cells was found with treatment of a similar methanol extract possibly containing triterpenoids. The corresponding activity involved reductions of p53 levels, Akt level, extracellular-signal-regulated kinase (Erk) level as well as the Bcl2/ Bcl-2-associated X protein (Bax) ratio [24].

Triterpenoid-rich extract extracted using ethanol were shown to induce apoptosis in platelet-derived growth factor (PDGF-BB)-activated rat hepatic stellate cells (HSC-T6) and it was mediated by down-regulation of cyclins D1 and D2, PDGFβR and Akt phosphorylation, up-regulation of JNK phosphorylation, and expression of α-SMA [25]. Ethanol extracts of triterpenoids from *Ganoderma lucidum* also induced apoptosis in human hepatocarcinoma Hep-3B and Hep-G2 cells [26, 27]. However, the underlying molecular mechanisms were not elucidated. In addition to hepatocarcinoma cells, ethanol extracts exhibited anti-proliferative activities on human breast cancer cells (MCF-7 and MDA-MB-231), myeloid leukemia cells (HL-60) and AGS human gastric carcinoma cells through induction of apoptosis [27, 28]. Induction of apoptosis in AGS human gastric carcinoma cells was associated with two distinct pathways including extrinsic plasma membrane death receptor-mediated pathway and intrinsic mitochondria-mediated pathway which corresponded to inactivation of Akt [28].

More recently, a triterpene-enriched extract was found to induce apoptosis in SW620 human colorectal carcinoma cells by activating caspase-3, up-regulating P53 and down-regulating Bcl2/Bax ratio [29].

Individual triterpenoid, ganoderic acid Me was reported to induce apoptosis in HCT-116 human colon carcinoma cells through mitochondrial mediated pathway. Increased expression of p53 and reduced Bcl-2/Bax ratio were reported [30]. The induction of apoptosis was also coupled with reduced mitochondria trans-membrane potential, released cytochrome c from mitochondria into the cytosol and increased caspase-3 activity. Following a similar mechanism induced by ganoderic acid Me in HCT-116 cells, a pair of position isomer, ganoderic acid Mf and ganoderic acid S were able to trigger apoptotic cell death in a human cervical carcinoma HeLa cells. The actions involved decreased Bcl-2/Bax ratio, activated caspase-3 and caspase-9, decreased mitochondria membrane potential and release of cytochrome c [31].

Autophagy and Senescence

Another type of programmed cell death is termed autophagy and it may be responsible for part of the cytotoxic properties and mechanisms attribute to the chemo-prevention properties of *Ganoderma lucidum* triterpenoids. Triterpenoids from *Ganoderm lucidum* induced autophagic cell death in HT-29 human colon cancer cells, which was associated with formation of autophagic vacuoles, up-regulation expression of Beclin-1 and LC-3 protein. These effects were suggested to be mediated by inhibition of p38 mitogen-activated protein kinase (p38 MAPK) [32].

When programmed cell death is blocked in cells, irreversible cell growth arrest, termed secescence has also been reported activated by *Ganoderma lucidum*. Ganoderiol F has been reported to induce senescence in HepG2 cells. The inhibition of DNA synthesis was presumably caused by the inhibition of topoisomerases activity and activation of mitogen-activated protein kinase EKR and up-regulation of cyclin-dependent kinase inhibitor p16 might contribute to the premature senescence induction [33].

Anti-Invasion and Anti-Metastasis

In addition to suppressing the growth of cells or existing tumors, preventing invasion and metastasis are also important mechanisms for treatment. Ganoderic acid A and ganoderic acid H were shown to exhibit anti-invasive effects on MDA-MB-231 breast cancer cells [34]. These effects were mediated by down-regulation of transcription factors activator protein (AP)-1 and NF-κB, subsequently suppressed expression of cyclin-dependent kinase (Cdk4) and secretion of urokinase-type plasminogen activator (uPA), respectively. A structure-activity relationship was also suggested. Ganoderic acid T was also demonstrated to effectively inhibit tumor metastasis in 95-D human highly metastatic lung tumor cells via blocking expression of matrix metalloproteinase MMP-2 and MMP-9 which could be mediated by inactivation of NF-κB [35]. Lucidenic acids A, B, C and N were found to possess anti-invasive activity on phorbol-12-myristate-13-acetate (PMA)-induced HepG2 cells by down regulating MMP-9 activity. Inhibition of ERK1/2 phosphorylation and reduction of DNA-binding activities of AP-1 and NF-kB were reported to be involve in this process [36].

Triterpenoids from *Ganoderma lucidum* have been reported to possess diverse bioactive properties and perhaps the most convincing evidence for bioactivity is the chemo-preventative properties. These triterpenoids may induce activity though activation of multiple programmed cell death pathways. However, elucidating a structure-activity relationship on specific cancer cell lines using individual isolated triterpenoids is still limited.

REFERENCES

[1] Dudhgaonkar, S.; Thyagarajan, A.; Sliva, D. Suppression of the inflammatory response by triterpenes isolated from the mushroom Ganoderma lucidum. *International Immunopharmacology* (2009), *9*, 1272-1280.

[2] Zhao, S.; Ye, G.; Fu, G.; Cheng, J. X.; Yang, B. B.; Peng, C. Ganoderma lucidum exerts anti-tumor effects on ovarian cancer cells and enhances their sensitivity to cisplatin. *International Journal of Oncology* (2011), *38*, 1319-1327.

[3] Li, Y. Q.; Wang, S. F. Anti-hepatitis B activities of ganoderic acid from Ganoderma lucidum. *Biotechnology Letters* (2006), *28*, 837-841.

[4] Iwatsuki, K.; Akihisa, T.; Tokuda, H.; Ukiya, M.; Oshikubo, M.; Kimura, Y.; Asano, T.; Nomura, A.; Nishino, H. Lucidenic Acids P and Q, Methyl Lucidenate P, and Other Triterpenoids from the Fungus Ganoderma lucidum and their Inhibitory Effects on Epstein-Barr Virus Activation. *Journal of Natural Products* (2003), *66*, 1582-1585.

[5] Gao, Y.; Zhou, S.; Wen, J.; Huang, M.; Xu, A. Mechanism of the antiulcerogenic effect of Ganoderma lucidum polysaccharides on indomethacin-induced lesions in the rat. *Life Sciences* (2002), *72*, 731-745.

[6] Nogami, M.; Tsuji, Y.; Kubo, M. Studies on Ganoderma lucidum. VI. Anti-allergic effect. *Yakugaku Zasshi* (1986), *106*, 594-599.

[7] Song, Y. S.; Kim, S. H.; Sa, J. H.; Jin, C.; Lim, C. J.; Park, E. H. Anti-angiogenic and inhibitory activity on inducible nitric oxide production of the mushroom Ganoderma lucidum. *Journal of Ethnopharmacology* (2004), *90*, 17-20.

[8] Meng, G.; Zhu, H.; Yang, S.; Wu, F.; Zheng, H.; Chen, E. E.; Xu, J. Attenuating effects of Ganoderma lucidum polysaccharides on myocardial collagen cross-linking relates to advanced glycation end product and antioxidant enzymes in high-fat-diet and streptozotocin-induced diabetic rats. *Carbohydrate Polymers* (2011), *84*, 180-185.

[9] Seto, S. W.; Lam, T. Y.; Tam, H. L.; Au, A. L. S.; Chan, S. W.; Wu, J. H.; Yu, P. H. F.; Leung, G. P. H.; Ngai, S. M.; Yeung, J. H. K.; Leung, P. S.; Lee, S. M. Y.; Kwan, Y. W. Novel hypoglycemic effects of Ganoderma lucidum water-extract in obese/diabetic (+db/+db) mice. *Phytomedicine* (2009), *16*, 426-436.

[10] Liu, J.; Shiono, J.; Shimizu, K.; Kondo, R. Ganoderic acids from Ganoderma lucidum: inhibitory activity of osteoclastic differentiation and structural criteria. *Planta Medica* (2010), *2*, 137-139.

[11] Kim, H. W.; Kim, B. K. Biomedicinal triterpenoids of Ganoderma lucidum (Curt.:Fr.) P. Karst. (Aphyllophoromycetideae). *Internation Journal of Medicinal Mushrooms* (1999), *1*, 121-138.

[12] Wang, J. L.; Li, Y. B.; Liu, R. M.; Zhong, J. J. A new ganoderic acid from Ganoderma lucidum mycelia. *Journal of Asian Natural Products Research* (2010), *12*, 727-730.

[13] Tschritter, O.; Fritsche, A.; Thamer, C.; Haap, M.; Shirkavand, F.; Rahe, S.; Staiger, H.; Maerker, E.; Haring, H.; Stumvoll, M. Plasma adiponectin concentrations predict insulin sensitivity of both glucose and lipid metabolism. *Diabetes* (2003), *52*, 239-243.

[14] Adams, M.; Christen, M.; Plitzko, I.; Zimmermann, S.; Brun, R.; Kaiser, M.; Hamburger, M. Antiplasmodial lanostanes from the Ganoderma lucidum mushroom. *Journal of Natural Products* (2010), *73*, 897-900.

[15] Lee, I.; Seo, J.; Kim, J.; Kim, H.; Youn, U.; Lee, J.; Jung, H.; Na, M.; Hattori, M.; Min, B.; Bae, K. Lanostane triterpenes from the fruiting bodies of Ganoderma lucidum and their inhibitory effects on adipocyte differentiation in 3T3-L1 Cells. *Journal of Natural Products* (2010), *73*, 172-176.

[16] Lee, I.; Kim, J.; Ryoo, I.; Kim, Y.; Choo, S.; Yoo, I.; Min, B.; Na, M.; Hattori, M.; Bae, K. Lanostane triterpenes from Ganoderma lucidum suppress the adipogenesis in 3T3-L1 cells through down-regulation of SREBP-1c. *Bioorganic & Medicinal Chemistry Letters* (2010), *20*, 5577-5581.

[17] Lee, I.; Kim, H.; Youn, U.; Kim, J.; Min, B.; Jung, H.; Na, M.; Hattori, M.; Bae, K. Effect of lanostane triterpenes from the fruiting bodies of Ganoderma lucidum on adipocyte differentiation in 3T3-L1 cells. *Planta Medica* (2010), *76*, 1558-1563.

[18] Shimojo, Y.; Kosaka, K.; Shirasawa, T. Effect of Ganoderma lucidum extract on adipocyte differentiation and adiponectin gene expression in the murine pre-adipocyte cell line, 3T3-L1. *Phytotherapy Research* (2011), *25*, 202-207.

[19] Miyamoto, I.; Liu, J.; Shimizu, K.; Sato, M.; Kukita, A.; Kukita, T.; Kondo, R. Regulation of osteoclastogenesis by ganoderic acid DM isolated from Ganoderma lucidum. *European Journal of Pharmacology* (2009), *602*, 1-7.

[20] Zhu H S; Yang X L; Wang L B; Zhao DX; Chen L Effects of extracts from sporoderm broken spores of Ganoderma lucidum on HeLa cells. *Cell Biology and Toxicology* (2000), *16*, 201-206.

[21] Wu, T. S.; Shi, L. S.; Kuo, S. C. Cytotoxicity of Ganoderma lucidum Triterpenes. *Journal of Natural Products* (2001), *64*, 1121-1122.

[22] Harhaji Trajkovic, L. M.; Mijatovic, S. A.; Maksimovic-Ivanic, D. D.; Stojanovic, I. D.; Momcilovic, M. B.; Tufegdzic, S. J.; Maksimovic, V. M.; Marjanovic, Z. S.; Stosic-Grujicic, S. D. Anticancer properties of Ganoderma lucidum methanol extracts in vitro and in vivo. *Nutr. Cancer* (2009), *61*, 696-707.

[23] Calvino, E.; Pajuelo, L.; Casas, J. A. O. D.; Manjon, J. L.; Tejedor, M. C.; Herraez, A.; Alonso, M. D.; Diez, J. C. Cytotoxic Action of Ganoderma lucidum on Interleukin-3 Dependent Lymphoma DA-1 Cells: Involvement of Apoptosis Proteins. *Phytotherapy Research* (2011), *25*, 25-32.

[24] Calvino, E.; Manjon, J. L.; Sancho, P.; Tejedor, M. C.; Herraez, A.; Diez, J. C. Ganoderma lucidum induced apoptosis in NB4 human leukemia cells: Involvement of Akt and Erk. *Journal of Ethnopharmacology* (2010), *128*, 71-78.

[25] Wang, G. J.; Huang, Y. J.; Chen, D. H.; Lin, Y. L. Ganoderma lucidum extract attenuates the proliferation of hepatic stellate cells by blocking the PDGF receptor. *Phytotherapy Research : PTR* (2009), *23*, 833-839.

[26] Chen, Y. K.; Kuo, Y. H.; Chiang, B. H.; Lo, J. M.; Sheen, L. Y. Cytotoxic activities of 9,11-dehydroergosteroi peroxide and ergosterol peroxide from the fermentation mycelia of Ganoderma lucidum cultivated in the medium containing leguminous plants on Hep 3B cells. *Journal of Agricultural and Food Chemistry* (2009), *57*, 5713-5719.

[27] Liu, Y. W.; Gao, J. L.; Guan, J.; Qian, Z. M.; Feng, K.; Li, S. P. Evaluation of antiproliferative activities and action mechanisms of extracts from two species of Ganoderma on tumor cell lines. *Journal of Agricultural and Food Chemistry* (2009), *57*, 3087-3093.

[28] Jang, K. J.; Han, M. H.; Lee, B. H.; Kim, B. W.; Kim, C. H.; Yoon, H. M.; Choi, Y. H. Induction of Apoptosis by Ethanol Extracts of Ganoderma lucidum in Human Gastric Carcinoma Cells. *JAMS Journal of Acupuncture and Meridian Studies* (2010), *3*, 24-31.

[29] Ji, Z.; Tang, Q.; Hao, R.; Zhang, J.; Pan, Y. Induction of apoptosis in the SW620 colon carcinoma cell line by triterpene-enriched extracts from Ganoderma lucidum through activation of caspase-3. *Oncology Letters* (2011), *2*, 565-570.

[30] Zhou, L.; Shi, P.; Chen, N. H.; Zhong, J. J. Ganoderic acid Me induces apoptosis through mitochondria dysfunctions in human colon carcinoma cells. *Process Biochemistry* (2011), *46*, 219-225.

[31] Liu, R. M.; Zhong, J. J. Ganoderic acid Mf and S induce mitochondria mediated apoptosis in human cervical carcinoma HeLa cells. *Phytomedicine* (2011), *18*, 349-355.

[32] Thyagarajan, A.; Jedinak, A.; Nguyen, H.; Terry, C.; Baldridge, L. A.; Jiang, J.; Sliva, D. Triterpenes from Ganoderma Lucidum induce autophagy in colon cancer through the inhibition of p38 mitogen-activated kinase (p38 MAPK). *Nutrition and Cancer* (2010), *62*, 630-640.

[33] Chang, U. M.; Li, C. H.; Lin, L. I.; Huang, C. P.; Kan, L. S.; Lin, S. B. Ganoderiol F, a ganoderma triterpene, induces senescence in hepatoma HepG2 cells. *Life Sciences* (2006), *79*, 1129-1139.

[34] Thyagarajan, A.; Jiang, J.; Hopf, A.; Adamec, J.; Sliva, D. Inhibition of oxidative stress-induced invasiveness of cancer cells by Ganoderma lucidum is mediated through the suppression of interleukin-8 secretion. *International Journal of Molecular Medicine* (2006), *18*, 657-664.

[35] Xu, K.; Liang, X.; Gao, F.; Zhong, J.; Liu, J. Antimetastatic effect of ganoderic acid T in vitro through inhibition of cancer cell invasion. *Process Biochemistry* (2010), *45*, 1261-1267.

[36] Weng, C. J.; Chau, C. F.; Hsieh, Y. S.; Yang, S. F.; Yen, G. C. Lucidenic acid inhibits PMA-induced invasion of human hepatoma cells through inactivating MAPK/ERK signal transduction pathway and reducing binding activities of NF-kappaB and AP-1. *Carcinogenesis* (2008), *29*, 147-156.

In: Saponins: Properties, Applications and Health Benefits ISBN: 978-1-62100-942-9
Editors: Rani Koh and Isaac Tay

Chapter 7

RECENT DEVELOPMENTS OF SOYASAPONINS FROM SOY (*GLYCINE MAX* (L.)) BIOACTIVITY IN CELL MODELS

Wei Zhang and David G. Popovich*
Department of Chemistry, National University of Singapore, Singapore

ABSTRACT

Soy bean (*Glycine max* (L.)) contains a class of phytochemicals known as soyasaponins which are oleanane triterpenoids. These molecules are diverse, structurally complex and can be classified into two main categories based on their respective soyasapogenols or aglycones. The two main groups of soyasaponins are group A and group B. In terms of biological activity far more in known about group B soyasaponins compared to group A. At the center of the biological activity of these molecules is cytotoxicity leading to apoptosis induction in cultured cancer cell models and it is this ability that has highlighted soy bean possible chemo-preventative properties. In this review the recent literature will be reviewed focusing on both group A and group B soyasaponins on reducing the cultured cancer cell growth and inducing apoptosis in various cancer cell lines. A probably structure function relationship between soyasaponins and cytotoxicity is emerging with the aglycones of both groups being the most cytotoxic than their related glycosides.

Recently, soy bean (*Glycine max* (L.)) extracts are under intensive study because of their potential beneficial health effects. Soyasaponins are oleanane triterpenoids and are one of main biological active components in soy bean. Studies indicate that soyasaponins can alter enzyme activities, lower cholesterol, interact with bile acids, and are chemo-preventative [1-3]. The biological activity of soyasaponins largely depends on their respective chemical structures as well as their polarity, acidity and hydrophobicity [3, 4]. Soyasaponins are classified in two groups, A and B, based on their respective

* Corresponding author.
Tel: (65) 6516-4695.
Fax: (65) 6775-7895.
E-mail address: chmpdg@nus.edu.sg.

soyasapogenols or aglycones [3]. Both bidesmosidic soyasaponin group A and monodesmosidic soyasaponin group B have varied biological activities. However, the exact mechanism of action and proof of a structure-function relationship of soyasaponins is still ongoing. In this review the reported biological activities of soyasaponins based on their structures classification and plausible mechanism of action will be reviewed.

Biological Activity of Group A Soyasaponins

Group A soyasaponins have a hydroxyl group at carbons 21 (Figure 1) and two glycosylation sites at carbon 3 and 22 on the oleanane ring structure. Group A soyasaponins can be further categorized into two additional groups as acetylated and deacetylated [1]. Less research is available regarding soyasaponins group A compared to group B. Soyasaponins A_2 combined with AOM (azoxymethane) significantly reduced more ODC activity (ornithine decarboxylase activity) and polyamine levels in the colonic mucosal tissue compared with those treated by AOM alone [5]. In addition, the combination of soyasaponin Ab and soyasaponin βg showed a strong active oxygen scavenging activity [5]. However, specific evidence of individual group A soyasaponins biological activity is very limited because of the lack of reliable methods for producing significant quantities of group A.

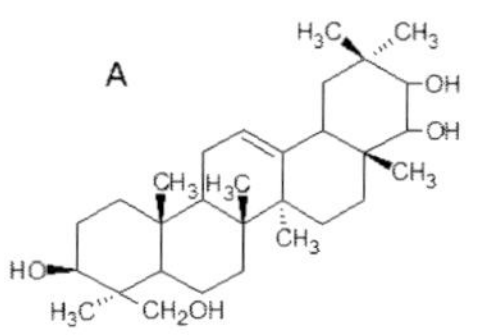

Group A Soyasaponins	Structure	MW	Formula
A1 (Ab)	glc(1→2)gal(1→2)glcU(1→3)-A-(22←1)ara(3←1)glc(2,3,4,6-tetra-O-Acetyl)	1463	$C_{67}H_{104}O_{33}$
A2 (Af)	gal(1→2)glcUA(1→3)-A-(22←1)ara(3←1)glc(2,3,4,6-tetra-O-Acetyl)	1274	$C_{61}H_{94}O_{28}$
A3 (Ah)	ara(1→2)glcUA(1→3)-A-(22←1)ara(3←1)glc(2,3,4,6-tetra-O-Acetyl)	1244	$C_{60}H_{92}O_{27}$
A4 (Aa)	glc(1→2)gal(1→2)glcU(1→3)-A-(22←1)ara(3←1)xyl(2,3,4-tri-O-Acetyl)	1364	$C_{64}H_{100}O_{31}$
A5 (Ae)	gal(1→2)glcUA(1→3)-A-(22←1)ara(3←1)xyl(2,3,4-tri-O-Acetyl)	1202	$C_{58}H_{90}O_{26}$
A6 (Ag)	ara(1→2)glcUA(1→3)-A-(22←1)ara(3←1)xyl(2,3,4-tri-O-Acetyl)	1172	$C_{57}H_{88}O_{25}$
Ac	rha(1→2)gal(1→2)glcUA(1→3)-A-(22←1)ara(3←1)glc(2,3,4,6-tetra-O-Acetyl)	1420	$C_{67}H_{104}O_{32}$
Ad	glc(1→2)ara(1→2)glcUA(1→3)-A-(22←1)ara(3←1)glc(2,3,4,6-tetra-O-Acetyl)	1390	$C_{66}H_{102}O_{31}$

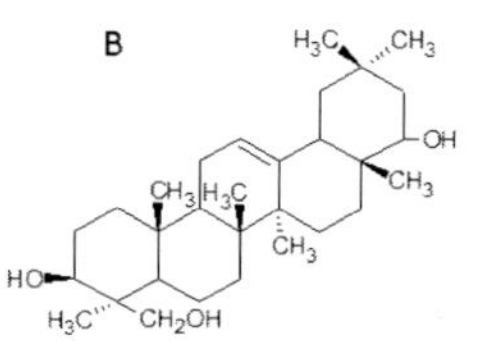

Group B Soyasaponins			
I (Bb)	rha(1→2)gal(1→2)glcUA(1→3)-B	942	$C_{48}H_{78}O_{18}$
II (Bc)	rha(1→2)ara(1→2)glcUA(1→3)-B	912	$C_{47}H_{76}O_{18}$
III (Bb')	gal(1→2)glcUA(1→3)-B	796	$C_{42}H_{68}O_{14}$
IV (Bc')	ara(1→2)glcUA(1→3)-B	766	$C_{41}H_{66}O_{13}$
V (Ba)	glc(1→2)gal(1→2)glcUA(1→3)-B	958	$C_{48}H_{78}O_{19}$
DDMP Group Soyasaponins			
βg	rha(1→2)gal(1→2)glcUA(1→3)-B-(22←2')-DDMP	1068	$C_{54}H_{84}O_{21}$
βa	rha(1→2)ara(1→2)glcUA(1→3)-B-(22←2')-DDMP	1038	$C_{53}H_{82}O_{20}$
γg	gal(1→2)glcUA(1→3)-B-(22←2')-DDMP	922	$C_{48}H_{74}O_{17}$
γa	ara(1→2)glcUA(1→3)-B-(22←2')-DDMP	892	$C_{47}H_{72}O_{16}$
αg	glc(1→2)gal(1→2)glcUA(1→3)-B-(22←2')-DDMP	1084	$C_{54}H_{84}O_{22}$

Figure 1. Chemical structure of oleanane triterpenoids found in soy.

Recently, we found specific acetyl group A soyasaponins showed different biological in three different cell lines. Group A soyasaponins treatment of colon cancer cells (Caco-2) resulted in lower IC50 concentration compared to hepatocarcinoma cells (Hep-G2), but no significant cytotoxicity in non-malignant murine fibroblast cells (3T3-L1) up to a concentration of 1 mg/mL (Figure 2). This may suggest that at least regarding the cytotoxic effect that there is cell specific target associated with group A soyasaponins. Group A soyasaponins have biological effects and possess antipoliferative and cytotoxic properties but the detailed mechanism is not presently clear. Moreover, simple and high efficient method for yielding group A soyasaponins is needed for further biological testing.

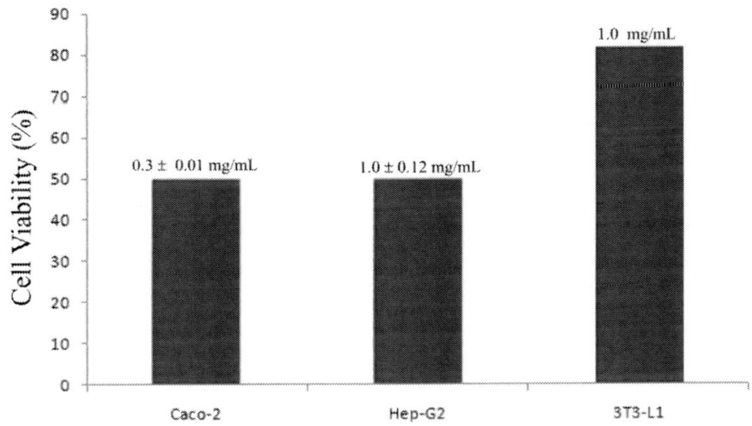

Unpublished data.

Figure 2. Variable IC50 of a group A soyasaponin extract in two human cancer cells, Caco-2 (intestinal) and Hep-G2 (hepatic-carcinoma) and a non-malignant murine fibroblast cells (3T3-L1). LC 50 values are expressed on top of the bars with the exception of 3T3-L1 which was not cytotoxic up to 1 mg/mL.

Biological Activity of Group B Soyasaponins

DDMP (2, 3-dihydro-2, 5-dihydroxy-6-methyl-4-pyrone) and non-DDMP conjugated soyasaponins are two main categories of group B soyasaponins, which have one glycosylation site on their aglycones (carbon 3) (Figure 1). The most abundant and naturally soyasaponins in soy bean was reported to be DDMP conjugated soyasaponins [6]. Non-DDMP soyasaponins have also been reported to be bioactive in many studies [7], especially for their ability to induced apoptosis in cultured cancer cell models. Apoptosis is a type of programmed cell death and typically represented as producing cellular DNA fragments that could be removed and cellular contents recycled. Once apoptosis is insufficient or suppressed, an uncontrolled cell proliferation may result in cancer development. Soyasaponin Bb was reported to inhibit esophageal cancer cell (Eca-9706) growth through inducing apoptosis by activating the caspase-3 pathway [8]. We have isolated soyasaponin I and III extracts from soy bean and examined their ability to induce apoptosis in Hep-G2 cancer cells [9], whereas DDMP soyasaponins extracts were found to induce cellular differentiation in the same cell lines without significant cytotoxicity [10] (Figure 2). Soyasaponins I and III apoptosis was confirmed by TUNEL and Multiple Caspase Apoptosis Detection assays [9]. The variety of the effects of DDMP and non-DDMP soyasaponins on Hep-G2 cells are proposed to be related to soyasaponins chemical structures. DDMP moiety will cause more polarity, while some evidence shows that bioactivity of soyasaponins increases as sugar moieties are removed from the structure to reduce polarity [11]. Disaccharide soyasaponins, soyasaponin III and IV, were reported to have stronger hepato-protective effects than soyasaponin I and II, and trisaccharide group [12]. Furthermore, soyasaponins that have a hexosyl unit shows a slightly greater ability than those with a pentosyl unit. The bioactivity related to chemical structure of group B soyasaponins is summarized in Figure 3. Nevertheless, more structure function evidence of soyasaponins metabolites released during cell treatment needs to be provided before definitive confirmation of the relationship between the biological activity and chemical structure.

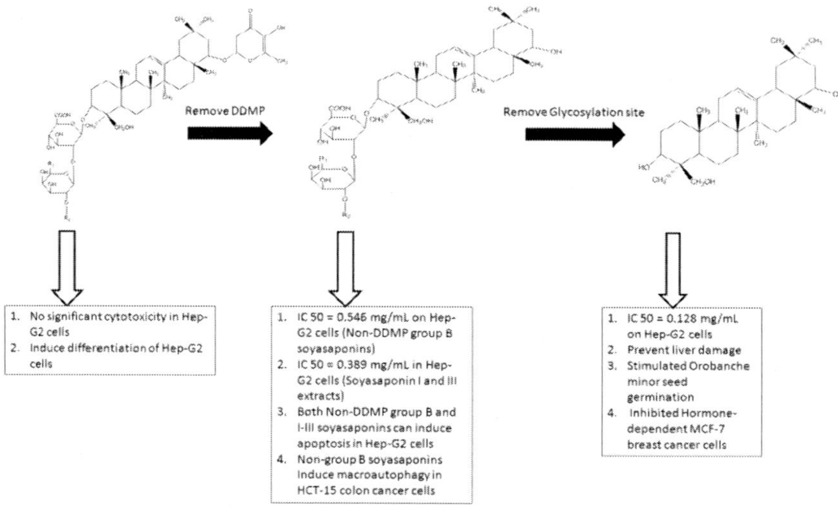

Figure 3. Relationship between biological activities of group B soyasaponins (DDMP, Non-DDMP and aglycone) and their chemical structures [9, 10, 13-16].

Biological Activity of Soyasapogenol

Soyasapogenol is the aglycone which does not contain any sugar moieties attached at glycosation sites. The aglycones are usually found as a result of soy bean product processing and are generally in very low amounts in soy bean (Figure 1). The aglycones have been reported to possess greater cytotoxicity compared to the respective soyasaponin glycosides. Soyasapogenol B was reported to inhibit hormone-dependent MCF-7 breast cancer cells, while soyasapogenol A stimulated this cell growth due to possible estrogenic activity [13]. We have reported that soyasapogenol A and B extracts inhibited Hep-G2 liver cancer cells and soyasapogenol A showed greater percentage of apoptotic cells compared to soyasapogenol B and mixture of group A soyasaponins [14]. We also found soyasapogenol B showed stronger cytotoxicity than their glycosides which is consistent with the literature [4].Soyasapogenol B derivatives bioactivity was increased with the replacement of the C-22 hydroxyl moiety with an acyloxy or alkyloxy group and by elimination all of hydroxyl group [15].

We speculate that future research with will fall into two research strategies, one is to purify soyasapogenols from soyasaponins for biological testing in sufficient amounts and another is to synthesis special modified soyasapogenols with enhanced biological activity. Overall soyasaponins are diverse and possess complex chemical structures that are often very similar to each other. The biological effects are diverse and tend to be dependent on chemical structure with minor changes in chemical composition can alter these effects. It seems that the soyasaponins may be important dietary components that can confer chemo-protective properties. More research is needed to fully characterize the individual biological effects of each of the main triterpenoids before we can fully understand if there is indeed a structure function relationship.

REFERENCES

[1] Yoshiki, Y.; Kudou, S.; Okubo, K. Relationship between chemical structures and biological activities of triterpenoid saponins from soybean. *Bioscience Biotechnology and Biochemistry* (1998), *62*, 2291-2299.

[2] Lasztity, R.; Hidevegi, M.; Bata, A. Saponins in food. *Food Reviews International* (1998), *14*, 371-390.

[3] Zhang, W.; Popovich, D. G. Chemical and Biological Characterization of Oleanane Triterpenoids from Soy. *Molecules* (2009), *14*, 2959-2975.

[4] Gurfinkel, D. M.; Rao, A. V. Soyasaponins: The Relationship Between Chemical Structure and Colon Anticarcinogenic Activity. *Nutrition and Cancer* (2003), *47*, 24-33.

[5] Yoshiki, Y.; Kinumi, M.; Kahara, T.; Okubo, K. Chemiluminescence of soybean saponins in the presence of active oxygen species. *Plant Science* (1996), *116*, 125-129.

[6] Shiraiwa, M.; Harada, K.; Okubo, K. Composition and structure of group B saponin in soybeen seed. *Agricultural and Biological Chemistry* (1991), *55*, 911-917.

[7] Zhang, W.; Popovich, D. G. Bioactivity of Oleanane Triterpenoids from Soy (*Glycine max* Merr) Depends on the Chemical Structure. In *Legumes: Properties, Consumption and Nutrition*, Nova Science Publishers : 2010; p in press.

[8] Pei, Y. Apoptosis effects on human esophageal cancer cells by soyasaponin Bb and its machanism. *Wei Sheng Yan Jiu* (2010), *39*, 444-446.

[9] Zhang, W.; Popovich, D. G. Group B Oleanane Triterpenoid Extract Containing Soyasaponins I and III from Soy Flour Induces Apoptosis in Hep-G2 Cells. *Journal of Agricultural and Food Chemistry* (2010), *58*, 5315-5319.

[10] Zhang, W.; Yeo, M. C.; Tang, F. Y.; Popovich, D. G. Bioactive responses of Hep-G2 cells to soyasaponin extracts differs with respect to extraction conditions. *Food and Chemical Toxicology* (2009), *47*, 2202-2208.

[11] Wink, M. Evolutionary advantage and molecular modes of action of multi-component mixtures used in phytomedicine. *Current Drug Metabolism* (2008), *9*, 996-1009.

[12] Kinjo, J.; Imagire, M.; Udayama, M.; Arao, T.; Nohara, T. Studies on the hepatoprotective drugs part 3 - Studies on the constituents of the leguminous plants part 56 - Structure-hepatoprotective relationships study of soyasaponins I-IV having soyasapogenol B as aglycone. *Planta Medica* (1998), *64*, 233-236.

[13] Rowlands, J. C.; Berhow, M. A.; Badger, T. M. Estrogenic and antiproliferative properties of soy sapogenols in human breast cancer cells in vitro. *Food and Chemical Toxicology* (2002), *40*, 1767-1774.

[14] Zhang, W.; Popovich, D. G. Effect of Soyasapogenol A and Soyasapogenol B Concentrated Extracts on Hep-G2 Cell Proliferation and Apoptosis. *Journal of Agricultural and Food Chemistry* (2008), *56*, 2603-2608.

[15] Sasaki, K.; Minowa, N.; Kuzuhara, H.; Nishiyama, S. Preventive effects of soyasapogenol B derivatives on liver injury in a concanavalin A-induced hepatitis model. *Bioorganic & Medicinal Chemistry* (2005), *13*, 4900-4911.

[16] Evidente, A.; Cimmino, A.; Fernández-Aparicio, M.; Rubiales, D.; Andolfi, A.; Melck, D. Soyasapogenol B and trans-22-dehydrocam- pesterol from common vetch (Vicia sativa L.) root exudates stimulate broomrape seed germination. *Pest Management Science* (2011), n/a.

In: Saponins: Properties, Applications and Health Benefits ISBN: 978-1-62100-942-9
Editors: Rani Koh and Isaac Tay

Chapter 8

OCCURRENCE AND PROPERTIES OF SAPONINS WITHIN THE FAMILY CHENOPODIACEAE

***Tiwatt Kuljanabhagavad*[*1] *and Michael Wink*[2]**

[1]Bioorganic Chemistry Research Laboratories, Faculty of Science and Technology, Suan Dusit Rajabhat University, Bangkok, Thailand

[2]Department of Biology, Institute of Pharmacy and Molecular Biotechnology, Heidelberg University, Heidelberg, Germany

1. INTRODUCTION

Saponins are a group of glycosides which is widely distributed in the plant kingdom [1-3]; however, certain lower marine animals such as sea cucumbers and starfish also contain these compounds [4-6]. They represent a diverse group of chemical compounds which are characterized by a steroid or triterpenoid nucleus to whichone or more carbohydrate chains are attached. The structural diversity of Saponins is reflected in their physicochemical and biological properties which areexploited in several traditions and industrial applications [7-11]. The plant extracts containing saponins have been widely used in food and industrial applications mainly as surface active and foaming agents [12]. The saponins in foods have traditionally been considered as antinutritional factors [13, 14] which as in quinoa (*Chenopodium quinoa* Willd.) have limited their use due to their bitter taste [15].

Saponins are classified as steroid or triterpenoid saponins depending upon the nature of the aglycone [16]. The aglycone of steroid saponins is usually a spirostanol or a furostanol [17]. Another class of saponins which are called basic steroid saponins (such as solanine) contain nitrogen analogues of steroid sapogenins as aglycones [18]. The hydrophilic parts of these compounds are carbohydrate chains, arranged either in a linear or branched fashion, attached to hydroxyl groups through an acetal linkage. The sites of carbohydrate chains attachment could be at C3; they are called monodesmosidic saponins [19]. When attached to both at C3 and C28 positions they aretermed bidesmosidic saponins [20]. Rarely, saponins

*Bioorganic Chemistry Research Laboratories, Faculty of Science and Technology, Suan Dusit Rajabhat University, 228-228/1-3 Sirithon Road, Bangplad District, Bangkok 10700, Thailand, E-mail address: ktiwatt@gmail.com

with three sugar chains at C3, C23, and C28 occur, the so-called tridesmosidic saponins [21, 22]. In some species of the genus *Chenopodium* such *Chenopodium ambrosioides* L. [23] and *C. anthelminticum* L. [24] have a carbohydrate chain attached at C22. The saponin type of Chenopodiaceae is almost completely based on β-amyrin. The most common aglycones in the family are; oleanolic acid, phytolaccagenic acid, hederagenin, serjanic acid, gypsogenin and echinocystic acid which carryhydroxyl and carboxylate groups at C3 and C28, respectively. In *C. quinoa* Willd., the saponin can be divided into three groups, the monodesmosides that contain a single oligosaccharide, typically attached with a glycosidic bond at C3 of phytolaccagenic acid (e.g. 3-*O*-β-D-Glucopyranosyl-(1→3)-α-L-arabinopyranosyl phytolaccagenic acid) (**42**) and the bisdesmosides that contain acetal- and ester-linked oligosaccharides, typically at C3 and C28 of gypsogenin (e.g. 3β-[(*O*-β-D-Glucopyranosyl-(1→3)-α-L-arabinopyranosyl)oxy]-23-oxo-olean-12-en-28-oic acid β-D-glucopyranoside (**66**) and the tridesmosides that contain three oligosaccharides, typically at C3, C23, and C28 of hederagenin (e.g. 3,23-bis(*O*-β-D-Glucopyranosyloxy) olean-12-en-28-oic acid 28-*O*-α-L-arabinopyanosyl (1→3) β-D-glucopyranosyl ester (**69**) (see Fig. 1).

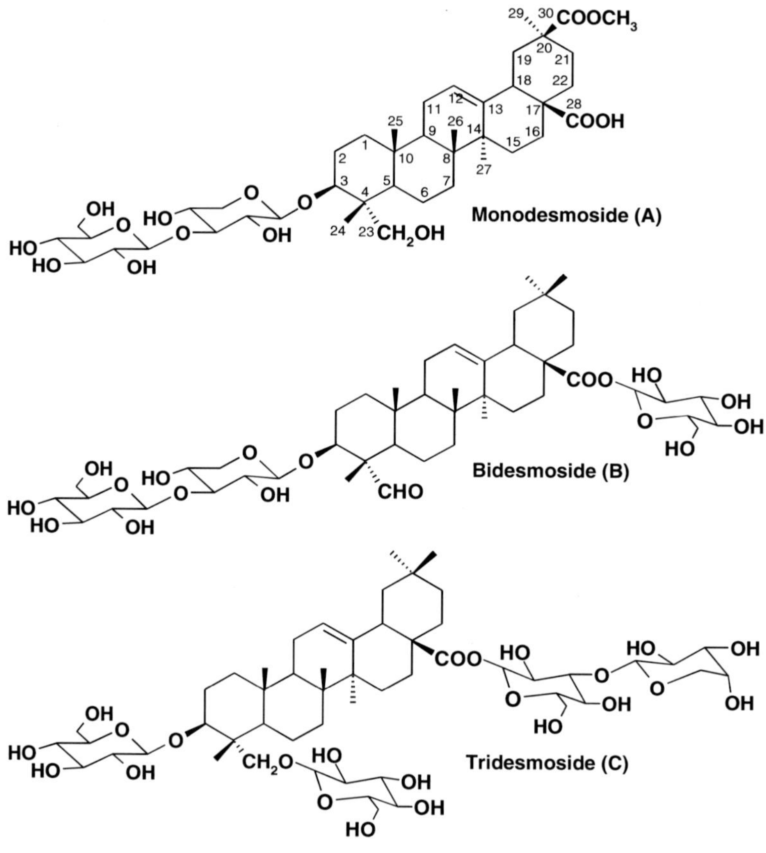

Figure 1. Monodesmosidic saponin(A); 3-*O*-β-D-Glucopyranosyl-(1→3)-α-L-arabinopyranosyl phytolaccagenic acid (**42**), Bidesmoside (B); 3β-[(*O*-β-D-Glucopyranosyl-(1→3)-α-L-arabinopyranosyl)oxy]-23-oxo-olean-12-en-28-oic acid β-D-glucopyranoside (**66**), and Tridesmoside (C); 3,23-bis(*O*-β-D-Glucopyranosyloxy) olean-12-en-28-oic acid 28-*O*-α-L-arabinopyanosyl-(1→3)-β-D-glucopyranosyl ester (**69**) saponins of *Chenopodium quinoa* Willd.

Members of Chenopodiaceae family are particularly successful in dry and saline areas [25]. They are common in temperate and tropical regions around the world. The family forms a close alliance with the mainly tropical Amaranthaceae [26]. Many plants of are often intimately involved with the daily life of people. Leafy vegetables and pseudocereals are present in this family, namely sugar beet (*Beta vulgaris* L.), spinach (*Spinacia oleracea* L.) and quinoa (*Chenopodium quinoa* Willd.), which are rich sources of essential amino acids, sugars, polyunsaturated fatty acids, vitamins, minerals, and trace elements [27]. Many plant species of this family synthesize triterpenoid saponins as part of their normal program of growth and development, often sequestering them in tissues where they protect the plant from herbivores and pathogens. Triterpenoid saponins-containing plants carry substances which can be toxic to animals. These plant glycosides form a soapy foam when shaken in water and act as emulsifying agents. Foam formation has been used for a long time to identify plants with saponins and for quantification of saponins.

All known classes of triterpenoid saponins have reported from the Chenopodiaceae. The main saponin-containing genus is *Chenopodium*, characterized by the predominant occurrence of triterpenoid saponins; other genera include *Kochia*, *Atriplex*, and *Spinacia*. Another excellent source of triterpenoid saponins is the genus *Salsola*. Many species in the genus *Chenopodium* contain triterpenoid saponins with oleanolic acid and hederagenin as the predominant aglycone. There are numerous structural derivatives of the oleanane skeleton and a number of these are shown in Table 1. A review article by Kokanova-Nedialkova and co-workers (2009) gives references and further examples, together with physical constants, of both oleananes and other triterpenes [28]. Mahato and co-workers have published lists of recently isolated triterpenes with their physical constants and plant sources [29, 30]. Oleanane triterpenes have been the subject of an update by Dinda and co-workers, covering various aspects of their occurrence, chemistry, and biological activities [31]. A review of recently reported data on the chemistry and biodiversity of the biologically active natural glycosides is provided by Dembitsky (2004) [32]. Another authoritative source of information on the saponins in food, feedstuffs and medicinal plants is the book written by Lacaille-Dubois (2000) [33].

Plant saponins include a large number of biologically and pharmacologically active compounds. Depending on their chemical and physical properties and the arrangement of the carbohydrate chains and types of sugar showed hemolytic, antibacterial, antifungal, membrane depolarizing antioxidant, apoptotic, anti-inflammatory, antinociceptive, and antiallergic activities [34-37]. The hemolytic and antifungal activities of monodesmosidic saponins of *C. quinoa* was reported by Woldemichael and Wink (2001). Apoptosis induction and cytotoxicity of bidesmosidic triterpenoid saponins and their aglycone (gypsogenin) from *C. quinoa* was reported by Kuljanabhagavad et al.,(2008) [20]. Anti-inflammatory activities of monodesmosidic triterpenoid saponins with oleanolic acid as aglycone was reported by Mujica as early as 1994 [38]. The antinociceptive, anti-inflammatory and antiallergic activities of monodesmosidic saponins from dried fruits of *Kochia scoparia* L. were reported by Matsuda and co-workers, 1997 [39]. From a medicinal point of view, the genera *Atriplex*, *Beta*, *Chenopodium*, *Kochia*, and *Spinacia* are the most important plants of the family Chenopodiaceae.

2. Molecular Properties

Plants produce a high diversity of structurally differing secondary metabolites that have advantageous ecological functions for the plants producing them, and many of these molecules also have nutritional, biological and pharmacological properties useful for humans and animals. Many secondary metabolites protect plant against herbivores and microbial pathogens.Triterpenoid saponins represent the largest and most diverse groups of plant natural products, with more than 5,000 known structures [40]. Several plants from the Chenopodiaceae are known for their medicinal value around the world [41] and several saponins have been isolated from this family with anti-edemic properties. Some plants such as *Chenopodium ambrosioides* L. and *C. multifidum* L., which contain some triterpenoid saponins and flavonoids glycosides, are used to treat diabetes and hypercholesterolemia [42].

In Chenopodiaceae family, the members of the family produce many glycosides plants including saponins and flavonoid glycosides [43, 44]. Triterpenoid saponins of the family possess one, two or three carbohydrate chains attached to the aglycone, and the terms monodesmosidic, bidesmosidic or tridesmosidic saponins have been given to them, respectively. The aglycone is called "sapogenin" or "genin" which are the non-polar part of the molecule, may have a triterpenoid or steroid backbone (see Fig. 2).

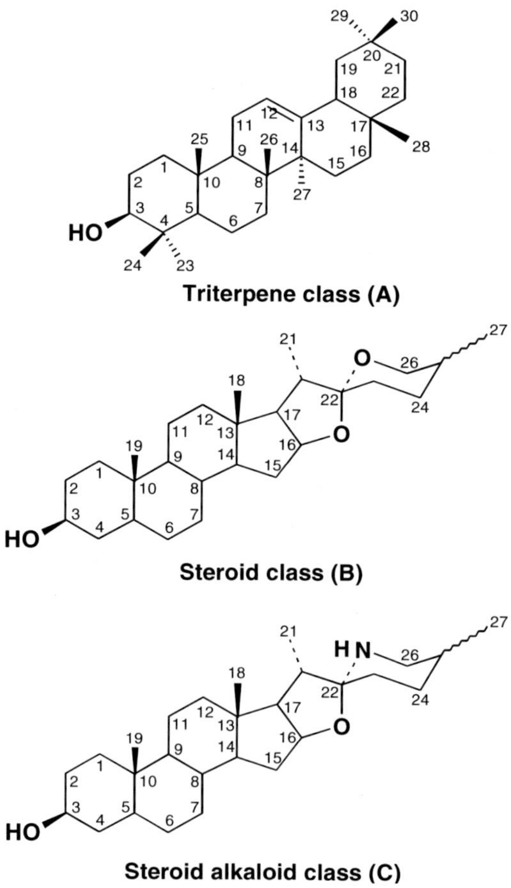

Figure 2. Structure of the genin present in the saponins (**A**), steroid (**B**) and steroid alkaloid (**C**).

Monodesmosidic saponins (**A**) and bidesmosidic saponins (**B**) are can be found in various species in the plant kingdom; tridesmosidic saponin (**C**) are rarely found in the nature (see Fig. 1). Tridesmosidic saponins have been detected in three plant species of the different families including *Medicago sativa* L. (Fabaceae), *Chenopodium quinoa* Willd. (Chenopodiaceae) and *Rhoiptelea chiliantha* Diels *et* Hand.-Mazz (Rhoipteleaceae). Six tridesmoside saponins such as zahnic acid were isolated from the aerial parts of *Medicago sativa* L. [22]; quinoside A was isolated from the seeds of *C. quinoa* Willd. [21]; rhoiptelesides A, B, C, and D were isolated from the leaves of *Rhoiptelea chiliantha* Diels *et* Hand.-Mazz, respectively [45, 46].

Triterpenoid saponin content depends on factors such as the cultivar, growing conditions, age and temperatures at harvest, and the geographical location of the plant. There can be considerable variation in composition and quantity of triterpenoid saponins in plant material from different places, as documented for *Chenopodium quinoa* (quinoa), *Chenopodium pallidicaule* (kañiwa) [47] and *Spinacia oleracea* (spinach) [48]. Considering triterpenoid saponins of quinoa, which are mainly oleanolic acid and oleanolic acid derivatives, they can be divided into seven major aglycone classes (see Fig. 3), including oleanolic acid (**I**), hederagenin (**II**), phytolaccagenic acid (**III**), serjanic acid (**IV**), 3β-hydroxy-23-oxo-olean-12-en -28-oic acid (=Gypsogenin) (**V**), 3β-hydroxy-27-oxo-olean-12-en-28-oic acid (**VI**), and 3β, 23α, 30β-trihydroxy-olean-12-en-28-oic acid (**VII**). The monodesmosidic saponins of *C. quinoa* Willd. carry a carbohydrate chain attached to C3 of the aglycone. Bidesmosides have two carbohydrate chains, most often with one attached through an ether linkage at C28. And also triterpenoid tridesmoside saponin can be found in this plant. Tridesmosidic saponins of quinoa have three carbohydrate chains linkage through glycoside, ether or ester bonds at the –OH or –COOH or –CH_2OH functional groups occurring on the aglycone. The most common monosaccharides appearing in the carbohydrate chains include: D-glucose (Glc), L-rhamnose (Rha), D-galactose (Gal), D-glucuronic acid (GlcUA), L-arabinose (Ara), D-xylose (Xyl) or D-fucose (Fuc). Because of the diversity of aglycones and carbohydrate side chains, many different saponin moleculars can be generated. Many plants of the family Chenopodiaceae produce complex mixtures of glycosides. The composition and the concentration can vary in various parts (roots, stems, leaves, flowers, fruits, and seeds) of the plant species and can be strongly influenced by multiple responses to environmental factor and the development the plant.

The complex mixtures of triterpenoid saponins can be changed during storage or processing, which in turn could modify their biological properties and pharmacologically activities. The glycosidic linkage of the carbohydrate chains to the aglycone by can be hydrolysed by-base/acidic treatment, using a reflux method or by enzymatic hydrolysis, resulting in the formation of aglycones, prosapogenins, carbohydrate residues or monosaccharides. The conventional alkaline hydrolysis, leads to cleavage of ester-linked carbohydrate chains to obtain prosapogenins, whereas under acid hydrolysis yields the aglycone and monosaccharides. The generation of monosaccharides or carbohydrate residues depends on the hydrolysis conditions. During enzymatic hydrolysis a specific cleavage of the glycosidic bond can be achieved. The solubility properties of the aglycone can be markedly different from the saponin due to its lipophilic nature. The solubility of saponins is affected by their composition, by pH, temperature, and the properties of the organic solvent. Mixtures of saponins or individual saponins can be extracted in water, alcohols such as methanol,

ethanol, and aqueous alcohols and organic solvents. Some oleanane saponins can be soluble in ether, chloroform, benzene, ethyl acetate, or glacial acetic acid. For the extraction of a complex crude triterpene saponin mixture of *Chenopodium quinoa* methanol water worked best.

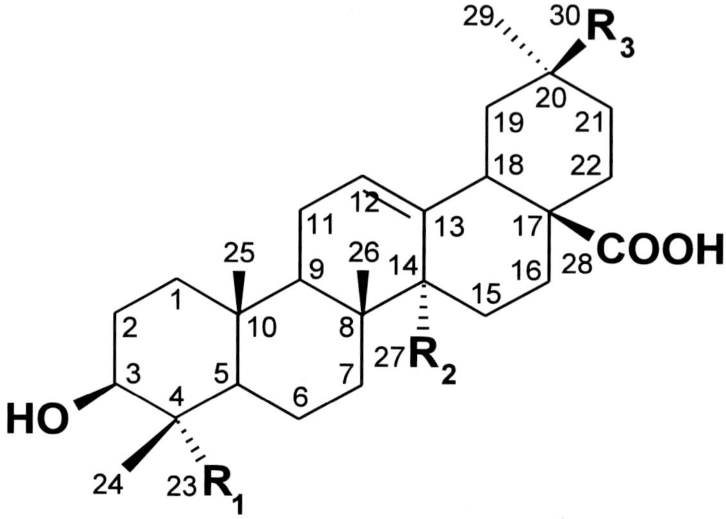

Aglycone	R_1	R_2	R_3	Formula	MW
Oleanolic acid (**I**)	CH_3	CH_3	CH_3	$C_{30}H_{48}O_3$	456
Hederagenin (**II**)	CH_2OH	CH_3	CH_3	$C_{30}H_{48}O_4$	472
Phytolaccagenic acid (**III**)	CH_2OH	CH_3	$COOCH_3$	$C_{31}H_{48}O_6$	516
Serjanic acid (**IV**)	CH_3	CH_3	$COOCH_3$	$C_{31}H_{48}O_5$	500
Gypsogenin (**V**)	CHO	CH_3	CH_3	$C_{30}H_{46}O_4$	470
3β-Hydroxy-27-oxo-olean-12-en-28-oic acid (**VI**)	CH_3	CHO	CH_3	$C_{30}H_{46}O_4$	470
3β,23α,30β-Trihydroxy-olean-12-en-28-oic acid (**VII**)	CH_2OH	CH_3	CH_2OH	$C_{30}H_{48}O_5$	488

Figure 3. Structure of the triterpene aglycones from *Chenopodium quinoa* Willd.

The amphiphilic nature of triterpenoid saponins is a dominant physical property in solution. Saponins exhibit a strong surface activity, form stable foams and act as emulsifying agents. They generally have a strong haemolytic and cytolytic activity and appear to form micelles with lipids in much the same way as detergents. These physical properties are exploited in most of the technological uses of saponins as in shampoos and carbonated drinks. Saponins are amphiphilic because they consist of a hydrophilic carbohydrate moiety and a hydrophobic genin or sapogenin. The presence of a carboxylic acid (–COOH) at C28 position in the triterpenoid saponins structure may strongly influence the surface activity because this functional group carries a negative charge under physiological conditions [49]. Triterpenoid saponins can possess from one to three straight or branched carbohydrate chains, the carbohydrate chains can contain one to several monosaccharide residues, and are usually attached at C3 position in monodesmosides. Monodesmosides, which are often poorly soluble in water in purified form, can be extracted readily due to the solubilizing effect of the co-occuring compounds [50]. The property of saponins to form micelles with lipids canaffect the solubilization of ingredients in cosmetic, food formulations or pharmaceutical preparations [51].

3. Occurrence and Properties

3.1. Family Chenopodiaceae

Saponins occur widely distributed in a large number of plant species, both wild plants and cultivated crops. Triterpenoid saponins dominate in dicotyledons while steroid saponins occur in monocotyledons. As mentioned earlier, steroid saponins have been detected inmembers of different families such as Agavaceae [52, 53], Dioscoraceae [54], Smilacaceae [55] and also other families. However, some plant species contain both steroid and triterpenoid saponins. Triterpenoid saponins are abundant in Araliaceae, Asteraceae, Caryophyllaceae, Chenopodiaceae, Fabaceae, Phytolaccaceae, Ranunculaceae, Rhamnaceae, Rhoipteleaceae, Sapindaceae as well as other families.

The Chenopodiaceae familyis one of the largest plant families and comprises 110 genera with more than 1,700 species which are widely distributed in tropical and subtropical area [56]. One of the great centers of diversity and richness of the family is Asia, especially China. The Chenopodiaceae are represented in the Flora of China by 42 genera and about 190 species [57]. This family mainly occurs in arid areas, desert, and coastal and saline habitats of North and South Africa, Asia, Australia, Europe, and North and South America. Most species of the Chenopodiaceae are annuals or subshrubs. Herbaceous perennials, shrubs, small trees, and lianas are restricted to only a few genera.

Chenopodiaceae include *Spinacia oleracea* L. and *Beta vulgaris* L. which are excellent vegetables. *Dysphania ambrosioides* L. and *Salsola collina* Pall. are used medicinally. *Agriophyllum squarrosum* (L.) Moq. is locally called sand-rice and is an edible plant. Seeds of *Corispermum declinatum* Steph. ex Iljin are used for producing gin. The ash of *Halogeton arachnoideus* Moq. and of some species of the genus *Salsola* contains soda which is used to make noodles. *Anabasis aphylla* L. can be used as an insecticide because it contains neurotoxic quinlizidine alkaloids. Many plants of this family are important as animal forage in desert, semidesert, and steppe regions, and some species are good windbreaks and soil binders. *Haloxylon ammodendron* C.A. Meyer has been used extensively in biological reconditioning of the desert. *Kochia scoparia* (L.) Schrader have also been employed for treatment of skin diseases in the Chinese medicine [39, 58] and for treatment of diabetes mellitus and rheumatoid arthritis in the Korean folk medicine in [59]. *Suaeda maritima* (L.) Dumort has been used against hepatitis [60]; it has antiviral activity due to the presence of triterpenoids and steroids [61]. In addition, Chenopodiaceae is a good source of many food plants, the mostly widely known species being *Chenopodium quinoa* (quinoa), which originated from South America but is cultivated in more than ten countries around the world (e.g. Argentina, Austria, Bolivia, Chile, Colombia, Equador, Germany, Mexico, Peru, Tibet, and United Kingdom).

Various alkaloids occur in the family Chenopodiaceae particularly in the tribe Salsoleae. Tetrahydroisoquinoline and β-carboline alkaloids have been reported from the dried plant of *Haloxylon articulatum* (Cav.) Bunge [62]. *Anabasis aphylla* L. produces quinolizidine alkaloids.Various flavonols and flavonoids have also been reported in genera of the family such as the *Anabasis*, *Atriplex*, *Beta*, *Chenopodium*, *Kochia*, and *Spinacia*. Members of Chenopodiaceae typically accumulate large quantities of oxalates and nitrates, which are sometimes converted into toxic nitrites [63, 64]. The spiny leaves and fruits, and the chemical constituents of other organs are known to cause skin irritation. The pollen of various weedy chenopods, such as the genus of *Ambrosia, Atriplex*, *Bassia*, and *Salsola* is known to be allergenic [65]. The genus *Chenopodium* is well-know for its application in the treatment of various ailments like pectoral complaints, cough, abdominal pain, pulmonary obstruction and nervous affections [66]. The high triterpenoid saponin content in Chenopodiaceae, such as from *Medicago sativa* L. can be interesting as a pharmaceutical against hypercholesterinaemia (Lucerne, alfalfa)[67].

The genus *Chenopodium* comprises about 250 species most of which are native to the Andean regions of South America and to Asia [68]. Some species are weed plants in Central America and many parts of Europe and Africa [69]. Leaves of some species of the genus *Chenopodium*, such as *Chenopodium murale* L. and *C. quinoa* Willd. are used for salads and vegetables respectively, while seeds of other *Chenopodium* species are used to improve the nutritional quality of snacks, bread, pastas, fermented drinks, and animal feed [70, 71]. In a breeding program of fifteen ecotypes of quinoa (*Chenopodium quinoa* Willd.) in the United Kingdom concentrations of three groups of the triterpenoid saponins have been analysed, including sapogenols, oleanolic acid, hederagenin and phytolaccagenic acid [72]. Furthermore, the occurrence and also chemical structures of triterpenoid saponins in many species of the genus *Chenopodium* have been reported in several chemical investigations such as for *Chenopodium ambrosioides* L. [23], *C. anthelminticum* L. [24], *C. album* L. [73], *C. ficifolium* Sm. [74], and *C. pallidicaule* Aellen [75].

The genus *Atriplex* withherbs or shrubs consists of about 250 species, which are widely distributed in temperate and tropical regions, often on saline and arid soils. Some are common weeds, like *Atriplex hortensis* L. Some species of the genus of this family such as *Atriplex nummularia* Lindley produce triterpenoid saponin [76, 77]. Moreover, the genus *Haloxylon* Bunge comprises of about 25 species [78]. They are distributed from Western Mediterranean region to Arabia, Iran, Mangolia, Burma, and Southwest of China [78]. In Saudi Arabia, *Haloxylon pericum* Bunge ex Boiss & Buhse. and *H. salicornicum* Bunge ex Boiss were reported in the documented to have folkloric uses [79]. *Haloxylon salicornicum* (Moq.) Bunge ex Bioss. has been used againstdiabetes [80], as an antiseptic and anti-inflammatory [81]. In Oman, the stems of *Haloxylon salicornicum* have been employed as a mordant for dyeing wool in traditional weaving [1]. In addition, *Hammada scoparia* Pomel. [=*Haloxylon articulatum*] have been used to treat eye disorders [82]. The Chenopodiaceae arerepresented in Egypt by 25 genera and about 300 species [83]. The genus *Salicornia*, especially the tetraploid species, was occasionally utilized as a vegetable in Europe. The seeds of *Salicornia bigelovii* Torr. from the United State are rich in oil that can be used on a large scale as a commercial source of vegetable oils.

3.2. Diversity of Saponins in the Family Chenopodiaceae

The wide chemical diversity of triterpene saponins detected in different species of the family Chenopodiaceae is documented in Table 1. Table 1 presents the extracted and characterized saponins from the last 40 years from nine genera such as *Atriplex*, *Bassia, Beta, Chenopodium, Climacoptera, Cornulaca, Kochia*, *Salsola*, and *Spinacia*. Triterpenoid saponins summarized in this table have been purified by different methods comprising liquid-liquid extractions with different organic solvents, solid phase extraction or chromatography (silica gel or an ion exchange resin), high performance liquid chromatography (HPLC) and high performance liquid chromatography-mass spectrometry (LC-MS). Mass spectrometry (MS)-based techniques and nuclear magnetic resonance (NMR) combined with chemical reactions and chemical evidence were used to elucidate the chemical structure of these saponins. More than 100 triterpenoid saponins have been reported from the Chenopodiaceae. From the viewpoint of triterpenoid saponins, note that the highly oxygenated 28,30-dicarboxyl-pentacyclic triterpenoids have been found in some genera of other families-such as *Phytolacca* (Phytolaccaceae) [84], *Mollugo* (Molluginaceae) [85], *Serjanica* [86] and *Talinum* (Portulacaceae) [87]. One triterpene aglycone i.e. gypsogenin has also been found in some genera such as *Arenaria* (Caryophyllaceae) [88], *Gypsophila* (Caryophyllaceae) [89], *Saponaria* (Caryophyllaceae) [90], *Anemone* (Ranunculaceae) [91], and *Akebia* (Lardizabalaceae) [92].

Table 1. Occurrence of monodesmosidic, bidesmosidic, and tridesmosidic triterpenoid saponins in species of the Chenopodiaceae

	Saponins	Plant part	References
Atriplex nummularia Lindley	*Monodesmosidic triterpenoid saponins*		
3β-*O* ← GlcUA	3-*O*-β-D-Glucuronopyranosyl hederagenin (**1**)	aerial part	[77]
3β-*O* ← GlcUA	3-*O*-β-D-Glucuronopyranosyl oleanolic acid (**2**)	aerial part	[77]
Atriplex semibaccata L.	*Monodesmosidic triterpenoid saponins*		
3β-*O* ← Gal^2 ← Glc	3-*O*-β-D-Glucopyranosyl-(1→2)-β-D-galactopyranosyl-11α-methoxy-23-hydroxylongispinogenin (**3**)	whole plant	[94]
3β-*O* ← Gal^2 ← Glc	3-*O*-β-D-Glucopyranosyl-(1→2)-β-D-galactopyranosyl-11α-methoxy-23,29-dihydroxylongispinogenin (**4**)	whole plant	[94]
3β-*O* ← Gal^2 ← Glc	3-*O*-β-D-Glucopyranosyl-(1→2)-β-D-galactopyranosyl-29-hydroxysaikogenin F (**5**)	whole plant	[94]
3β-*O* ← Gal^2 ← Glc	3-*O*-β-D-Glucopyranosyl-(1→2)-β-D-galactopyranosyl saikogenin F (**6**)	whole plant	[94]
Bassia muricata (L.) Murr.	*Monodesmosidic triterpenoid saponins*		
3β-*O* ← GlcUA	3-*O*-β-D-Glucuronopyranosyl oleanolic acid (**7**)	aerial part	[95]
Bassia muricata (L.) Murr.	*Bidesmosidic triterpenoid saponins*		
3β-*O* ← GlcUA 28-*O* ← Glc	3-*O*-β-D-Glucuronopyranosyl oleanolic acid 28-*O*-β-D-glucopyranosyl ester (**8**)	aerial part	[95]
3β-*O* ← GlcUA(6-OMe) 28-*O* ← Glc	3-*O*-β-D-Glucuronopyranosyl-6-*O*-methyl oleanolic acid 28-*O*-β-D-glucopyranosyl ester (**9**)	aerial part	[95]
3β-*O* ← Glc 28-*O* ← Glc	3-*O*-β-D-Glucopyranosyl oleanolic acid 28-*O*-β-D-glucopyranosyl ester (**10**)	aerial part	[95]
Beta vulgaris L.	*Monodesmosidic triterpenoid saponins*		
3β-*O*←GlcUA	3-*O*-β-D-Glucuronopyranosyl oleanolic acid (**11**)	beet molasses	[96]
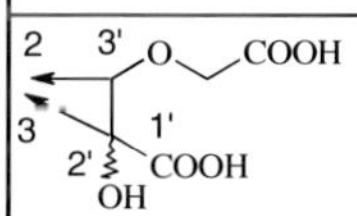 3β-*O* ← GlcUA	Betavulgarosides II (**12**)	root	[97]
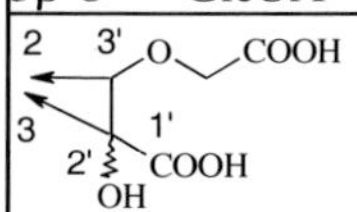 3β-*O* ← GlcUA	Betavulgarosides IV (**13**)	root	[97]

Table 1. (Continued)

	Saponins	Plant part	References
Beta vulgaris L.	*Monodesmosidic triterpenoid saponins*		
3β-*O* ← GlcUA^2 ← Glc ^{3}↑ Xyl	3-*O*-[β-D-Glucopyranosyl-(1→2)-(β-D-xylopyranosyl-(1→3))-β-D-glucuronopyranosyl-3β-hydroxyolean-12-en-28-oic acid (**14**)	beet molasses	[96]
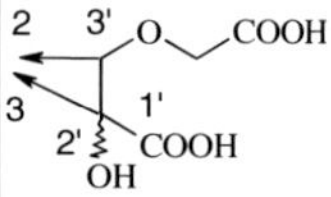 3β-*O* ← GlcUA	Betavulgarosides VII (**15**)	leaves, root	[98]
Beta vulgaris L.	*Bidesmosidic triterpenoid saponins*		
3β-*O* ← GlcUA^2 ← Glc ^{3}↑ Xyl 28-*O* ← Glc	3-*O*-[β-D-Glucopyranosyl-(1→2)-(β-D-xylopyranosyl-(1→3))-β-D-glucuronopyranosyl]-28-*O*-β-D-glucopyranosyl-3β-hydroxyolean-12-en-28-oic acid (**16**)	beet molasses	[96]
3β-*O* ← GlcUA 28-*O* ← Glc	3-*O*-β-D-Glucuronopyranosyl oleanolic acid 28-*O*-β-D-glucopyranosyl ester (**17**)	root	[97]
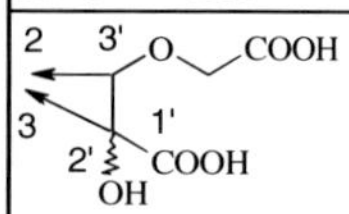 3β-*O* ← GlcUA 28-*O* ← Glc	Betavulgarosides I (**18**)	root	[97]
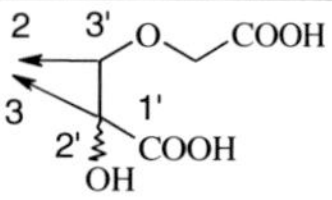 3β-*O* ← GlcUA 28-*O* ← Glc	Betavulgarosides III (**19**)	root	[97]
3β-*O* ← GlcUA^3 ← Xyl 28-*O* ← Glc	3-*O*-β-D-Xylopyranosyl-(1→3)-β-D-glucuronopyranosyl 29-exo-methylene-akebinoate 28-*O*-β-D-glucopyranosyl ester (**20**)	leaves, root	[98]
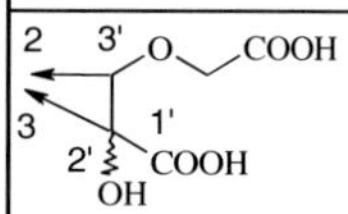 3β-*O* ← GlcUA 28-*O* ← Glc	Betavulgarosides VI (**21**)	leaves, root	[98]
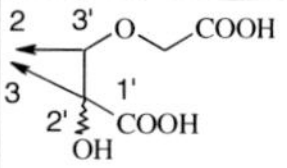 3β-*O* ← GlcUA 28-*O* ← Glc	Betavulgarosides VIII (**22**)	leaves, root	[98]
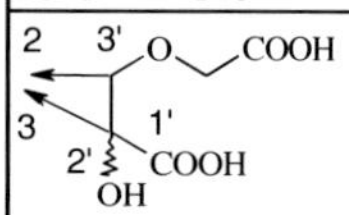 3β-*O* ← GlcUA ^{2}↑ Xyl 28-*O* ← Glc	Betavulgarosides IX (**23**)	leaves, root	[98]

	Saponins	Plant part	References
Beta vulgaris L.	*Bidesmosidic triterpenoid saponins*		
3β-*O* ← GlcUA^3 ← Xyl 28-*O* ← Glc	3-*O*-β-D-Xylopyranosyl-(1→3)-β-D-glucuronopyranosyl oleanolate 28-*O*-β-D-glucopyranosyl ester (**24**)	leaves, root	[98]
Chenopodium album L.	*Monodesmosidic triterpenoid saponins*		
3β-*O* ← GlcUA	3-*O*-β-D-Glucuronopyranosyl oleanolic acid (**25**)	root	[73]
3β-*O* ← GlcUA ← (3′-*O*-(2″-*O*-glycolyl)-glyoxylyl)	3-*O*-[3′-*O*-(2″-*O*-Glycolyl)-glyoxylyl β-D-glucuronopyranosyl] oleanolic acid (**26**)	root	[73]
Chenopodium album L.	*Bidesmosidic triterpenoid saponins*		
3β-*O* ← GlcUA 28-*O* ← Glc	3-*O*-β-D-Glucuronopyranosyl oleanolic acid 28-*O*-β-D-glucopyranosyl ester (**27**)	root	[73]
3β-*O* ← GlcUA^3 ← Ara 28-*O* ← Glc	3-*O*-α-L-Arabinopyranosyl-(1→3)-β-D-glucuronopyranosyl hederagenin 28-*O*-β-D-glucopyranosyl ester (**28**)	seed	[75]
3β-*O* ← Glc^4 ← Glc 28-*O* ← Glc	3-*O*-β-D-Glucopyranosyl-(1→4)-β-D-glucopyranosyl phytolaccagenic acid 28-*O*-β-D-glucopyranosyl ester (**29**)	seed	[75]
3β-*O* ← Glc^4 ← Glc^4 ← Glc 28-*O* ← Glc	3-*O*-β-D-Glucopyranosyl-(1→4)-β-D-glucopyranosyl)-(1→4)-β-D-gluconopyranosyl phytolaccagenic acid 28-*O*-β-D-glucopyranosyl ester (**30**)	seed	[75]
3β-*O* ← Glc 28-*O* ← Glc	3-*O*-β-D-Glucopyranosyl phytolaccagenic aid 28-*O*-β-D-glucopyranosyl ester (**31**)	seed	[75]
Chenopodium anthelminticum L.	*Monodesmosidic triterpenoid saponins*		
3β-*O* ← Xyl^6 ← Glc^2 ← Ara	3-*O*-β-D-Xylopyranosyl-(1→6)-β-D-glucopyranosyl-(1→2)-α-L-arabinopyranosyl echinocystic acid ester (**32**)	root	[24]
Chenopodium anthelminticum L.	*Bidesmosidic triterpenoid saponins*		
3β-*O* ← Ara^2 ← Glc^6 ← Xyl 28-*O* ← Glc^4 ← Rha	3-*O*-β-D-Xylopyranosyl (1→6)-β-D-glucopyranosyl-(1→2)-α-L-arabinopyranosyl echinocystic acid 28-*O*-β-D-glucopyranosyl-(1→4)-α-L-rhamnopyranosyl ester (**33**)	root	[24]
Chenopodium ficifolium Sm.	*Bidesmosidic triterpenoid saponins*		
3β-*O* ← GlcUA 28-*O* ← Glc	3-*O*-β-D-Glucuronopyranosyl oleanolic acid 28-*O*-β-D-glucopyranosyl ester (**34**)	aerial part	[74]
3β-*O* ← Glc 28-*O* ← GlcUA^2 ← Glc	3-*O*-β-D-Glucopyranosyl oleanolic acid 28-*O*-β-D-glucopyranosyl-(1→2)-β-D-glucuronopyranosyl ester (**35**)	aerial part	[74]
Chenopodium quinoa Willd.	*Monodesmoside triterpenoid saponins*		
3β-*O* ← GlcUA	3-*O*-β-D-Glucuronopyranosyl oleanolic acid (**36**)	seed	[99]
3β-*O* ← Glc	3-*O*-β-D-Glucopyranosyl oleanolic acid (**37**)	seed	[100]
3β-*O* ← GlcUA(6-OMe)^3 ← Xyl	3-*O*-β-D-Xylopyranosyl-(1→3)-6-*O*-methyl-β-D-glucuronopyranosyl oleanolic acid (**38**)	seed	[100]
3β-*O* ← GlcUA^3 ← Xyl	3-*O*-β-D-Xylopyranosyl-(1→3)-β-D-glucuronopyranosyl oleanolic acid (**39**)	seed	[100]
3β-*O* ← Glc	3-*O*-β-D-Glucopyranosyl hederagenin (**40**)	seed coat, seed, flower, fruit	[93]

Table 1. (Continued)

	Saponins	Plant part	References
Chenopodium quinoa Willd.	*Monodesmoside triterpenoid saponins*		
3β-*O* ← Ara^3 ← Glc	3-*O*-β-D-Glucopyranosyl-(1→3)-α-L-arabinopyranosyl hederagenin (**41**)	seed	[99]
3β-*O* ← Ara^3 ← Glc	3-*O*-β-D-Glucopyranosyl-(1→3)-α-L-arabinopyranosyl phytolaccagenic acid (**42**)	seed	[19, 99]
Chenopodium quinoa Willd.	*Bidesmosidic triterpenoid saponins*		
3β-*O* ← Ara^3 ← Glc^2 ← Glc 28-*O* ← Glc	3-*O*-β-D-Glucopyranosyl-(1→2)-β-D-glucopyranosyl-(1→3)-α-L-arabinopyranosyl oleanolic acid 28-*O*-β-D-glucopyranosyl ester (**43**)	seed coat, seed, flower, fruit seed coat seed	[20] [101] [99, 102]
3β-*O* ← Ara^3 ← Glc 28-*O* ← Glc	3-*O*-β-D-Glucopyranosyl-(1→3)-α-L-arabinopyranosyl oleanolic acid 28-*O*-β-D-glucopyranosyl ester (**44**)	seed coat, seed, flower, fruit seed coat seed	[20] [101] [99, 103]
3β-*O* ← GlcUA^3 ← Xyl 28-*O* ← Glc	3-*O*-β-D-Xylopyranosyl-(1→3)-β-D-glucuronopyranosyl oleanolic acid 28-*O*-β-D-glucopyranosyl ester (**45**)	seed coat, seed, flower, fruit seed	[20] [101, 102]
3β-*O* ← GlcUA 28-*O* ← Glc	3-*O*-β-D-Glucuronopyranosyl oleanolic acid 28-*O*-β-D-glucopyranosyl ester (**46**)	seed coat, seed, flower, fruit seed	[20] [19, 101, 104]
3β-*O* ← GlcUA^3 ← Ara 28-*O* ← Glc	3-*O*-α-L-Arabinopyranosyl-(1→3)-β-D-glucuronopyranosyl oleanolic acid 28-*O*-β-D-glucopyranosyl ester (**47**)	seed	[99, 101, 104]
3β-*O* ← Ara^3 ← Glc 28-*O* ← Glc	3-*O*-β-D-Glucopyranosyl-(1→3)-α-L-arabinopyranosyl hederagenin 28-*O*-β-D-glucopyranosyl ester (**48**)	seed coat, seed, flower, fruit seed	[20] [19, 99, 101] [105-107]
3β-*O* ← Gal^3 ← Glc 28-O ← Glc	3-*O*-β-D-Glucopyranosyl-(1→3)-α-L-galactopyranosyl hederagenin 28-*O*-β-D-glucopyranosyl ester (**49**)	seed coat, seed, flower, fruit seed	[20] [99, 101, 102]
3β-*O* ← GlcUA 28-*O* ← Glc	3-*O*-β-D-Glucuronopyranosyl hederagenin 28-*O*-β-D-glucopyranosyl ester (**50**)	seed coat, seed, flower, fruit seed	[20] [101, 102]
3β-*O* ← Ara 28-*O* ← Glc	3-*O*-α-L-Arabinopyranosyl hederagenin 28-*O*-β-D-glucopyranosyl ester (**51**)	seed coat, seed, flower, fruit seed	[20] [19, 101, 102]
3β-*O* ← GlcUA^3 ← Xyl 28-*O* ← Glc	3-*O*-β-D-Xylopyranosyl-(1→3)-β-D-glucuronopyranosyl hederagenin 28-*O*-β-D-glucopyranosyl ester (**52**)	seed	[101, 102]
3β-*O* ← Glc^4 ← Glc^4 ← Glc 28-*O* ← Glc	3-*O*-β-D-Glucopyranosyl-(1→4)-β-D-glucopyranosyl-(1→4)-β-D-glucopyranosyl hederagenin 28-*O*-β-D-glucopyranosyl ester (**53**)	seed	[101, 105]
3β-*O* ← Ara^3 ← Glc 28-*O* ← Glc	3-*O*-β-D-Glucopyranosyl-(1→3)-α-L-arabinopyranosyl phytolaccagenic acid 28-*O*-β-D-glucopyranosyl ester (**54**)	seed coat, seed, flower, fruit seed	[20] [19, 21, 99] [101, 103, 105] [107]

	Saponins	Plant part	References
Chenopodium quinoa Willd.	*Bidesmosidic triterpenoid saponins*		
3β-*O* ← Ara 28-*O* ← Glc	3-*O*-α-L-Arabinopyranosyl phytolaccagenic acid 28-*O*-*β*-D-glucopyranosyl ester (**55**)	seed coat, seed, flower, fruit seed	[20] [19, 99, 101, 104, 107]
3β-*O* ← Ara³ ← Glc² ← Glc 28-*O* ← Glc	3-*O*-β-D-Glucopyranosyl-(1→2)-β-D-glucopyranosyl-(1→3)-α-L-arabinopyranosyl phytolaccagenic acid 28-*O*-β-D-glucopyranosyl ester (**56**)	seed coat, seed, flower, fruit seed	[20] [101, 103, 107]
3β-*O* ← Gal³ ← Glc 28-*O* ← Glc	3-*O*-β-D-Glucopyranosyl-(1→3)-β-D-galactopyranosyl phytolaccagenic acid 28-*O*-β-D-glucopyranosyl ester (**57**)	seed coat, seed, flower, fruit seed	[20] [101, 107]
3β-*O* ← Glc⁴ ← Glc⁴ ← Glc 28-*O* ← Glc	3-*O*-β-D-Glucopyranosyl-(1→4)-β-D-glucopyranosyl-(1→4)-β-D-glucopyranosyl phytolaccagenic acid 28-*O*-β-D-glucopyranosyl ester (**58**)	seed coat, seed, flower, fruit seed	[20] [101, 105]
3β-*O* ← Glc² ← Xyl³ ← Glc 28-*O* ← Glc	3-*O*-β-D-Glucopyranosyl-(1→3)-β-D-xylopyranosyl-(1→2)-β-D-glucopyranosyl phytolaccagenic acid 28-*O*-β-D-glucopyranosyl ester (**59**)	seed	[101-103]
3β-*O* ← GlcUA³ ← Ara 28-*O* ← Glc	3-*O*-α-L-Arabinopyranosyl-(1→3)-β-D-glucuronopyranosyl phytolaccagenic acid 28-*O*-β-D-glucopyranosyl ester (**60**)	seed	[103, 105]
3β-*O* ← Ara³ ← Glc² ← Glc 28-*O* ← Glc	3-*O*-β-D-Glucopyranosyl-(1→2)-β-D-glucopyranosyl-(1→3)-α-L-arabinopyranosyl serjanic acid 28-*O*-β-D-glucopyranosyl ester (**61**)	seed coat, seed, flower, fruit seed	[20] [99, 102, 103]
3β-*O* ← Ara³ ← Glc 28-*O* ← Glc	3-*O*-β-D-Glucopyranosyl-(1→3)-α-L-arabinopyranosyl serjanic acid 28-*O*-β-D-glucopyranosyl ester (**62**)	seed coat, seed, flower, fruit seed	[20] [99, 101, 104]
3β-*O* ← Ara 28-*O* ← Glc	3-*O*-α-L-Arabinopyranosyl serjanic acid 28-*O*-β-D-glucopyranosyl ester (**63**)	seed coat, seed, flower, fruit	[20]
3β-*O* ← GlcUA 28-*O* ← Glc	3-*O*-β-D-Glucuronopyranosyl serjanic acid 28-*O*-β-D-glucopyranosyl ester (**64**)	seed coat, seed, flower, fruit	[20]
3β-*O* ← GlcUA³ ← Ara 28-*O* ← Glc	3-*O*-α-L-Arabinopyranosyl-(1→3)-β-D-glucuronopyranosyl serjanic acid 28-*O*-β-D-glucopyranosyl ester (**65**)	seed	[105]
3β-*O* ← Ara³ ← Glc 28-*O* ← Glc	3β-[(*O*-β-D-Glucopyranosyl-(1→3)-α-L-arabinopyranosyl)oxy]-23-oxo-olean-12-en-28-oic acid β-D-glucopyranoside (**66**)	seed coat, seed, flower, fruit	[20]
3β-*O* ← Ara³ ← Glc 28-*O* ← Glc	3β-[(*O*-β-D-Glucopyranosyl-(1→3)-α-L-arabinopyranosyl)oxy]-27-oxo-olean-12-en-28-oic acid β-D-glucopyranoside (**67**)	seed coat, seed, flower, fruit	[20]
3β-*O* ← Ara³ ← Glc 28-*O* ← Glc	3-*O*-β-D-Glucopyranosyl-(1→3)-α-L-arabinopyranosyl-3, 23, 30-trihydroxyolean 12 en-28-oic acid 28-*O*-β-D-glucopyranosyl ester (**68**)	seed coat, seed, flower, fruit seed	[20] [101]

Table 1. (Continued)

	Saponins	Plant part	References
Chenopodium quinoa Willd.	*Tridesmosidic triterpenoid saponins*		
3β-*O* ← Glc 23α-*O* ← Glc 28-*O* ← Ara^3 ← Glc	3,23-bis(*O*-β-D-Glucopyranosyloxy) olean-12-en-28-oic acid 28-*O*-α-L-arabinopyanosyl-(1→3)-β-D-glucopyranosyl ester (**69**)	seed	[21]
Chenopodium pallidicaule Aellen	*Bidesmosidic triterpenoid saponins*		
3β-*O* ← GlcUA^3 ← Ara 28-*O* ← Glc	Hederagenin 3-*O*-[α-L-arabinopyranosyl-(1→3)-β-D-glucuronopyranosyl]-28-*O*-β-D-glucopyranoside (**70**)	seed	[75]
3β-*O* ← Glc^4 ← Glc ^{4}↑ Glc 28-*O* ← Glc	Phytolaccagenic acid 3-*O*-[β-D-glucopyranosyl-(1→4)-β-D-glucopyranosyl]-28-*O*-β-D-glucopyranoside (**71**)	seed	[75]
3β-*O* ← Glc^4 ← Glc^4 ← Glc 28-*O* ← Glc	Phytolaccagenic acid 3-*O*-[β-D-glucopyranosyl-(1→4)-β-D-glucopyranosyl-(1→4)-β-D-glucopyranosyl]-28-*O*-β-D-glucopyranoside (**72**)	seed	[75]
3β-*O* ← Glc 28-*O* ← Glc	Phytolaccagenic acid-3-*O*-β-D-glucopyranosyl-28-*O*-β-D-glucopyranoside (**73**)		[75]
3β-*O* ← Glc^2 ← Glc ^{4}↑ Glc 28-*O* ← Glc	Oleanolic acid 3-*O*-[2′-4′-di-*O*-(β-D-glucopyranosyl)-β-D-glucopyranosyl]-28-*O*-β-D-glucopyranoside (**74**)	seed	[75]
3β-*O* ← GlcUA^3← Ara 28-*O* ← Glc	Oleanolic acid 3-*O*-[α-L-arabinopyranosyl-(1→3)-β-D-glucuronopyranosyl]-28-*O*-β-D-glucopyranoside (**75**)	seed	[75]
3β-*O* ← Glc 28-*O* ← Glc	Oleanolic acid 3-*O*-β-D-glucopyranosyl-28-*O*-β-D-glucopyranoside (**76**)	seed	[75]
Climacoptera aralensis (Iljin) Botsch.	*Bidesmosidic triterpenoid saponins*		
3β-*O* ← GlcUA^2 ← Xyl ^{3}↑ Xyl 28-*O* ← Glc	Oleanolic acid 3-*O*-[β-D-xylopyranosyl-(1→2)-[β-D-xylopyranosyl-(1→3)]-β-D-glucuronopyranosyl-28-*O*-β-D-glucopyranoside (**77**)	aerial part	[108]
Climacoptera obtusifolia (Schrenk) Botsch.	*Bidesmosidic triterpenoid saponins*		
3β-*O* ← Xyl^3 ← Glc 28-*O* ← Glc	3-*O*-β-D-Xylopyranosyl-(1→3)-β-D-glucopyranosyl gypsogenin-28-*O*-β- D-glucopyranosyl ester (**78**)	aerial part	[109]
3β-*O* ← Xyl^3 ← Glc 28-*O* ← Glc	3-*O*-β-D-xylopyranosyl-(1→3)-β-D-glucopyranosyl hederagenin-28-*O*-β-D-glucopyranosyl ester (**79**)	aerial part	[109]
Climacoptera lanata (Schrenk.) Botsch.	*Bidesmosidic triterpenoid saponins*		
3β-*O* ← GlcUA^2 ← Xyl ^{3}↑ Xyl 28-*O* ← Glc	Oleanolic acid 3-*O*-[β-D-xylopyranosyl-(1→2)-[β-D-xylopyranosyl-(1→3)]-β-D-glucuronopyranosyl-28-*O*-β-D-glucopyranoside (**80**)	aerial part	[108]

	Saponins	Plant part	References
Climacoptera transoxana (Iljin) Botsch.	*Monodesmosidic triterpenoid saponins*		
3β-*O*←GlcUA	3-*O*-β-D-Glucuronopyranosyl hederagenin (**81**)	epigeal part	[110]
3β-*O* ← Xyl^2 ← Glc	3-*O*-β-D-Glucopyranosyl-(1→2)-β-D-xylopyranosyl hederagenin (**82**)	epigeal part	[110]
Climacoptera transoxana (Iljin) Botsch.	*Bidesmosidic triterpenoid saponins*		
3β-*O*←GlcUA 28-*O*←Glc	3-*O*-β-D-Glucuronopyranosyl gypsogenic acid 28-*O*-β-D-glucopyranosyl ester (**83**)	epigeal part	[111]
3β-*O* ← Xyl^2 ← GlcUA 28-*O* ← Glc	3-*O*-β-D-Glucuronopyranosyl-(1→2)-β-D-xylopyranosyl gypsogenic acid 28-*O*-β-D-glucopyranosyl ester (**84**)	epigeal part	[111]
3β-*O* ← Xyl^2 ← GlcUA 28-*O* ← Glc	3-*O*-β-D-Glucuronopyranosyl-(1→2)-β-D-xylopyranosyl hederagenin 28-*O*-β-D-glucopyranosyl ester (**85**)	epigeal part	[112]
3β-*O* ← Xyl^4 ← GlcUA 28-*O* ← Glc	3-*O*-β-D-Glucuronopyranosyl-(1→4)-β-D-xylopyranosyl-(1→2)-β-D-xylopyranosyl oleanolic acid 28-*O*-β-D-glucopyranosyl ester (**86**)	epigeal part	[113]
3β-*O* ← Xyl^2 ← Xyl^4 ← Glc 28-*O* ← Glc	3-*O*-β-D-Glucopyranosyl-(1→4)-β-D-xylopyranosyl-(1→2)-β-D-xylopyranosyl hederagenin 28-*O*-β-D-glucopyranosyl ester (**87**)	epigeal part	[113]
Cornulaca monacantha Delile	*Monodesmosidic triterpenoid saponins*		
3β-*O* ← $GlcUA^3$ ← Xyl	3-*O*-[β-Xylopyranosyl-(1→3)-β-glucuronopyranosyl]-30-methyl phytolaccagenate (**88**)	aerial part	[114]
Cornulaca monacantha Delile	*Bidesmosidic triterpenoid saponins*		
3β-*O* ← $GlcUA^3$ ← Xyl 28-*O* ← Glc	3-*O*-[β-Xylopyranosyl-(1→3)-β-glucuronopyranosyl]-30-methyl phytolaccagenate 28-*O*-β-glucopyranoside (**89**)	aerial part	[114]
3β-*O* ← $GlcUA^3$ ← Xyl 28-*O* ← Glc	3-*O*-[β-Xylopyranosyl-(1→3)-β-glucuronopyranosyl]-30-methyl serjanate 28-*O*-β-glucopyranoside (**90**)	aerial part	[114]
Kochia scoparia (L.) Schrader	*Monodesmosidic triterpenoid saponins*		
3β-*O* ← $GlcUA^2$ ← Rib	3-*O*-β-D-ribopyranosyl-(1→2)-β- D-glucuronopyranosyl oleanolic acid (**91**)	fruits	[115]
3β-*O* ← GlcUA	3-*O*-β-D-Glucuronopyranosyl oleanolic acid (**92**)	fruit	[59, 116] [117]
3β-*O* ← GlcUA(6-OMe)	3-*O*-β-D-Glucuronopyranosyl-6-*O*-methyl oleanolic acid (**93**)	fruit	[59, 117]
3β-*O*←GlcUA	3-*O*-β-D-Glucuronopyranosyl 22α-hydroxyoleanolic acid (**94**)	fruit	[116]
3β-*O*←$GlcUA^3$ ← Ara	3-*O*-α-L-Arabinopyranosyl-(1→3)-β-D-glucuronopyranosyl oleanolic acid (**95**)	fruit	[116]
3β-*O* ← $GlcUA^2$ ← Glc ^{3}↑ Xyl	3β-[(*O*-β-D-Glucopyranosyl (1→2)][β D xylopyranosyl-(1→3)] β-D-Glucuronopyranosyl morolic acid (**96**)	fruit	[116]
3β-*O* ← $GlcUA^3$ ← Xyl	3-*O*-β-D-Xylopyranosyl-(1→3)-β-D-glucuronopyranosyl-3β,12α-dihydroxyolean-28,13β-olide (**97**)	fruit	[116]

Table 1. (Continued)

	Saponins	Plant part	References
Kochia scoparia (L.) Schrader	*Monodesmosidic triterpenoid saponins*		
3β-*O* ← GlcUA^{3} ← Xyl	3-*O*-β-D-Xylopyranosyl-(1→3)-β-D-glucuronopyranosyl betulinic acid (**98**)	fruit	[116]
3β-*O* ← GlcUA^{3} ← Xyl	3-*O*-β-D-Xylopyranosyl-(1→3)-β-D-glucuronopyranosyl oleanolic acid (**99**)	fruit	[116]
3β-*O* ← GlcUA(6-OMe)^{3} ← Xyl	3-*O*-β-D-Xylopyranosyl-(1→3)-6-*O*-methyl-β-D-glucuronopyranosyl oleanolic acid (**100**)	fruit	[116]
3β-*O* ← GlcUA^{2} ← Glc ^{3}↑ Xyl	3β-[(*O*-β-D-Glucopyranosyl-(1→2)][β-D-xylopyranosyl-(1→3)] β-D-Glucuronopyranosyl oleanolic acid (**101**)	fruit	[116]
Kochia scoparia (L.) Schrader	*Bidesmosidic triterpenoid saponins*		
3β-*O* ← GlcUA^{3} ← Xyl 28-*O* ← Glc	3-*O*-β-D-Xylopyranosyl-(1→3)-β-D-glucuronopyranosyl oleanolic acid 28-*O*-β-D-glucopyranosyl ester (**102**)	fruit	[116]
3β-*O* ← GlcUA(6-OMe)^{3} ← Xyl 28-*O* ← Glc	3β-*O*-[6-*O*-methyl-β-D-glucuronopyranosyl]-oleanolic acid 28-*O*-β-D-glucopyranosyl ester (**103**)	fruit	[116]
3β-*O* ← GlcUA^{2} ← Glc ^{3}↑ Xyl 28-*O* ← Glc	3β-[(*O*-β-D-Glucopyranosyl-(1→2)][β-D-xylopyranosyl-(1→3)] β-D-Glucuronopyranosyl oleanolic acid 28-*O*-β-D-glucopyranosyl ester (**104**)	fruit	[116]
Salsola imbricata Pall.	*Bidesmosidic triterpenoid saponins*		
3β-*O* ← GlcUA^{2} ← Xyl 28-*O* ← Glc	3-*O*-β-D-Xylopyranosyl-(1→2)-*O*-β-D-glucuronopyranosyl akebonic acid 28-*O*-β-D-glucopyranosyl ester (**105**)	root	[118]
3β-*O* ← GlcUA^{2} ← Xyl 28-*O* ← Glc	3-*O*-β-D-Xylopyranosyl-(1→2)-*O*-β-D-glucuronopyranosyl-29-hydroxy oleanolic acid-28-*O*-β-D-glucopyranosyl ester (**106**)	root	[118]
3β-*O* ← GlcUA^{2} ← Xyl 28-*O* ← Glc	3-*O*-β-D-Xylopyranosyl-(1→2)-*O*-β-D-glucuronopyranosyl oleanolic acid 28-*O*-β-D-glucopyranosyl ester (**107**)	root	[118]
3β-*O* ← GlcUA 28-*O* ← Glc	3-*O*-β-D-Glucuronopyranosyl oleanolic acid 28-*O*-β-D-glucopyranosyl ester (**108**)	root	[118]
3β-*O* ← GlcUA 28-*O* ← Glc	3-*O*-[β-D-Glucuronopyranosyl]-30-norolean 12,20(29)-dien-28-*O*-[β-D- glucopyranosyl] ester (**109**)	root	[118]
Salsola micranthera Botsch.	*Bidesmosidic triterpenoid saponins*		
3β-*O* ← Glc^{2} ← Xyl^{4} ← GlcUA 28-*O* ← Glc	3-*O*-β-D-Glucuronopyranosyl-(1→4)-β-D-xylopyranosyl-(1→2)-β-D-glucopyranosyl oleanolic acid 28-*O*-β-D-glucopyranosyl ester (**110**)	epigeal part	[119]
3β-*O* ← Xyl^{4} ← GlcUA 28-*O* ← Glc	3-*O*-β-D-Glucuronopyranosyl-(1→4)-β-D-xylopyranosyl oleanolic acid 28-*O*-β-D-glucopyranosyl ester (**111**)	epigeal part	[120]
3β-*O* ← Xyl^{4} ← GlcUA 28-*O* ← Glc	3-*O*-β-D-Glucuronopyranosyl-(1→4)-β-D-xylopyranosyl hederagenin 28-*O*-β-D-glucopyranosyl ester (**112**)	epigeal part	[120]
Spinacia oleracea L.	*Monodesmosidic triterpenoid saponins*		
3β-*O* ← GlcUA^{3} ← Glc	3-*O*-β-D-Glucopyranosyl-(1→3)-β-D-glucuronopyranosyl oleanolic acid (**113**)	root	[121]
3β-*O* ← GlcUA^{3} ← Glc	3-*O*-β-D-Glucopyranosyl-(1→3)-β-D-glucuronopyranosyl hederagenin (**114**)	root	[121]

	Saponins	Plant part	References
Spinacia oleracea L.	*Bidesmosidic triterpenoid saponins*		
3β-*O*←GlcUA 28-*O*←Glc	3-*O*-β-D-Glucuronopyranosyl oleragenin 28-*O*-β-D-glucopyranosyl ester (**115**)	leaf , stem	[48]

The most evident inter-specific difference that can be highlighted among the genus *Chenopodium* are based on the presence of phytolaccagenic acid and serjanic acid. Two genera of the family such *Climacoptera* and *Cornulaca* are related to the genus *Chenopodium* and contain triterpene aglycones such as serjanic acid and oleanolic acid. *Chenopodium pallidicaule* has similarbidesmosidic triterpenoid saponins as *Chenopodium quinoa* with phytolaccagenic acid, hederagenin, and oleanolic acid as aglycones. Other aglycones found are saikogenin F in the genus *Atriplex*, betulinic acid in the genus *Kochia*, oleragenin in the genus *Spinacia*, and akebonic acid in the genus *Salsola* etc. The large number of different triterpenoid saponins within a species as well as the intra-individual variations in saponin mixtures raises the question of the functions of these molecules. *Chenopodium quinoa* accumulates more than 33 different saponins [93]. A single plant species may contain a complex mixture of saponins. For example, the saponins of *Chenopodium pallidicaule* Aellen include three groups of aglycones: oleanolic acid, phytolaccagenic acid, and hederagenin (see Fig. 3). As mentioned before, *C. quinoa* Willd. contains oleanolic acid, phytolaccagenic acid, hederagenin, serjanic acid, gypsogenin and also other aglycones (see Fig. 1). Some species of the Chenopodiaceae contain gypsogenin as the aglycone such as members of *Chenopodium* and *Climacoptera*. In addition, the gypsogenin is well known as an aglycone of many species in Caryophyllaceae.

3.3. Biosynthesis of Saponins in Chenopodiaceae

Saponins are secondary metabolite, and more than 5,000 different saponins and related compounds have been isolated from higher plants [40]. The presence of saponins have been reported in more than 100 plant families and some marine animal sources such as star fish and sea cucumber [122, 123]. The large complexity of saponins arise from the variability of the aglycone structure, the nature of the side chains and the position of attachment of these moieties on the aglycone [124].

Triterpenoid saponins are characterized by the presence of a skeleton derived from the C30 precursor squalene. Squalene is oxidized to oxidosqualene, and this is converted to cyclic derivatives. The type of cyclase that is involved in the cyclization reaction primarily determines which skeleton is formed. The cyclization of oxidosqualene to saponins can proceed in two ways, either via the "chair-chair-chair" or via the "chair-boat-chair" conformation. An important difference between the two resulting skeletons lies in their stereochemistry. Triterpenoids originate from the "chair chair-chair" conformation, while steroids arise from the "chair-boat-chair" conformation [125]. Their production and accumulation are frequently stimulated in response to environmental challenges. For this reason of the most important roles of saponins and other secondary metabolites in plants is to protect them from herbivore and pathogenic microorganisms.

4. Structural Determination of Triterpenoid Saponins

4.1. General Strategy for Structure Elucidation

The chemical structure of saponins can be determined by spectroscopic methods however, base and acid hydrolysis and other chemical reactions are sometimes found to be necessary for the elucidation of complex structures [126]. The complete structural characterization of complex saponins typically requires purification of the aglycones and their glycosides, liberation of the carbohydrate unit from the remaining aglycone in some instances, and determination of the following structural aspects of the complete structure of a saponin: (i) the structure of the aglycone, (ii) the monosaccharide composition, (iii) the sequence and the anomeric configurations of each glycosidically linked monosaccaharide unit, (iv) the positions of glycosidic linkages between the carbohydrates. The identification and structural elucidation of saponins can be divided into the following steps.

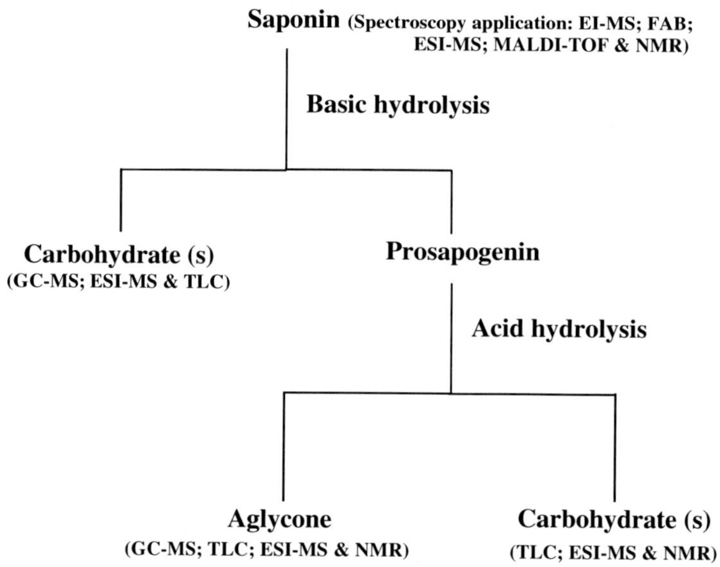

Figure 4. The steps involved in the identification and structural elucidation of saponins. The conventional method of structural identification starts with alkaline hydrolysis to obtain a prosapogenin after cleavage of an ester linkage. The acid hydrolysis of the pure saponin can be used to identify the aglycone and individual carbohydrate residues. The carbohydrate residues can be identified by comparison with authentic standards. The aglycone of saponins are pentacyclic triterpenes, which can be identified by comparing their ^{1}H and ^{13}C NMR data with reported values. The carbohydrate residues at the C3 and C28 positions can be deduced from the chemical shifts of both carbons, with a downfield chemical shift of the C3 by approx. 5–12 ppm and an upfield shift of C28 from 179–180 ppm to 175–177 ppm for the carbon to the corresponding signal in pentacyclic triterpene and was subsequently confirmed by 2D NMR experiments. One- and two-dimensional NMR techniques are used for the identification of individual carbohydrate residues, their anomeric configuration, interglycosidic linkages, their sequence and the site of any appended group.

4.2. The Identification of Aglycones

The ^{1}H- and ^{13}C-NMR spectroscopy is a useful tool for the structure determination of triterpenoid saponins without chemical degradation provided that^{1}H- and ^{13}C-NMR spectral data of the aglycone [127] and monosaccharides are available [128].

The assignments of chemical shift of aglycones are generally made by the comparison with ^{13}C-NMR spectral data of reported compounds. For instance, the ^{13}C NMR spectral data of oleanane- and phytolaccagenan-type aglycones present in triterpenoid saponins of *Chenopodium quinoa* have been reported [103-105]. The methyl and olefinic signals in ^{1}H-NMR spectra, support the structure of oleanane- and phytolaccagenane-type aglycones. The mass fragments observed due to loss of (M+H^{+}-carbohydrate chains) in ESI-MS^{+} positive mode ion mass spectrum can be used to determine the molecular formula of the aglycone moiety. The chemical structure of prosapogenins elucidated by spectroscopic means can be confirmed by alkaline hydrolysis whereas the aglycone can be confirmed by acid hydrolysis of saponins. Acid hydrolysis of saponins is generally achieved with 2 N hydrochloric acid (HCl) with good results [129].

For instance, the ^{1}H-NMR spectrum of oleanolic acid showed signals due to 7 tertiary methyl groups at 0.76, 0.78, 0.90, 0.92, 0.93, 0.98 and 1.13 ppm, one hydroxyl bearing *ax-eq* methine proton at δ 3.22 (1H, *dd*, J = 11.3, 4.4 Hz, H3), an olefinic proton at δ 5.29 (1H, *t*, J = 3.4 H12) ppm. The carbon-13 NMR spectrum showed 30 signals, seven due to methyls groups, ten due to methylenes, five due to methines, leaving eight quaternary carbons. In ^{13}C-NMR spectrum showed a carbon bearing a hydroxyl group showed a chemical shift at δ 183.5 ppm. Chemical shifts at δ 122.8 (C12) and 143.6 (C13) ppm confirm the Δ^{12} oleanene skeleton through the resonances of trisubstituted olefinic carbons. ^{1}H- and ^{13}C-NMR spectra of oleanolic acid and hederagenin have also been reported by Seebacher *et al.*, 2003 and Joshi *et al.*, 1999, respectively [130, 131].

4.3. The Identification of Monosaccharide Units

As regards the monosaccharide units, hexoses such β-D-glucose, β-D-galactose, β-D-glucuronic acid, and pentoses such α-L-arabinose and β-D-xylose, in are commonly found in triterpenoid saponins. The carbohydrates obtained from the hydrolysates, after acid hydrolysis can be identified on TLC by comparing them with authentic samples (R_f value).

The ^{13}C-NMR chemical shift of carbohydrate chains can deduce the β-D-/β-L-/α-L-, pyranosyl or furanosyl. The anomeric signals in ^{13}C-NMR spectra of triterpenoid saponins indicate the number of pyranose and furanose carbohydrate residues and show that carbohydrates attached to aglycone have either α- or β-configurations. ^{13}C-NMR studies of saponins indicated that anomeric signals in pyranose carbohydrate residues, appeared at 94–96 ppm when they are attached by an ester bond [132] and at 98–108 ppm when they are attached by an ester linkage, while the anomeric signals in furanose carbohydrate residues appeared at 109–111 ppm [128, 133].

The symbol of α or β which designated the anomeric configuration of monosaccharide unit can be determined by ^{1}H-NMR spectrum of triterpenoid saponins. The anomeric proton signals shows a doublet with J = 7 Hz, assignable to that of β-D-glucopyranosyl, α-L-arabinopyranosyl etc. because of the *trans* diaxial relationship of the protons at C1 and C2 of pyranose carbohydrate residues. However, the anomeric proton doublet appeared with J = 1–3 Hz assignable for α-L-rhamnopyranosyl etc. suggesting atdiequatorial oraxial equatorial orientation of the C1 and C2 protons.

4.4. Determination of the Inter-Glycosidic Linkage and Carbohydrate Sequences

The carbohydrate linkage and sequence can be established by ^{13}C-NMR and positive mode electron spray ionization mass spectrometry. The overlapped ^{13}C-NMR assignments of the carbohydrate chains with corresponding methyl glycosides, point out the terminal carbohydrate chains. The linkage between terminal to inner carbohydrate chains and inner carbohydrate chains to aglycone can also be determined through ^{13}C-NMR measurements in which the upfield shifts of β-carbons and downfield shift of α-carbons are characteristic for the establishment of attachments. The upfield shifts of β-carbons and downfield shifts of α-carbons of aglycone and monosaccharide chains are determined by comparison with the ^{13}C-NMR chemical shift of corresponding saponins and methyl glycosides using the following formula reported in literature for aglycone moiety [134, 135].

$$\Delta^{S}A = \delta\text{ (triterpene glycoside)} - \delta\text{ (triterpene)}$$

And for carbohydrate chains

$$\Delta\delta = \delta\text{ (triterpene glycoside)} - \delta\text{ (methyl glycoside)}$$

The symbol δ and Δδ represent the chemical shift and glycosidation shift values. The glycosidation shifts, can be defined by ^{13}C-NMR chemical shifts from aglycone to glycoside and carbohydrate to glycoside.

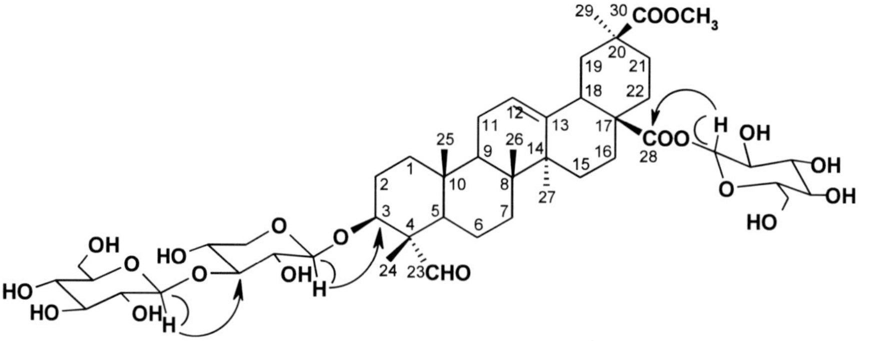

Figure 5. Selected HMBC (→) and HSQC (—) correlations of 3β-[(O-β-D-glucopyranosyl-(1→3)-α-L-arabinopyranosyl)oxy]-23-oxo-olean-12-en-28-oic acid β-D-glucopyranoside (**66**).

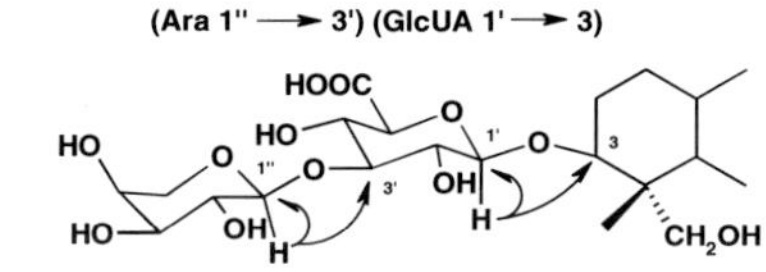

3-*O*-[α-L-arabinopyranosyl-(1″→3′)-β-D-glucuronopyranosyl]-phytolaccagenic acid 28-*O*-β-D-glucopyranoside (**1**)

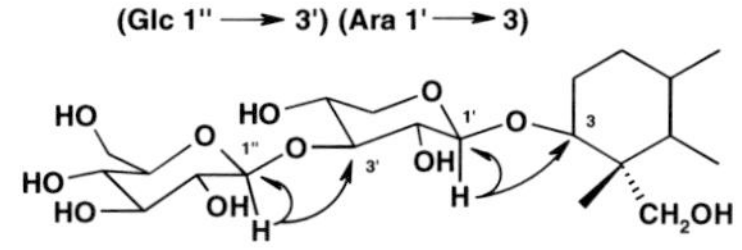

3-*O*-[β-D-glucopyranosyl]-(1″→3′)-α-L-arabinopyranosyl]-phytolaccagenic acid 28-*O*-β-D-glucopyranoside (**2**)

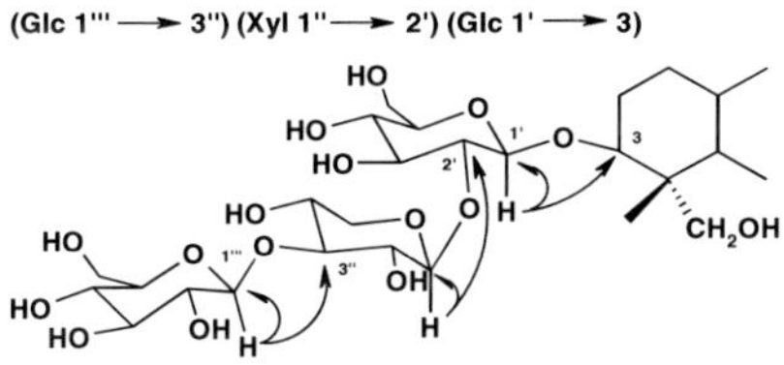

3-*O*-[β-D-glucopyranosyl]-(1‴→3″)-β-D-xylopyranosyl-(1″→2′)-β-D-glucopyranosyl]-phytolaccagenic acid 28-*O*-β-D-glucopyranoside (**3**)

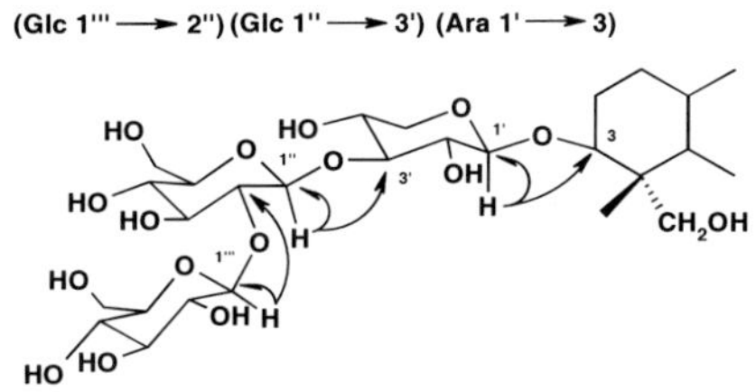

3-*O*-[β-D-glucopyranosyl]-(1‴→2″)-β-D-glucopyranosyl-(1″→3′)-α-L-arabinopyranosyl]-phytolaccagenic acid 28-*O*-β-D-glucopyranoside (**4**)

Figure 6. Selected HMBC (→) and HMQC (⇀) correlations in **1–4**. The interglycosidic linkage and the sequential arrangement of the trisaccharide moiety linked at C3 of the aglycone were determined by ^{13}C NMR and HMBC spectra. The ^{13}C showed significant glycosidation shifts: for the C2′ (+8 ppm), the C1′ (–2 ppm), and the C3′ (–2.7 ppm) of the Glc_{inner} moiety; and for the C3″ (+8 ppm), the C2″ (–2.2 ppm), and the C4″ (–2 ppm) of the Xyl moiety. In the HMBC experiment carried out to confirm a position of glycosyl bond were observed diagnostic HMBC cross-peaks between the anomeric proton (H1‴) of a terminal $glucose_{outer}$ at δ = 4.64 (1H, *d*, *J* = 7.7 Hz) and the xylose (C3″) signal at δ = 86.1 as well as between the xylose (H1″) signal at δ = 4.42 (1H, *d*, *J* = 7.7 Hz) and the signal (C2′) at δ = 83.5 ($Glc2_{inner}$), and between the glucose (H1′) signal at δ = 4.64 (1H, *d*, *J* = 7.7 Hz) and signal (C3) at δ = 85.1 (aglycone C3), indicating linkage of a terminal glucose via its anomeric carbon to Xyl3 linked to Glc2 and linkage of the latter with the 3-hydroxy group of phytolaccagenic acid (Source: adapted from Woldemichael & Wink; J. Agric. Food Chem. 2001, 49; 2327–2332; Dini *et al.*; J. Agric. Food Chem. 2001, 49: 741–746)

Basic hydrolysis of a saponin liberates glucose. Further acid hydrolysis of the prosapogenin formed provided arabinose. These findings indicated that arabinose was a monosaccharide residue at the C3 hydroxy group whereas glucose was esterified with C28 position. The positions of monosaccharide moiety can be further defined by the HMBC experiment. Attachment of the carbohydrate chain at C3 is indicated by the significant downfield shift (δ 81.8 ppm) relative to the corresponding signal in similar compounds, for example 3β-hydroxy-23-oxo-olean-12-en-28-oic acid (=Gypsogenin) (δ 79.1 ppm), and was subsequently confirmed by 2D NMR experiments.

A cross peak due to long-rang correlations between C3 (δ 81.8 ppm) of the aglycone and H1 of the arabinose (δ 4.99 ppm) indicated that arabinose was pentose residue linked to C3 of the aglycone. Further conformation was obtained from ^{1}H,^{1}H COSY spectrum with cross peaks arising from H3 (δ 4.28 ppm) of the aglycone and H1 of arabinose. Similarly, H1 of the glucose residue was seen to cross peak with C28 of the aglycone in HMBC spectrum.

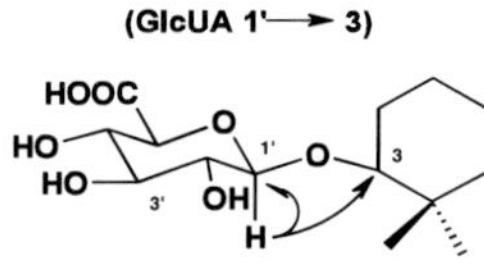

3-*O*-[β-D-glucuronopyranosyl]-oleanolic acid 28-*O*-β-D-glucopyranoside (**5**)

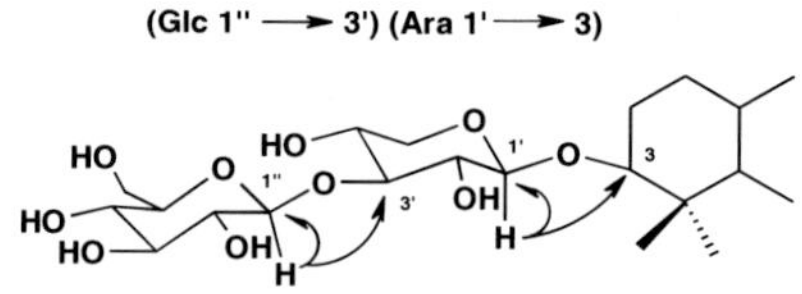

3-*O*-[β-D-glucopyranosyl]-(1″→3′)-α-L-arabinopyranosyl]-oleanolic acid 28-*O*-β-D-glucopyranoside (**6**)

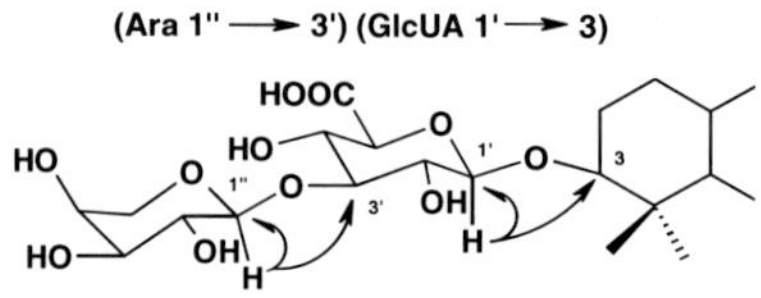

3-*O*-[α-L-arabinopyranosyl-(1″→3′)-β-D-glucuronopyranosyl]-oleanolic acid 28-*O*-β-D-glucopyranoside (**7**)

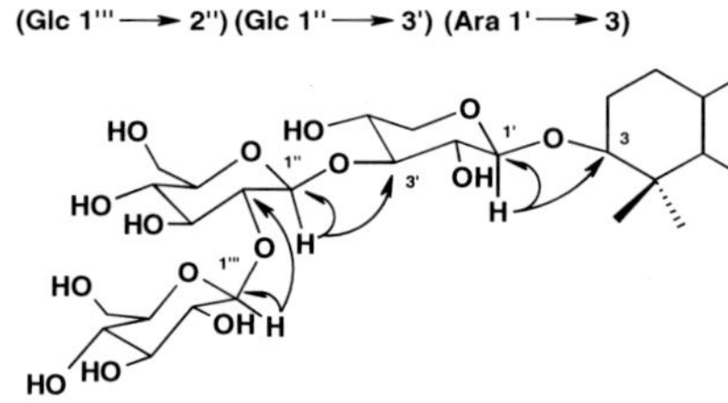

3-*O*-[β-D-glucopyranosyl]-(1‴→2″)-β-D-glucopyranosyl-(1″→3′)-α-L-arabinopyranosyl]-oleanolic acid 28-*O*-β-D-glucopyranoside (**8**)

Figure 7. Selected HMBC (→) and HMQC (→) correlations in **5–8**. (**5**); In ^{1}H NMR spectrum showed signals for seven methyl groups at δ 0.82, 0.92, 0.95, 1.00, 1.08, 1.22, and 1.27, a trisubstituted olefinic proton at δ 5.40 (1H, *m*, H12) ppm, and a methine proton signal at δ 3.36 (1H, *dd*, *J*) 11.7, 4.0 Hz, H3) in the aglycone, which are characteristic of an oleanene-type triterpene. The ^{13}C-NMR spectrum confirmed the oleanene nature through the shifts for C12 and C13 at δ 122.8 and 144.1, respectively. The anomeric ^{13}C signals at δ 107.2 and 95.7 ppm and their corresponding protons at δ 5.03 (1H, *d*, *J* = 7.6 Hz) and 6.31 (1H, *d*, *J* = 7.9 Hz), respectively, were strongly indicative of two hexoses. The HMQC and HMBC spectra allowed the identification of the spin systems of the two monosaccharide residues. (**6–8**); The interglycosidic linkage and the sequential arrangement of the trisaccharide moiety linked at C3 of the aglycone was determined by ^{13}C-NMR and HMBC spectra. The ^{13}C showed significant glycosidation shifts: for the C2′ (+8 ppm), the C1′ (–2 ppm), and the C3′ (–2.7 ppm) of the Glc_{inner} moiety; and for the C3″ (+8 ppm), the C2″ (–2.2 ppm), and the C4″ (–2 ppm) of the Xyl moiety. In the HMBC experiment carried out to confirm a position of glycosyl bond diagnostic HMBC cross-peaks were observed between the anomeric proton (H1‴) of a terminal $glucose_{outer}$ at δ = 4.64 (1H, *d*, *J* = 7.7 Hz) and the xylose (C3″) signal at δ = 86.1 as well as between the xylose (H1″) signal at δ = 4.42 (1H, *d*, *J* = 7.7 Hz) and the signal (C2′) at δ = 83.5 ($Glc2_{inner}$), and between the glucose (H1′) signal at δ = 4.64 (1H, *d*, *J* = 7.7 Hz) and signal (C3) at δ = 85.1 (aglycone C3), indicating linkage of a terminal glucose via its anomeric carbon to Xyl3 linked to Glc2 and linkage of the latter with the 3β-hydroxy group of oleanolic acid aglycone. (Source: adapted from Woldemichael & Wink; J. Agric. Food Chem. 2001, 49; 2327–2332; Dini *et al.*; J. Agric. Food Chem. 2001, 49: 741–746; Dini *et al.*; J. Agric. Food Chem. 2001, 49: 3976–3981).

Triterpenoid saponins containing carbohydrate chain(s) at C3 and/or C28 positions are common in higher plants. Some plant species were reported oleanane-type saponins to possess a carbohydrate chain on C23. The gypsogenin is example secondary metabolites of triterpenoid as aglycone found in the closed family with Chenopodiaceae family. The relative stereochemistry of each of the monocarbohydrate was determined as β-D-glucopyranosyl at C28 and α-L-arabinopyranosyl at C3 base on the characteristic $J_{1,2}$ coupling constants. The anomeric proton of α-L-arabinopyranosyl at C3 appeared as a doublet with J = 7.2 Hz. The anomeric proton of β-D-glucopyranosyl at C28 appeared at δ 6.31 (*d*, J = 7.9) ppm.

5. Biological and Pharmacological Activities

Triterpenoid saponins show a broad spectrum of biological activities; earlier studies were limited only to crude extracts, which contained both saponins and other constituents. Recently, due to advanced methods of extraction, purification and structure determination individual constituents were studied in adition to characterized extracts. A large number of triterpenoid saponins are extremely toxic in cold-blooded animals, whereas their oral toxicity to mammals is much lower [103, 105]. In addition, many triterpenoid saponins are being used as food additives and feedstuffs. A number of reviews have been published describing the various biological activities of saponins *viz* antibacterial antifungal, antiviral, hypocholesterolemic, antitumor, analgesic properties etc.; however, the application of these secondary metabolites as therapeutic agents has not been very successful due to limited supply of the compounds. Recently bioactive triterpenoid saponins, including the monodesmoside 3-*O*-β-D-Glucuronopyranosyl oleanolic acid (**36**) have been reported from the roots of *Cyathula officinalis* Kuan (Amaranthaceae) [136] and have also beenisolated from the root barks of *Aralia armata* (Wall.) Seem. (Araliaceae) [137]. The potent spermicidal saponin of 3-*O*-β-D-Glucuronopyranosyl oleanolic acid (**36**) was isolated from*Sesbania sesban* Merrill (Fabaceae) [138]. Furthermore, 3-*O*-β-D-Glucuronopyranosyl oleanolic acid (**36**); momordin Ic is a derivative of oleanolic acid strongly reduced serum glucose levels [139]. Also anti-neoplastic effect and spermicidal activity been reported for monodesmosidic triterpene saponins [140, 141].

Whereas monodesmosides of triterpenoid saponins exhibit a broad spectrum of activities against bacteria, fungi, viruses, and fish, bidesmosides are generally inactive [142-146]. In addition, the number, kind, and sequence of the carbohydrate residues significantly modify antifungal effects of triterpenoid saponins [147, 148].

Interestingly, monodesmoside triterpenoid saponins can dive into biomembranes with their lipophilic side chain and complex cholesterol, whereas their hydrophilic carbohydrate chain binds to extracellular glycoproteins and glycolipids. This inter action disturbs the fluidity and permeability of biomembranes [4]. Monodesmoside triterpenoid saponins showed higher haemolytic activity than bidesmoside triterpenoid saponins because only monodesmosidic saponins act as emulsifying agents and can lyse biomembranes. Several reports have shown that the carbohydrate composition and type of linkage are also directly related to the activity of the saponins. Chwalek and co-workers demonstrated that the (1→4) linkage in hederagenin diglycosides had a higher hemolytic activity than the (1→6) linkage. Moreover, the β-linkage configuration in hederagenin diglycosides also showed a higher hemolytic activity than the α-linkage configuration [149]. Triterpenoid saponins confer protection to the plants producing them due to their antibacterial, antifungal, membrane depolarizing antioxidant, anti-inflammatory, antinociceptive, and antiallergic activities. Interestingly, the bidesmoside triterpenoid saponin, 3-*O*-β-D-Glucuronopyranosyl oleanolic acid 28-*O*-β-D-glucopyranosyl ester (**46**) has been reported from the roots of *Chenopodium ficifolium* Sm. (Chenopodiaceae); this compound was also found in the rhizomes of *Panax japonicus* C.A. Meyer (Araliaceae) [150] and also in the roots of *Beta vulgaris* L. (Chenopodiaceae) [151]. The bidesmoside triterpenoid saponin can be found in three common species with different qualities in each plant; *Panax ginseng* C.A. Meyer (Asian ginseng), *Panax quinquefolius* C.A. Meyer (American ginseng), and *Panax japonicus* (Japanese ginseng).

Chikusetsusaponin Iva (**46**) shows a wide range of biological activities. This bidesmoside has been discovered in quinoa, in the flowers of *Calendula officinalis* L. (Asteraceae) [185, 186], the epigeal part of *Silphium perfoliatum* L. (Asteraceae) [187], the aerial parts of *Cynara cardunculus* L. (Asteraceae) [188], the rhizomes of *Panax pseudo-ginseng* subs *himalaicus* var. *angustifolius* (Araliaceae) [189], the dried roots and rhizomes of *Panax zingiberensis* (Araliaceae) [190], the aerial parts of *Aralia continentalis* (Araliaceae) [191], species of *Panax* (ginseng) have been to contain bidesmoside saponins as chikusetsusaponin Iva; the rhizomes of *Panax japonicus* C. A. Meyer (Araliaceae) [150, 192], the roots of *Panax japonicus* C.A. Meyer. (Araliaceae) [193], the rhizomes of *Panax stipuleanatus* (Araliaceae) [194], the roots of *Panax japonicus* var. *major* (Araliaceae) [195], the rhizomes of *Panax pseudo-ginseng* subsp. *himalaicus* (Araliaceae) [196], the dried roots of *Achyranthes fauriei* (Amaranthaceae) [197], the roots of *Pfaffia iresinoides* (Amaranthaceae) [198], the fresh leaves of *Ilex rotunda* Thunb. (Aquifoliaceae) [199], the fresh aerial parts of *Basella rubra* L. (Basellaceae) [200], the leaves of *Boussingaultia baselloides* (Basellaceae) [201], the rhizomes of *Hemsleya macrosperma* (Cucurbitaceae) [202], the roots of *Ilex pubescens* Hook et Arn. (Ilexaceae) [203], the seeds of *Dolichos lablab* L. (Leguminosae) [204], the aerial parts of *Dumasia truncate* (Leguminosae) [205], the leaves of *Swartzia simplex* (Leguminosae) [206], the leaves of *Pisonia umbellifera* (Nyctaginaceae) [207], the roots of *Talinum triangulare* (Portulacaceae) [87].

Some interesting results have been reported in the literature on the biological activities of triterpenoid saponins of the Chenopodiaceae family, which are summarized below.

5.1. Hypocholesterolemic Activity

The pericarp of the quinoa seeds contains saponins that significantly decreased serum and liver cholesterol levels in mice [152]. The *C. quinoa* Willd. grain supplementation diet can temporally reduce food intake and prevent growth [153]. The protein fraction of pericarp from quinoa seeds significantly reduced the plasma cholesterol concentration even though the mice were fed a cholesterol-supplemented diet [154]. Various studies of the flour or protein hydrolysate of *C. quinoa* Willd. have been shown to lower blood pressure [155].

A methanolic extract of the fruit of Japanese *Kochia scoparia* (L.) Schrader (Summer-cypress) was shown to inhibit the increase in serum glucose in glucose-loaded rats. The active principles shown inhibit glucose and ethanol absorption in rats were 3-*O*-β-D-Xylopyranosyl-(1→3)-β-D-glucuronopyranosyl oleanolic acid (**99**); momordin Ic and its 2′-*O*-β-D-glucopyranoside together with three triterpenoid saponins named scoparianosides A, B and C [151]. The 50% ethanolic extract of *Salicomia herbacea* L. was found to prevent the onset of the hyperglycemia and hyperlipidemia induced by high fat diet in ICR mice [156].

5.2. Antidiabetic Activity

The extracts of *Beta vulgaris* var. *cicla* L. inhibited the nonenzymatic glycosylation of skin proteins and increase of blood glucose. These results demonstrated the ability of the plant in preventing or at least retarding the development of some diabetic complications [157]. The monodesmosidic and bidesmosidic triterpenoid saponins such as betavulgarosides I (**18**), II (**12**), III (**19**), IV (**13**) with oleanolic acid oligoglycosides were isolated from root together with betavulgarosides VI (**21**), VII (**15**), VIII (**22**) from the roots and leaves of *Beta vulgaris* L. Three triterpenoid saponins named betavulgarosides II (**12**) (monodesmoside), betavulgarosides III (**19**) (bidesmoside) and betavulgarosides IV (**13**) (monodesmoside) produced hypoglycaemic effects that were improvement by an oral glucose tolerance test in rats [97]. In a study of 31 desert plants that were collected from different Egyptian localities, oral administration of an extract from *Haloxylon salicorlicum* Bunge (Chenopodiaceae) to normoglycaemic rats produced an hypoglycaemic effects comparable to that of Daonil [158].

Oral administration of an extract from *Arthrocnemum glaucum* Delile (Chenopodiaceae) to normoglycaemic rats produced a persistent hypoglycaemic effect. In addition, in alloxanised diabetic rats, this extract showed a hypoglycaemic effect that was more potent than that of Daonil [158]. The methanolic extract of the Japanese fruit *Kochia scoparia* (L.) Schrader inhibited the increase in serum glucose in glucose-loaded rats. The active principles were 3-*O*-β-D-Xylopyranosyl-(1→3)-β-D-glucuronopyranosyl oleanolic acid (**39**); momordin Ic and its 2′-*O*-β-D-glucopyranoside together with three saponins 3-*O*-β-D-xylopyranosyl (1→3)-β-D-glucopyranosiduronic acid 22α-hydroxyoleanolic acid; scoparianosides A, 3β-hydroxyolean-18-en-28-oic acid (morolic acid), 3-*O*-β-D-xylopyranosyl (1→3)-β-D-glucopyranosiduronic acid; scoparianosides B and 3β-hydroxyolean-13(18)-en-28-oic acid, 3-*O*-β-D-xylopyranoxyl(1→3)-β-D-glucopyranosiduronic acid; scoparianosides C [151].

5.3. Immunomodulatory Activity

Triterpenoid saponins from quinoa seeds can potentiate specific IgG and IgA antibody responses to the co-administered antigen cholera toxin or ovalbuminin serum, intestinal and lung secretions. The antigen specific IgG antibodies were characterized by an increase of the IgG_1 subclass which is associated with the stimulation of $CD4^+$ T cells of the Th_2 subset, which prime for the production of secretory IgA responses at mucosal sites [159]. The production of systemic and mucosal immune responses by oral or intranasal immunization requires the repeated administration of large amounts of antigen [160]. The potentiating effect of the triterpenoid saponins appeared, to some extent, mediated by an increased permeability of the mucosa, allowing an enhanced uptake of the polar antigen. Hence, saponins acted as immunological adjuvants [161].

5.4. Anti-Inflammatory Activity

Several triterpenoid saponins of quinoa appear to possess anti-inflammatory activities [38]. One compound, the monodesmoside 3-*O*-β-D-glucopyranosyl oleanolic acid (**37**) which was isolated from the seeds of *Randia dumetornm* Lam. (Rubiaceae) showed significant anti-inflammatory activity in the exudative and proliferative phases of inflammation in the doses of 25 and 100 mg/kg (with LD_{50} values of 3,600 mg/kg in mice and 1,500 mg/kg in rats) [162]. A similaractivity has been reported for monodesmoside saponins from *C. quinoa* Willd. The bidesmoside triterpenoid saponin known as chikusetsusaponin IVa; 3-*O*-β-D-Glucuronopyranosyl oleanolic acid 28-*O*-β-D-glucopyranosyl ester (**46**) was found to be effective in the hypercoagulable state [163]. Bidesmoside triterpenoid saponins which are closely related to chikusetsusaponin V (3-*O*-β-D-Glucuronopyranosyl-(1→2)-β-D-glucopyranosyl oleanolic acid 28-*O*-β-D-glucopyranosyl ester). This compound has been reported antiinflammatory effects which differ from ginsenosides Rb_1 and Rg_1 responsible for adaptogenic effects of ginseng. Also several species of Amaranthaceae family such as *Achyranthes bidentata* Blume have been isolated the monodesmoside triterpenoid saponin as Chikusetsusaponin V from the roots [164]. and *Achyranthes fauriei* H. Lev. & Vaniot have been isolated the same compound from the roots [165].

Furthermore, the bidesmoside triterpenoid saponin known as Chikusetsusaponin V has been found wide occurrence from *Panax* species as well as many other plants [166]. *Panax ginseng* C. A. Meyer is the most famous Chinese herb being. It is rich in dammarane saponins such ginsenoside Ro emerges as the unique oleanane saponin [167]. The chemical structural of the bidesmosidic ginsenoside Ro represents a typical saponin termed glucuronide oleanane-type triterpene carboxylic acid 3, 28-*O*-bisdesmoside [31]. Such a structure shows no hemolytic or cytotoxic activities [168, 169]. However, this bidesmoside is an effective solubilizer for hydrophobic compounds in water [170]. Interestingly, ginsenoside Ro exhibited significant antithrombic, anti-inflammatory, and anti-hepatitis activities in experimental models [163, 171, 172].

Triterpenoid saponins have been tested in several applications by now. *Hedera colchica* (K. Koch) K. Koch, was found to be quite effective in preventing inflammation in acute and chronic. A crude (CSE) and purified (SPE) extract of *H. colchica* in carrageenan- and cotton pellet-induced acute and chronic inflammation models in rats revealed anti-inflammatory properties. The presence of a free carboxylic acid group of hederagenin monodesmosides appears to be responsible for the anticomplement activity [173]. The extract of dried leaves of *Chenopodium ambrosioides* L. (300–700 mg kg-1, p.o.) produced a dose dependent inhibition of carrageenan-induced paw oedema and cotton pellet-induced granuloma in rats [174]. In the Middle East, *Salsola baryosma* (R. & S.) Dandy is used against inflammations and as a diuretic agent [175]. The methanolic extract of leaves from *C. ambrosioides* inhibited the carrageenan-induced rat paw oedema [219]. Some saponins have structures, which resemble those of anti-inflammatory glycocorticoids, such as cortisol. Therefore, it could be possible that some saponins function as cortisol mimics.

5.5. Antioxidant Activity

Several triterpenid saponins from *Hedera colchica* (K. Koch) K. Koch (Araliaceae) have been isolated and structurally characterized by Gülçin and co-workers (2006). The monodesmoside 3-*O*-β-D-glucopyranosyl hederagenin (**40**) from ivy berries showed antioxidant activity [176]. A similar to antioxidant activity was recorded for 3-*O*-β-D-glucopyranosyl hederagenin (**40**) of different plant parts of *C. quinoa* Willd. such as seeds, seed coats, and flowers. *Salicornia herbacea* L. (Chenopodiaceae) has been used as a seasoned vegetable and also have showed antioxidant effects [156]. In the recently present, Letelier and co-workers has been reported antioxidant properties of the extract of seed coats from *Chenopodium quinoa* [177]. The plant species of the genus *Salsola* have been reported to have medicinal properties. In Namibia and South Africa have been used in traditional medicine as an oral contraceptive by Bushmen women. In Middle East, *Salsola baryosma* (R. & S.) Dandy have been reported to possess antioxidant effects [178] and CNS depressant activity [179].

5.6. Hepatoprotective and other Activities

Mode of action for the hypoglycemic activity of monodesmoside triterpenoid saponin as 3-*O*-β-D-Xylopyranosyl-(1→3)-β-D-glucuronopyranosyl oleanolic acid (**99**); momordin Ic showed inhibited gastric emptying in rats and inhibited glucose uptake in the small intestine *in vitro* [215]. The dried fruits of *Kochia scoparia* (L.) Schrader are usedin traditional Chinese medicine for the treatment of diseases of the skin, urinary tract, and eyes. The isolated monodesmoside triterpenoid saponin momordin Ic applied orally and topically. The monodesmoside triterpenoid saponin was found to inhibit ethanol- and indomethacin-induced gastric mucosal lesions [216]. However, the bidesmoside triterpenoid saponin chikusetsusaponin IVa; 3-*O*-β-D-Glucuronopyranosyl oleanolic acid 28-*O*-β-D-glucopyranosyl ester (**46**) showed hepatoprotective activity on rat primary hepatocyte cultures [217].

5.7. Antipuritic Activity

Ethanolic extract of the fruits from *Chenopodium album* L. inhibited the scratching behavior induced by 5-HT [218].

5.8. Antiallergic Activity

Antiallergic activity of monodesmosidic triterpenoid saponins from dried fruits of *Kochia scoparia* (L.) Schrader was reported by Matsuda and co-workers (1997) [39].

5.9. Antifungal Activity

Monodesmoside triterpenoid saponins such as 3-*O*-β-D-glucopyranosyl hederagenin (**40**) of the roots of *Medicago hybrida* (Pourret) Trautv. (Fabaceae) showed a strong inhibition of mycelium growth of *Botrytis tulipae* [208]. Also the triterpenoid saponins from quinoa have antifungal activity. The crude saponin mixture showed inhibited the growth of *Candida albicans* at 50 μg/ml, whereas the pure bidesmoside triterpenoid saponins exhibited very low activity [19]. Similarly, the monodesmoside 3-*O*-β-D-glucopyranosyl hederagenin shows substantial fungitoxic activity against many plant pathogens. These saponins occur in fruits of *Hedera helix* L. (Araliaceae) [209], stems and bark of *Hedera nepalensis* K. Koch. (Araliaceae) [210], two species of Cucurbitaceae (fruits of *Luffa cylindrical* Roem. [211] dry roots of *Momordica dioica* Roxb. [212]), and the roots of *Dolichos kilimandscharicus* (Fabaceae) [213]. In contrast, the bidesmosidic triterpenoid glycoside of hederagenin exhibit very low activity because they cannot interfere with fungal biomembranes in a similar way than monodesmosides.

5.10. Antibacterial Activity

Saponins from *Chenopodium ambrosioides* L. exhibit significant antimicrobial activity against the drug resistant strain (CCK028469V) of *Mycobacterium tuberculosis* at concentration of 0.1 mg/ml have been reported [220]. The leaves of *Spinacia oleracea* are practically free of saponins, the roots contain the monodesmoside triterpenoid saponin A and B, the aglycones of which are oleanolic acid and hederagenin [221].

5.11. Antiviral Activity

A number of bidesmoside triterpene saponins are known to possess antiviral activity, such as chikusetsusaponin IVa (**46**) was isolated from the whole plant of *Alternanthera philoxeroides* (Mart.) Griseb (Amaranthaceae) showed significant antiviral activity against HSV-1, HSV-2, human cytomegalovirus, measles virus, and mumps virus with selectivity indices (CC_{50}/IC_{50}) of 29, 30, 73, 25, and 25, respectively [180]. The same activity is related to the bidesmoside triterpenoid saponin in different plant parts (seed coats, seeds, flowers, and fruits) of *C. quinoa* Willd. and isolated compound from the aerial part of *Bassia muricata* (L.) Murr. [95]. Moreover, the same bidesmosidic saponin has been reported from the roots of *Achyranthes fauriei* H. Lev. & Vaniot (Amaranthaceae) [181]. And this compound isolated of the aerial parts from *Galium rivale* (Sibth. and Sm.) Griseb. (Rubiaceae) [182]. Bidesmoside triterpenoid saponin known as chikusetsusaponin IVa of oleanolic acid-type [182] or taraxeryl acetate of taraxerane-type was purified from aerial part of *Laggera pterodonta* (DC.) Benth. (Asteraceae) showed significant antiviral activity against HSV-1, HSV-2 of different methods for testing antiviral activity [183]. And a mixture of saponins from *Chenopodium anthelminticum* L., were reported to activate human type A influenza viruses [184].

5.12. Anti-Anthelmintic Activity

Anti-anthelmintic activity of the *Chenopodium ambrosioides* L. has been reported [223]. Decoctions containing up to 300 mg dry plant material per kg body weight are active against ascariasis. Some plants of this genus have been reported to have anthelmintic properties [224].

5.13. Cytogenetic Activity

The aqueous extract of the aerial part of the *Chenopodium multifidum* L. shown possess cytogenetic activity have been reported [222].

5.14. Mollucicidal Activity

Atriplex nummularia Lindley (Chenopodiaceae) is a species of saltbush which has been reported two monodesmoside triterpenoid saponins as 3-*O*-*β*-D-Glucuronopyranosyl hederagenin (**1**) and 3-*O*-β-D-Glucuronopyranosyl oleanolic acid (**2**). The monodesmoside triterpenoid saponins have been reported to be potent molluscicides possess strong molluscicidal activity against the schistosomiasis-transmitting snail *Biomphalaria glabrata* [214].

CONCLUSION

In the family Chenopodiaceae triterpenoid saponins are common. They include a diverse group of compounds characterized by triterpenoid aglycone and one or more carbohydrate branches. The aglycones are oleanolic acid and oleanolic derivatives. Their physicochemical and biological properties are increasingly being exploited in cosmetic and pharmaceutical industries. Especially rich in triterpene saponins, are genera such as *Atriplex*, *Bassia, Beta, Chenopodium*, *Climacoptera, Cornulaca, Kochia*, *Salsola*, and *Spinacia*. Some species are good candidates for food and beverage industries, cosmetic and further drug discovery. Triterpenoid saponins of the Chenopodiaceae exert a plethora of biological activities including anti-inflammatory, antioxidant, apoptotic, anticholesterolemic and antiallergic properties. The use of saponins as therapeutic agents has become a fascinating challenge. Saponins have potential health benefits for humans, and plants with saponin have been used in traditional medicine around the world. Isolation, separation, detection, and structure elucidation of triterpenoid saponins has improved considerably recently in resolution and flexibility. The purification and analysis of triterpenoid saponins is still challenging due to their structural complexity, polar amphiphilic properties and also lack of a chromophore. However, since structurally divergent triterpenoid saponins show different biological and pharmacological activities, large quantities of purified triterpenoid saponins are required for future investigations.

REFERENCES

[1] Mahato, S. B.; Nandy, A. K., Triterpenoid saponins discovered between 1987 and 1989. *Phytochemistry* 1991, 30, (5), 1357–1390.

[2] Tan, N.; Zhou, J.; Zhao, S., Advances in structural elucidation of glucuronide oleanane-type triterpene carboxylic acid 3,28-*O*-bisdesmosides (1962–1997). *Phytochemistry* 1999, 52, (2), 153–192.

[3] Vincken, J. P.; Heng, L.; de Groot, A.; Gruppen, H., Saponins, classification and occurrence in the plant kingdom. *Phytochemistry* 2007, 68, (3), 275–297.

[4] Prokof'eva, N. G.; Chaikina, E. L.; Kicha, A. A.; Ivanchina, N. V., Biological activities of steroid glycosides from starfish. *Comparative Biochemistry and Physiology* 2003, 134, (4), 695–701.

[5] Avilov, S. A.; Silchenko, A. S.; Antonov, A. S.; Kalinin, V. I.; Kalinovsky, A. I.; Smirnov, A. V.; Dmitrenok, P. S.; Evtushenko, E. V.; Fedorov, S. N.; Savina, A. S.; Shubina, L. K.; Stonik, V. A., Synaptosides A and A_1, triterpene glycosides from the sea cucumber *Synapta maculata* containing 3-*O*-methylglucuronic acid and their cytotoxic activity against tumor cells. *Journal of Natural Products* 2008, 71, (4), 525–531.

[6] Findlay, J. A.; He, Z. Q.; Blackwell, B., Minor saponins from the starfish *Asterias forbesi*. *Canadian Journal of Chemistry* 1990, 68, (7), 1215–1217.

[7] Fenwick, G. R.; Price, K. R.; Tsukamoto, C.; Okubo, K., Saponins. In *Toxic Substances in Crop Plants*, J. P. F. D'Mello, et al., Ed. The Royal Society of Chemistry: Cambridge, 1991.

[8] Hostettmann, K.; Marston, A., Saponins In *Chemistry and pharmacology of natural products*, Cambridge University Press: New York, 1995; p 548.

[9] Oakenfull, D., Saponins in food — a Review. *Food Chemistry* 1981, 7, (1), 19–40.

[10] Oakenfull, D.; Sidhu, G. S., Saponins. In *Toxicants of plant origin, vol. II glycosides*, Cheeke, P. R., Ed. CRC Press, Inc. Boca Raton: Florida, 1989.

[11] Price, K. R.; Johnson, I. T.; Fenwick, G. R., The chemistry and biological significance of saponins in foods and feedingstuffs. *Critical Reviews in Food Science and Nutrition* 1987, 26, (1), 27–135.

[12] San Martin, R.; Briones, R., Industrial uses and sustainable supply of *Quillaja saponaria* (Rosaceae) saponins. *Economic Botany* 1999, 53, (3), 302–311.

[13] Thompson, L. U., Potential health benefits and problems associated with antinutrients in foods. *Food Research International* 1993, 26, (2), 131–149.

[14] Dini, I.; Tenore, G. C.; Dini, A., Nutritional and antinutritional composition of kancolla seeds: An interesting and underexploited andine food plant. *Food Chemistry* 2005, 92, (1), 125–132.

[15] Ridout, C. L.; Price, K. R.; Dupont, M. S.; Parker, M. L.; Fenwick, G. R., Quinoa saponins-analysis and preliminary investigations into the effects of reduction by processing. *Journal of the Science of Food and Agriculture* 1991, 54, (2), 165–176.

[16] Francis, G.; Kerem, Z.; Makkar, H. P. S.; Becker, K., The biological action of saponins in animal systems: A review. *British Journal of Nutrition* 2002, 88, (6), 587–605.

[17] Agrawal, P. K.; Jain, D. C.; Gupta, R. K.; Thakur, R. S., Carbon-13 NMR spectroscopy of steroidal sapogenins and steroidal saponins. *Phytochemistry* 1985, 24, (11), 2479–2496.

[18] Mahato, S. B.; Ganguly, A. N.; Sahu, N. P., Steroid saponins. *Phytochemistry* 1982, 21, (5), 959–978.

[19] Woldemichael, G. M.; Wink, M., Identification and biological activities of triterpenoid saponins from *Chenopodium quinoa*. *Journal of Agricultural and Food Chemistry* 2001, 49, (5), 2327–2332.

[20] Kuljanabhagavad, T.; Thongphasuk, P.; Chamulitrat, W.; Wink, M., Triterpene saponins from *Chenopodium quinoa* Willd. *Phytochemistry* 2008, 69, (9), 1919–1926.

[21] Meyer, B. N.; Heinstein, P. F.; Burnouf-Radosevich, M.; Delfel, N. E.; McLaughlin, J. L., Bioactivity-directed isolation and characterization of quinoside A: One of the toxic/bitter principles of quinoa seeds (*Chenopodium quinoa* Willd.). *Journal of Natural Products* 1990, 38, (1), 205–208.

[22] Oleszek, W.; Jurzysta, M.; Ploszynski, M.; Colquhoun, I. J.; Price, K. R.; Fenwick, G. R., Zahnic acid tridesmoside and other dominant saponins from alfalfa (*Medicago sativa* L.) aerial parts. *Journal of Agricultural and Food Chemistry* 1992, 40, (2), 191–196.

[23] Bogacheva, N. G.; Kogan, L. M.; Libizov, N. I., Triterpene glycosides of *Chenopodium ambrosioides*. *Chemistry of Natural Compounds* 1974, 8, (3), 392.

[24] Chirva, V. Y.; Cheban, P. L.; Kintya, P. K.; Bobeiko, V. A., Structure of the triterpene glycosides from the roots of *Chenopodium anthelminticum*. *Chemistry of Natural Compounds* 1971, 7, (1), 23–25.

[25] Pyankov, V. I.; Artyusheva, E. G.; Edwards, G. E.; Black, C. C., Jr.; Soltis, P. S., Phylogenetic analysis of tribe Salsoleae (Chenopodiaceae) based on ribosomal ITS sequences: Implications for the evolution of photosynthesis types. *American Journal of Botany* 2001, 88, (7), 1189–1198.

[26] Kadereit, G.; Gotzek, D.; Jacobs, S.; Freitag, H., Origin and age of Australian Chenopodiaceae. *Organisms Diversity & Evolution* 2005, 5, (1), 59–80.

[27] Souci, S. W.; Fachmann, W.; Kraut, H., *Food composition and nutrition tables*. CRC Press: Stuttgart, 2000.

[28] Kokanova-Nedialkova, Z.; Nedialkov, P. T.; Nikolov, N. S., The genus *Chenopodium*: Phytochemistry, ethnopharmacology and pharmacology. *Pharmacognosy Reviews* 2009, 3, (6), 280–306.

[29] Das, J. L.; Mahato, S. B., Triterpenoids. *Phytochemistry* 1983, 22, 1071–1095.

[30] Mahato, S. B.; Nandy, A. K.; Roy, G., Triterpenoids. *Phytochemistry* 1992, 31, (7), 2199–2249.

[31] Dinda, B.; Debnath, S.; Mohanta, B. C.; Harigaya, Y., Naturally occurring triterpenoid saponins. *Chemistry & Biodiversity* 2010, 7, (10), 2327–2580.

[32] Dembitsky, V. M., Chemistry and biodiversity of the biologically active natural glycosides. *Chemistry & Biodiversity* 2004, 1, (5), 673–781.

[33] Lacaille-Dubois, M. A., Biologically and pharmacologically active saponins from plants: Recent advances. In *Saponins in food, feedstuffs and medicinal plants*, Marston, A.; Oleszek, W., Eds. Kluwer: Dordrecht, 2000; pp 205–218.

[34] Lacaille-Dubois, M. A.; Wagner, H., A review of the biological and pharmacological activities of saponins. *Phytomedicine* 1996, 2, (4), 363–386.

[35] Lacaille-Dubois, M. A., Bioactive saponins from plants: recent developments. In *Handbook of medicinal plants*, Yaniv, Z.; Bachroch, U., Eds. The Haworth Medicinal Press (HMP): New York, 2005; pp 399–428.

[36] Lacaille-Dubois, M. A.; Wagner, H., Bioactive saponins from plants: An update. In *Studies in natural products chemistry*, Atta-Ur-Rahman, Ed. Elsevier: Amsterdam, 2000; Vol. 21, pp 633–687.

[37] Rao, A. V.; Gurfinkel, D. M., The bioactivity of saponins: Triterpenoid and steroidal glycosides. *Drug Metabolism and Drug Interactions* 2000, 17, (1–4), 211–235.

[38] Mujica, A., Andean grains and legumes. In: Neglected crops: 1492 from a different perspective. In *Plant Production and Protection*, Bermejo, J. E. H. Leon, J. , Ed. FAO Rome, 1994.

[39] Matsuda, H.; Dai, Y.; Ido, Y.; Ko, S.; Yoshikawa, M.; Kubo, M., Studies on *Kochiae fructus*. III. antinociceptive and anti-inflammatory effects of 70% ethanol extract and its component, momordin Ic from dried fruits of *Kochia scoparia* L. *Biological & Pharmaceutical Bulletin* 1997, 20, (10), 1086–1091.

[40] Wink, M., Phytochemical diversity of secondary metabolites. In *Encyclopedia of plant & crop science*, Marcel Dekker: New York, 2004; pp 915–919.

[41] Corio-Costet, M. F.; Chapuis, L.; Delbecque, J. P., *Chenopodium album* L. (Fat Hen): In vitro cell culture, and production of secondary metabolites (Phytosteroid and ecdysteroids). In *Biotechnology in Agriculture and Forestry*, Bajaj, Y. P. S., Ed. Springer: Berlin, 1998; Vol. 41, pp 97–118.

[42] de Feo, V.; Senatore, F., Medicinal plants and phytotherapy in the Amalfitan Coast, Salerno Province, Campania, southern Italy. *Journal of Ethnopharmacology* 1993, 39, (1), 39–51.

[43] Al-Jaber, N. A. A.; Mujahid, T. G.; Al-Hazmi, H. M. G., Secondary meabolites of Chenopodiaceae species. *Journal of the Chemical Society of Pakistan* 1992, 14, (1), 76–83.

[44] Sanderson, S. C.; Chu, G. L.; McArthur, E. D.; Stutz, H. C., Evolutionary loss of flavonoids and other chemical characters in the Chenopodiaceae. *Biochemical Systematics and Ecology* 1988, 16, (2), 143–149.

[45] Jiang, Z. H.; Tanaka, T.; Kouno, I., Euphane-type triterpene tridesmosides from the leaves of *Rhoiptelea chiliantha. Chemical & Pharmaceutical Bulletin* 1999, 47, (1), 101–103.

[46] Jiang, Z. H.; Tanaka, T.; Hirata, H.; Fukuoka, R.; Kouno, I., The first euphane-type triterpene tridesmosides and bisdesmoside from *Rhoiptelea chiliantha. Tetrahedron* 1997, 53, (50), 16999–17008.

[47] Repo-Carrasco, R.; Espinoza, C.; Jacobsen, S. E., Nutritional value and use of the Andean crops quinoa (*Chenopodium quinoa*) and kañiwa (*Chenopodium pallidicaule*). *Food Reviews International* 2003, 19, (1–2), 179–189.

[48] Mithöfer, A.; Jakupovic, J.; Weiler, E. W., A Triterpenoid glycoside from *Spinacia oleracea. Natural Product Research* 1999, 14, (1), 5–10.

[49] Voutquenne, L.; Lavaud, C.; Massiot, G.; Men-Olivier, L. L., Structure-activity relationships of haemolytic saponins. *Pharmaceutical Biology* 2002, 40, (4), 253–262.

[50] Kimata, H.; Nakashima, T.; Kokubun, S.; Nakayama, K.; Mitoma, Y.; Kitahara, T.; Yata, N.; Tanaka, O., Saponins of pericarps of *Sapindus mukurossi* Gaertn. and solubilization of monodesmosides by bidesmosides. *Chemical & Pharmaceutical Bulletin* 1983, 31, (6), 1998–2005.

[51] Shirakawa, Y.; Itoh, M.; Koyama, K.; Minowa, Y. Aqueous preparation containing vitamin E and saponins. U.S. Patent. 1986.

[52] Eskander, J.; Lavaud, C.; Harakat, D., Steroidal saponins from the leaves of *Agave macroacantha*. *Fitoterapia* 2010, 81, (5), 371–374.

[53] Yokosuka, A.; Jitsuno, M.; Yui, S.; Yamazaki, M.; Mimaki, Y., Steroidal glycosides from *Agave utahensis* and their cytotoxic activity. *Journal of Natural Products* 2009, 72, (8), 1399–1404.

[54] Lin, J. T.; Yang, D. J., Determination of steroidal saponins in different organs of yam (*Dioscorea pseudojaponica* Yamamoto). *Food Chemistry* 2008, 108, (3), 1068–1074.

[55] Ivanova, A.; Mikhova, B.; Batsalova, T.; Dzhambazov, B.; Kostova, I., New furostanol saponins from *Smilax aspera* L. and their in vitro cytotoxicity. *Fitoterapia* 2011, 82, (2), 282–287.

[56] Zhu, G. L., Origin, differentiation, and geographic distribution of the Chenopodiaceae. *Acta Phytotaxonomica Sinica* 1995, 34, (5), 486–504.

[57] Zhu, G. L.; Mosyakin, S. L.; Clemants, S. E., Chenopodiaceae. *Flora of China* 2003, 5, 351–414.

[58] Matsuda, H.; Dai, Y.; Ido, Y.; Yoshikawa, M.; Kubo, M., Studies on kochiae fructus. IV. anti-allergic effects of 70% ethanol extract and its component, momordin Ic from dried fruits of *Kochia scoparia* L. *Biological & Pharmaceutical Bulletin* 1997, 20, (11), 1165–1170.

[59] Choi, J.; Lee, K. T.; Jung, H.; Park, H. S.; Park, H. J., Anti-rheumatoid arthritis effect of the *Kochia scoparia* fruits and activity comparison of momordin Ic, its prosapogenin and sapogenin. *Archives of Pharmacal Research* 2002, 25, (3), 336–342.

[60] Bandaranayake, W. M., Bioactivies bioactive compounds and chemical constituents of mangrove plant. *Wetlands Ecology and Management* 2002, 10, 421.

[61] Ghosh, A.; Misra, S.; Dutta, A. K.; Choudhury, A., Pentacyclic triterpenoids and sterols from seven species of mangrove. *Phytochemistry* 1985, 24, (8), 1725–1727.

[62] El-Shazly, A.; Wink, M., Tetrahydroisoquinoline and b-carboline alkaloids from *Haloxylon articulatum* (Cav.) Bunge (Chenopodiaceae). *Zeitschrift fur Naturforschung C* 2003, 58, (7–8), 477–480.

[63] Hegnauer, R., *Chemotaxonomie der Pflanzen. Band 3.* . Basel and Stuttgart, 1964; p 743.

[64] McWorter, C. D.; Paul, R. N.; Ouzts, J. C., Bicellular trichomes of Johnson grass (*Sorghum halepense*) leaves: Morphology, histochemistry and function. *Weed Science* 1995, 43, (2), 201–208.

[65] Lewis, W. H.; Imber, W. E., Allergy epideminology in the Sant Lous, Missouriarea. IV. weeds. *Ann Allergy* 1975, 35, (3), 180–187.

[66] Yadav, N.; Neeru, V.; Sumitra, S.; S., S. K., Medicinal properties of genus *Chenopodium* Linn. *Natural Product Radiance* 2007, 6, (2), 131–134.

[67] Ueda, H.; Ohshima, M.; Akimoto, I., Nutritive value and hypocholesterolemic effect of alfalfa leaf protein concentrates prepared from two different varieties in chicks. *Japanese Journal of Zootechnical Science* 1987, 58, (4), 347–355.

[68] Risic, J.; Galwey, N. W., *The Chenopodium grains of the Andes: Inca crops for modern agriculture*. Academic Press: London, 1984.

[69] Ruas, P. M.; Bonifacio, A.; Ruas, C. F.; Fairbanks, D. J.; Andersen, W. R., Genetic relationship among 19 accessions of six species of *Chenopodium* L., by random amplified polymorphic DNA fragments (RAPD). *Euphytica* 1999, 105, (1), 25–32.

[70] Ando, H.; Chen, Y. C.; Tang, H. J.; Shimizu, M.; Watanabe, K.; Mitsunaga, T., Food components in fractions of quinoa seed. *Food Science and Technology Research* 2002, 8, (1), 80–84.

[71] Bhargava, A.; Shukla, S.; Ohri, D., *Chenopodium quinoa* — an Indian perspective. *Industrial Crops and Products* 2006, 23, (1), 73–87.

[72] Ng, K. G.; Price, K. R.; Fenwick, G. R., A TLC method for the analysis of quinoa (*Chenopodium quinoa*) saponins. *Food Chemistry* 1994, 49, (3), 311–315.

[73] Lavaud, C.; Voutquenne, L.; Bal, P.; Pouny, I., Saponins from *Chenopodium album*. *Fitoterapia* 2000, 71, (3), 338–340.

[74] Gohar, A. A.; Maatooq, G. T.; Niwa, M.; Yoshiaki, T., A new triterpene saponin from *Chenopodium ficifolium*. *Zeitschrift fur Naturforschung C* 2002, 57, (7–8), 597–602.

[75] Rastrelli, L.; de Simone, F.; Schettino, O.; Dini, A., Constituents of *Chenopodium pallidicaule* (Cañihua) seeds: Isolation and characterization of new triterpene saponins. *Journal of Agricultural and Food Chemistry* 1996, 44, (11), 3528–3533.

[76] Bylka, W.; Stobiecki, M.; Frański, R., Sulphated flavonoid glycosides from leaves of *Atriplex hortensis*. *Acta Physiologiae Plantarum* 2001, 23, (3), 285–290.

[77] Christensen, S. B.; Omar, A. A., *Atriplex nummularia*, a Source for the two molluscicide saponins: Hederagenin-3-*O*-β-D-glucuronopyranoside and calenduloside E. *Journal of Natural Products* 1985, 48, (1), 161–161.

[78] Mabberley, D. J., *The Plant-Book, A portable dictionary of the vascular plants*. Cambridge University Press: UK, 1997; p 326.

[79] Shaukat, A. C., *Flora of the Kingdom of Saudi Arabia' Illustrsated*. Riyadh: Saudi Arabia, 2000; Vol. I, p 180–181.

[80] Ajabnoor, M. A.; Al-Yahya, M. A.; Tariq, M.; Jayyab, A. A., Antidiabetic activity of *Hammada salicornicum*. *Fitoterapia* 1984, LV, 107–109.

[81] Al-Shanawani, M. A. A., *Plant used in Saudi folk medicine*. Riyadh: 1996.

[82] Salah, H. B.; Raoudha, J.; Marie-Thérèse, M.; Nigel, C. V.; Renée, J. G.; Monique, S. J. S.; Mohamed, D., Flavonol triglycosides from the leaves of *Hammada scoparia* (POMEL). *Chemical & Pharmaceutical Bulletin* 2002, 50, (9), 1268–1270.

[83] Tackholm, V., *Student Flora of Egypt*. Caieo University: Caieo, 1974.

[84] Escalante, A. M.; Santecchia, C. B.; Lopez, S. N.; Gattuso, M. A.; Gutierrez Ravelo, A.; Delle Monache, F.; Gonzalez Sierra, M.; Zacchino, S. A., Isolation of antifungal saponins from *Phytolacca tetramera*, an Argentinean species in critic risk. *Journal of Ethnopharmacology* 2002, 82, (1), 29–34.

[85] Sahu, N. P.; Koike, K.; Banerjee, S.; Achari, B.; Nikaido, T., Triterpenoid saponins from *Mollugo spergula*. *Phytochemistry* 2001, 58, (8), 1177–1182.

[86] Woo, W. S.; Kang, S. S.; Yamasaki, K.; Tanaka, O., Carbon-13 NMR spectra of phytolaccagenin and its glycosides. *Archives of Pharmacal Research* 1978, 1, (1), 21–25.

[87] Kohda, H.; Yamaoka, Y.; Morinaga, S.; Ishak, M.; Darise, M., Saponins from *Talinum triangulare*. *Chemical & Pharmaceutical Bulletin* 1992, 40, (9), 2557–2558.

[88] Soliman, H. S.; Elgamal, M. H.; Simon, A.; G, T. t.; Horvath, G.; Duddeck, H., A new gypsogenin saponin from *Arenaria filicaulis*. *Journal of Natural Products* 1999, 62, (6), 885–888.

[89] Chen, Q.; Luo, J. G.; Kong, L. Y., New triterpenoid saponins from the roots of *Gypsophila perfoliata* Linn. *Carbohydrate Research* 2011, 346, (14), 2206–2212.

[90] Szakiel, A.; Henry, M., Analysis of gypsogenin saponins in homeopathic tinctures. *Acta Biochemica Polonica* 2007, 54, (4), 853–856.

[91] Ding, Y.; Tang, H. F.; Wang, J. B.; Liu, D.; Tian, X. R.; Wang, X. Y.; Zhou, X. M., Triterpenoid saponins from *Anemone rivularis* var. *flore-minore*. *Biochemical Systematics and Ecology* 2011, 39, (3), 236–239.

[92] Choi, J.; Jung, H. J.; Lee, K. T.; Park, H. J., Antinociceptive and anti-inflammatory effects of the saponin and sapogenins obtained from the stem of *Akebia quinata. Journal of Medicinal Food* 2005, 8, (1), 78–85.

[93] Kuljanabhagavad, T.; Wink, M., Biological activities and chemistry of saponins from *Chenopodium quinoa* Willd. *Phytochemistry Reviews* 2009, 8, (2), 473–490.

[94] Shaker, K. H.; Dockendorff, K.; Seifert, K., Titerpenoid saponins from *Atriplex semibaccata. Zeitschrift fur Naturforschung C* 2003, 58, (7–8), 485–489.

[95] Kamel, M. S.; Mohamed, K. M.; Hassanean, H. A.; Ohtani, K.; Kasai, R.; Yamasaki, K., Acylated flavonoid glycosides from *Bassia muricata. Phytochemistry* 2001, 57, (8), 1259–1262.

[96] Ridout, C. L.; Price, K. R.; Parkin, G.; Dijoux, M. G.; Lavaud, C., Saponins from sugarbeet and the floc problem. *Journal of Agricultural and Food Chemistry* 1994, 42, (2), 273–282.

[97] Yoshikawa, M.; Murakami, T.; Kadoya, M.; Matsuda, H.; Muraoka, O.; Yamahara, J.; Murakami, N., Medicinal foodstuff. III. sugar beet. (1): Hypoglycemic oleanolic acid oligoglycosides, betavulgarosides I, II, III, and IV, from the root of *Beta vulgaris* L. (Chenopodiaceae). *Chemical & Pharmaceutical Bulletin* 1996, 44, (6), 1212–1217.

[98] Yoshikawa, M.; Murakami, T.; Kodoya, M.; Yamahara, J.; Matsuda, H., Medicinal foodstuffs. XV. Sugar beet. (2): Structures of betavulgarosides V, VI, VII, VIII, IX, and X from the roots and leaves of sugar beet (*Beta vulgaris* L., Chenopodiaceae). *Chemical & Pharmaceutical Bulletin* 1998, 46, (11), 1758–1763.

[99] Zhu, N. Q.; Sheng, S. Q.; Sang, S. M.; Jhoo, J. W.; Bai, N. S.; Karwe, M. V.; Rosen, R. T.; Ho, C. T., Triterpene saponins from debittered quinoa (*Chenopodium quinoa*) seeds. *Journal of Agricultural and Food Chemistry* 2002, 50, (4), 865–867.

[100] Ma, W. W.; Heinstein, P. F.; McLaughlin, J. L., Additional toxic, bitter saponins from the seeds of *Chenopodium quinoa. Journal of Natural Products* 1989, 52, (5), 1132–1135.

[101] Madl, T.; Sterk, H.; Mittelbach, M., Rechberger, G. N., Tandem mass spectrometric analysis of a complex triterpene saponin mixture of *Chenopodium quinoa. Journal of The American Society for Mass Spectrometry* 2006, 17, (6), 795–806.

[102] Mizui, F.; Kasai, R.; Ohtani, K.; Tanaka, O., Saponins from bran of quinoa, *Chenopodium quinoa* Willd.II. *Chemical & Pharmaceutical Bulletin* 1990, 38, (2), 375–377.

[103] Dini, I.; Schettino, O.; Simioli, T.; Dini, A., Studies on the constituents of *Chenopodium quinoa* seeds: Isolation and characterization of new triterpene saponins. *Journal of Agricultural and Food Chemistry* 2001, 49, (2), 741–746.

[104] Dini, I.; Tenore, G. C.; Dini, A., Oleanane saponins in "kancolla", a sweet variety of *Chenopodium quinoa. Journal of Natural Products* 2002, 65, (7), 1023–1026.

[105] Dini, I.; Tenore, G. C.; Schettino, O.; Dini, A., New oleanane saponins in *Chenopodium quinoa. Journal of Agricultural and Food Chemistry* 2001, 49, (8), 3976–3981.

[106] Ruales, J.; Nair, B. M., Saponins, phytic acid, tannins and protease inhibitors in quinoa (*Chenopodium quinoa*, Willd.) seeds. *Food Chemistry* 1993, 48, (2), 137–143.

[107] Mizui, F.; Kasai, R.; Ohtani, K.; Tanaka, O., Saponins from brans of quinoa, *Chenopodium quinoa* Willd. I. *Chemical & Pharmaceutical Bulletin* 1988, 36, (4), 1415–1418.

[108] Eskalieva, B. K.; Akhmed, A.; Burasheva, G. S.; Abilov Zh, A.; Akhmad, V. U., Biologically active compounds from *Climacoptera*. *Chemistry of Natural Compounds* 2004, 40, (1), 87–88.

[109] Yeskaliyeva, B.; Mesaik, M. A.; Abbaskhan, A.; Kulsoom, A.; Burasheva, G.; Abilov Zh, A.; Choudhary, M. I.; Atta ur, R., Bioactive flavonoids and saponins from *Climacoptera obtusifolia*. *Phytochemistry* 2006, 67, (21), 2392–2397.

[110] Annaev, C.; Isamukhamedova, M.; Abubakirov, N. K., Triterpene glycosides of *Climacoptera transoxana* I. *Chemistry of Natural Compounds* 1983, 19, (2), 190–194.

[111] Annaev, C.; Abubakirov, N. K., Triterpene glycosides of *Climacoptera transoxana* IV. structures of copterosides G and H. *Chemistry of Natural Compounds* 1983, 20, (1), 56–60.

[112] Annaev, C.; Isamukhamedova, M.; Abubakirov, N. K., Triterpene glycosides of *Climacoptera transoxana*. II. The structure of copteroside D. *Chemistry of Natural Compounds* 1983, 19, (4), 425–428.

[113] Annaev, C.; Isaev, M. I.; Abubakirov, N. K., Triterpene glycosides of *Climacoptera transoxana*. III. the structures of copterosides E and F. *Chemistry of Natural Compounds* 1983, 19, (5), 560–564.

[114] Kamel, M. S.; Ohtani, K.; Hassanean, H. A.; Khalifa, A. A.; Kasai, R.; Yamasaki, K., Triterpenoidal saponins from *Cornulaca monacantha*. *Die Pharmazie* 2000, 55, (6), 460–462.

[115] Whang, W. K.; Hahn, D. R., Saponins from fructus of *Kochia scopria*. *Archives of Pharmacal Research* 1991, 14, (2), 176–180.

[116] Yoshikawa, M.; Dai, Y.; Shimada, H.; Morikawa, T.; Matsumura, N.; Yoshizumi, S.; Matsuda, H.; Matsuda, H.; Kubo, M., Studies on Kochiae fructus. II. on the saponin constituents from the fruit of Chinese *Kochia scoparia* (Chenopodiaceae): Chemical structures of kochianosides I, II, III, and IV. *Chemical & Pharmaceutical Bulletin* 1997, 45, (6), 1052–1055.

[117] Wen, Y.; Chen, Y.; Cui, Z.; Li, J.; Wang, Z., Triterpenoid glycosides from the fruits of *Kochia scoparia*. *Planta Medica* 1995, 61, (5), 450–452.

[118] Hamed, A. J.; Masullo, M.; Sheded, M. G.; Mahalel, U. A.; Tawfik, M. M.; Perrone, A.; Piacente, S., Triterpene saponins from *Salsola imbricata*. *Phytochemistry Letters* 2011, 4, (3), 353–356.

[119] Annaev, C.; Isamukhamedova, M.; Abubakirov, N. K., Triterpene glycosides of *Salsola micranthera*. II. the strucutre of salsoloside E. *Chemistry of Natural Compounds* 1964, 20, (1), 60–64.

[120] Annaev, C.; Isamukhamedova, M.; Abubakirov, N. K., Triterpene glycosides of *Salsola micranthera*. I. structures of salsolosides C and D. *Chemistry of Natural Compounds* 1983, 19, (6), 691–695.

[121] Tschesche, R.; Rehkämper, H.; Wulff, G., Über Triterpene, XXVIII[1]) Über die saponine des spinats (*Spinacia oleracea* L.). *Justus Liebigs Annalen der Chemie* 1969, 726, (1), 125–135.

[122] Girard, M.; Bélanger, J.; ApSimon, J. W.; Garneau, F. X.; Harvey, C.; Brisson, J. R., Frondoside A. A novel triterpene glycoside from the holothurian *Cucumaria frondosa*. *Canadian Journal of Chemistry* 1990, 68, (1), 11–18.

[123] Garneau, F. X.; Simard, J. L.; Harvey, O., The structure of psoluthurin A, the major triterpene glycoside of the sea cucumber *Psolus fabricii*. *Canadian Journal of Chemistry* 1983, 61, (7), 1465–1471.

[124] Güçlü-Üstündağ, Ö.; Mazza, G., Saponins: properties, applications and processing. *Critical Reviews in Food Science and Nutrition* 2007, 47, (3), 231–258.

[125] Henry, M., Saponins and phylogeny: Example of the ''gypsogenin group'' saponins. *Phytochemistry Reviews* 2005, 4, (2–3), 89–94.

[126] Massiot, G.; Lavaud, C., Structural elucidation of saponins. In *Studies in Natural Products Chemistry*, Atta-ur-Rahman, Ed. Elsevier Science: 1995; Vol. 15, pp 187–224.

[127] Mahato, S. B.; Kundu, A. P., ^{13}C NMR spectra of pentacyclic triterpenoids — a Compilation and some salient features. *Phytochemistry* 1994, 37, (6), 1517–1575.

[128] Agrawal, P. K., NMR Spectroscopy in the structural elucidation of oligosaccharides and glycosides. *Phytochemistry* 1992, 31, (10), 3307–3330.

[129] Larhsini, M.; Marston, A.; Hostettmann, K., Triterpenoid saponins from the roots of *Silene cucubalus*. *Fitoterapia* 2003, 74, (3), 237–241.

[130] Seebacher, W.; Simic, N.; Weis, R.; Saf, R.; Kunert, O., Complete assignments of ^{1}H and ^{13}C NMR resonances of oleanolic acid, 18α-oleanolic acid, ursolic acid and their 11-oxo derivatives. *Magnetic Resonance in Chemistry* 2003, 41, (8), 636–638.

[131] Joshi, B. S.; Singh, K. L.; Roy, R., Complete assignments of ^{1}H and ^{13}C NMR spectra of the pentacyclic triterpene hederagenin from *Nigella sativa* Linn. *Magnetic Resonance in Chemistry* 1999, 37, (4), 295–298.

[132] Seo, S.; Tomita, Y.; Tori, K.; Yoshimura, Y., Determination of the absolute configuration of a secondary hydroxy group in a chiral secondary alcohol using glycosidation shifts in carbon-13 nuclear magnetic resonance spectroscopy. *Journal of the American Chemical Society* 1978, 100, (11), 3331–3339.

[133] Panov, V. P.; Zhbankov, R. G., NMR conformational analysis of saccharides and polysaccharides. *Journal of Applied Spectroscopy* 1973, 18, (6), 809–822.

[134] Tori, K.; Seo, S.; Shimaoka, A.; Tomita, Y., Carbon-13 NMR spectra of olean-12-enes. Full signal assignments including quaternary carbon signals assigned by use of indirect ^{13}C, ^{1}H spin couplings. *Tetrahedron Letters* 1974, 15, (48), 4227–4230.

[135] Tori, K.; Seo, S.; Yoshimura, Y.; Arita, H.; Tomita, Y., Glycosidation shifts in carbon-13 NMR spectroscopy: Carbon-13 signal shifts from aglycone and glucose to glucoside. *Tetrahedron Letters* 1977, 18, (2), 179–182.

[136] Zhou, R.; Li, B. G.; Zhang, G. L., Glycosides from roots of *Cyathula officinalis* Kuan. *Journal of Integrative Plant biology* 2005, 47, (3), 368–374.

[137] Hu, M.; Ogawa, K.; Sashida, Y.; Xiao, P. G., Triterpenoid glucuronide saponins from root bark of *Aralia armata*. *Phytochemistry* 1995, 39, (1), 179–184.

[138] Das, N.; Chandran, P.; Chakraborty, S., Potent spermicidal effect of oleanolic acid 3-beta-D-glucuronide, an active principle isolated from the plant *Sesbania sesban* Merrill. *Contraception* 2011, 83, (2), 167–175.

[139] Murakami, N.; Murakami, T.; Kadoya, M.; Matsuda, H.; Yamahara, J.; Yoshikawa, M., New hypoglycemic constituents in "gymnemic acid" from *Gymnema sylvestre*. *Chemical & Pharmaceutical Bulletin* 1996, 44, (2), 469–471.

[140] Furtado, R. A.; Rodrigues, E. P.; Araujo, F. R.; Oliveira, W. L.; Furtado, M. A.; Castro, M. B.; Cunha, W. R.; Tavares, D. C., Ursolic acid and oleanolic acid suppress

preneoplastic lesions induced by 1,2-dimethylhydrazine in rat colon. *Toxicologic Pathology* 2008, 36, (4), 576–580.

[141] Ovesná, Z.; Vachálková, A.; Horváthová, K.; Tóthová, D., Pentacyclic triterpenoic acids: New chemoprotective compounds minireview. *Neoplasma* 2004, 51, (5), 327–333.

[142] Sparg, S. G.; Light, M. E.; van Staden, J., Biological activities and distribution of plant saponins. *Journal of Ethnopharmacology* 2004, 94, (2–3), 219–243.

[143] Parkhurst, R. M.; Thomas, D. W.; Skinner, W. A.; Cary, L. W., Molluscicidal saponins of *Phytolacca dodecandra*: Lemmatoxin. *Canadian Journal of Chemistry* 1974, 52, (5), 702–705.

[144] Schenkel, E. P.; Werner, W.; Schulte, K. E., Die saponine aus *Thinouia coriacea. Planta Medica* 1991, 57, (5), 463–467.

[145] Favel, A.; Steinmetz, M. D.; Regli, P.; Vidal-Ollivier, E.; Elias, R.; Balansard, G., In vitro antifungal activity of triterpenoid saponins. *Planta Medica* 1994, 60, (1), 50–53.

[146] Lee, M. W.; Kim, S. U.; Hahn, D. R., Antifungal activity of modified hederagenin glycosides from the leaves of *Kalopanax pictum* var. *chinense*. *Biological & Pharmaceutical Bulletin* 2001, 24, (6), 718–719.

[147] Mshvildadze, V.; Favel, A.; Delmas, F.; Elias, R.; Faure, R.; Decanosidze, G.; Kemertelidze, E.; Balansard, G., Antifungal and antiprotozoal activities of saponins from *Hedera colchica. Die Pharmazie* 2000, 55, (4), 325–326.

[148] Zhang, J. D.; Cao, Y. B.; Xu, Z.; Sun, H. H.; An, M. M.; Yan, L.; Chen, H. S.; Gao, P. H.; Wang, Y.; Jia, X. M.; Jiang, Y. Y., In vitro and in vivo antifungal activities of the eight steroid saponins from *Tribulus terrestris* L. with potent activity against fluconazole-resistant fungal pathogens. *Biological & Pharmaceutical Bulletin* 2005, 28, (12), 2211–2215.

[149] Chwalek, M.; Lalun, N.; Bobichon, H.; Ple, K.; Voutquenne-Nazabadioko, L., Structure-activity relationships of some hederagenin diglycosides: Haemolysis, cytotoxicity and apoptosis induction. *Biochimica et Biophysica Acta (BBA) - General Subjects* 2006, 1760, (9), 1418–1427.

[150] Lin, T. D.; Kondo, N.; Shoji, J., Studies on the constituents of *Panacis japonici* rhizoma V.1 the structure of chikusetsusaponin I, Ia, Ib, Iva and glycoside P_1. *Chemical & Pharmaceutical Bulletin* 1976, 24, 253–261.

[151] Yoshikawa, M.; Shimada, H.; Morikawa, T.; Yoshizumi, S.; Matsumura, N.; Murakami, T.; Matsuda, H.; Hori, K.; Yamahara, J., Medicinal foodstuffs. VII. On the saponin constituents with glucose and alcohol absorption-inhibitory activity from a food garnish "Tonburi", the fruit of Japanese *Kochia scoparia* (L.) Schrader: Structures of scoparianosides A, B, and C. *Chemical & Pharmaceutical Bulletin* 1997, 45, (8), 1300–1305.

[152] Konishi, Y.; Arai, N.; Umeda, J.; Gunji, N.; Saeki, S.; Takao, T.; Minoguchi, R.; Kensho, G., Cholesterol lowering effect of the methanol insoluble materials from the quinoa seed pericarp. In *Hydrocolloids Part 2*, Nishinari, K., Ed. Elsevier Science: B.V., 2000; pp 417–422.

[153] Ogawa, H.; Watanabe, K.; Mitsunaga, T.; Meguro, T., Effect of quinoa on blood pressure and lipid metabolism in diet induced hyperlipidemic spontaneously hypertensive rats (SHR). *Journal of Japan Society of Nutrition and Food Sciences* 2001, 54, (4), 221–227.

[154] Takao, T.; Watanabe, N.; Yuhara, K.; Itoh, S.; Suda, S.; Tsuruoka, Y.; Nakatsugawa, K.; Konishi, Y., Hypocholesterolemic effect of protein isolated from quinoa (*Chenopodium quinoa* Willd.) seeds. *Food Science and Technology Research* 2005, 11, (2), 161–167.

[155] Aluko, R. E.; Monu, E., Functional and bioactive properties of quinoa seed protein hydrolysates. *Journal of Food Science* 2003, 68, (4), 1254–1258.

[156] Park, S. H.; Ko, S. K.; Choi, J. G.; Chung, S. H., *Salicornia herbacea* prevents high fat diet-induced hyperglycemia and hyperlipidemia in ICR mice. *Archives of Pharmacal Research* 2006, 29, (3), 256–264.

[157] Tunali, T.; Yarat, A.; Yanardag, R.; Ozcelik, F.; Ozsoy, O.; Ergenekon, G.; Emekli, N., The effect of chard (*Beta vulgaris* var. *cicla* L.) on the skin of streptozotocin induced diabetic rats. *Die Pharmazie* 1998, 53, (9), 638–640.

[158] Shabana, M. M.; Mirhom, Y. W.; Genenah, A. A.; Aboutabl, E. A.; Amer, H. A., Study into wild Egyptian plants of potential medicinal activity. ninth communication: Hypoglycaemic activity of some selected plants in normal fasting and alloxanised rats. *Archiv Für Experimentelle Veterinarmedizin* 1990, 44, (3), 389–394.

[159] Kramer, D. R.; Sutherland, R. M.; Bao, S.; Husband, A. J., Cytokine mediated effects in mucosal immunity. *Immunology and Cell Biology* 1995, 73, (5), 389–396.

[160] de Aizpurua, H. J.; Russell-Jones, G. J., Oral vaccination identification of classes of proteins that proke an immune response upon oral feeding. *Journal of Experimental Medicine* 1988, 167, (2), 440–451.

[161] Estrada, A.; Li, B.; Laarveld, B., Adjuvant action of *Chenopodium quinoa* saponins on the induction of antibody responses to intragastric and intranasal administered antigens in mice. *Comparative Immunology, Microbiology and Infectious Diseases* 1998, 21, (3), 225–236.

[162] Ghosh, D.; Thejomoorthy, P.; Veluchamy, Anti-inflammatory and analgesic activities of oleanolic acid 3-/3-glucoside (RDG-1) from *Randia dumetorum* (Rubiaceae). *Indian Journal of Pharmacology* 1983, 15, (4), 331–342.

[163] Matsuda, H.; Samukawa, K.; Kubo, M., Anti-inflammatory activity of ginsenoside Ro. *Planta Medica* 1990, 56, (1), 19–23.

[164] Marouf, A.; Desbene, S.; Khanh, T. C.; Wagner, H.; Correia, M.; Chauffert, B.; Lacaille-Dubois, M. A., Triterpene saponins from the roots of *Achyranthes bidentata*. *Pharmaceutical Biology* 2001, 39, (4), 263–267.

[165] Ando, H.; Fukumura, M.; Hori, Y.; Hirai, Y.; Toriizuka, K.; Kuchino, Y.; Ida, Y., Two new glucuronide saponins, achyranthosides G and H, from *Achyranthes fauriei* root. *Journal of Natural Medicines* 2008, 62, (1), 57–62.

[166] Tanaka, O.; Kasai, R., Saponins of ginseng and related plants. In *Progress in the chemistry of organic natural products*, Herz, W.; Grisebach, H.; Kirby, G. W.; Tamm, C., Eds. Springer-Verlag: New York, 1984; Vol. 46, pp 1–76.

[167] Leung, K. W.; Wong, A. S., Pharmacology of ginsenosides: A literature review. *Chinese Medicine* 2010, 5, (1), 20.

[168] Oda, K.; Matsuda, H.; Murakami, T.; Katayama, S.; Ohgitani, T.; Yoshikawa, M., Adjuvant and haemolytic activities of 47 saponins derived from medicinal and food plants. *Biological Chemistry* 2000, 381, (1), 67–74.

[169] Atopkina, L. N.; Malinovskaya, G. V.; Elyakov, G. B.; Uvarova, N. I.; Woerdenbag, H. J.; Koulman, A.; Pras, N.; Potier, P., Cytotoxicity of natural ginseng glycosides and semisynthetic analogues. *Planta Medica* 1999, 65, (1), 30–34.

[170] Zhou, X. H.; Kasai, R.; Yoshikawa, M.; Kitagawa, I.; Tanaka, O., Solubilization of saponins of *Bupleuri radix* with ginseng saponins: Effect of malonyl-ginsenosides on water solubility of saikosaponin-b_1. *Chemical & Pharmaceutical Bulletin* 1991, 39, (5), 1250–1252.

[171] Matsuda, H.; Namba, K.; Fukuda, S.; Tani, T.; Kubo, M., Pharmacological study on *Panax ginseng* C. A. Meyer. IV. Effects of red ginseng on experimental disseminated intravascular coagulation. (3). effect of ginsenoside-Ro on the blood coagulative and fibrinolytic system. *Chemical & Pharmaceutical Bulletin* 1986, 34, (5), 2100–2104.

[172] Lee, Y. M.; Saito, H.; Takagi, K.; Shibata, S.; Shoji, J.; Kondo, N., Pharmacological studies of *Panacis Japonici* rhizoma II. *Chemical & Pharmaceutical Bulletin* 1977, 25, (6), 1391–1398.

[173] Oh, S. R.; Kinjo, J.; Shii, Y.; Ikeda, T.; Nohara, T.; Ahn, K. S.; Kim, J. H.; Lee, H. K., Effects of triterpenoids from *Pueraria lobata* on immunohemolysis: beta-D -glucuronic acid plays an active role in anticomplementary activity *in vitro*. *Planta Medica* 2000, 66, (6), 506–510.

[174] Ibironke, G. F.; Ajiboye, K. I., Studies on the anti-inflammatory and analgesic properties of *Chenopodium ambrosioides* leaf extract in rats. *International Journal of Pharmacology* 2007, 3, (1), 111–115.

[175] Al-Saleh, F. S.; Ali, H.; Mirza, M., Chemical constituents of some medicinal plants growing in Bahrain. *Fitoterapia* 1993, 64, 251–256.

[176] Gülçin, I.; Mshvildadze, V.; Gepdiremen, A.; Elias, R., The antioxidant activity of a triterpenoid glycoside isolated from the berries of *Hedera colchica*: 3-*O*-(beta-D-glucopyranosyl)-hederagenin. *Phytotherapy Research* 2006, 20, (2), 130–134.

[177] Letelier, M. E.; Rodríguez-Rojas, C.; Sánchez-Jofré, S.; Aracena-Parks, P., Surfactant and antioxidant properties of an extract from *Chenopodium quinoa* Willd seed coats. *Journal of Cereal Science* 2011, 53, (2), 239–243.

[178] Ahmad, Z.; Mehmood, S.; Fatima, I.; Malik, A.; Ifzal, R.; Afza, N.; Iqbal, L.; Latif, M.; Nizami, T. A., Structural determination of salsolins A and B, new antioxidant polyoxygenated triterpenes from *Salsola baryosma*, by 1D and 2D NMR spectroscopy. *Magnetic Resonance in Chemistry* 2008, 46, (1), 94–98.

[179] Woo, W. S.; Lee, E. B.; Chi, H. J., Biological evaluation of some Saudi Arabian plants. *Journal of the Pharmaceutical Society of Korea* 1977, 21, 141–145.

[180] Rattanathongkom, A.; Lee, J. B.; Hayashi, K.; Sripanidkulchai, B.; Kanchanapoom, T.; Hayashi, T., Evaluation of chikusetsusaponin IVa isolated from *Alternanthera philoxeroides* for its potency against viral replication. *Planta Medica* 2009, 75, (8), 829–835.

[181] Yoo, H. H.; Kwon, S. W.; Park, J. H., The cytotoxic saponin from heat-processed *Achyranthes fauriei* roots. *Biological & Pharmaceutical Bulletin* 29, (5), 1053–1055.

[182] de Rosa, S.; Iodice, C.; Mitova, M.; Handjieva, N.; Popov, S.; Anchev, M., Triterpene saponins and iridoid glucosides from *Galium rivale*. *Phytochemistry* 2000, 54, (8), 751–756.

[183] Kuljanabhagavad, T.; Suttisri, R.; Pengsuparp, T.; Ruangrungsi, N., Chemical structure and antiviral activity of aerial part from *Laggera pterodonta*. *Journal of Health Research* 2009, 23, (4), 175–177.

[184] Vichkanova, S. A.; Goryunova, L. V., Antiviral activity of some saponins. *Tr Vses Nauch-Issled Inst Lek Rast.* 1971, 14, 204–212.

[185] Vidal-Ollivier, E.; Babadjamian, A.; Maillard, C.; Elias, R.; Balansard, G., Identification et dosage par chromatographie liquide haute performance de six saponosides dans les fleurs de *Clendula officinalis*. *Pharmaceutica Acta Helvetiae* 1989, 64, 156–159.

[186] Vidal-Ollivier, E.; Balansard, G.; Faure, R.; Babadjamian, A., Revised sructures of triterpenoid saponins from the flowers of *Calendula officinalis*. *Journal of Natural Products* 1989, 52, (5), 1156–1159.

[187] Davidyants, É. S.; Putieva, Z. M.; Bandyukova, V. A.; Abubakirov, N. K., Triterpene glycosides of *Silphium perfoliatum* II. *Chemistry of Natural Compounds* 1984, 20, (5), 636–636.

[188] Shimizu, S.; Ishihara, N.; Umehara, K.; Miyase, T.; Ueno, A., Sesquiterpene glycosides and saponins from *Cynara cardunculus* L. *Chemical & Pharmaceutical Bulletin* 1988, 36, (7), 2466–2474.

[189] Shukla, Y. N.; Thakur, R. S., Saponins and other constituents from the rhizomes of *Panax pseudo-ginseng* subs *himalaicus* var. *angustifolius*. *Phytochemistry* 1986, 25, (9), 2201–2203.

[190] Tran, Q. L.; Than, M. M.; Tezuka, Y.; Banskota, A. H.; Kouda, K.; Watanabe, H.; Zhu, S.; Komatsu, K.; Thet, M. M.; Swe, T.; Maruyama, Y.; Kadota, S., Wild ginseng grows in Myanmar. *Chemical & Pharmaceutical Bulletin* 2003, 51, (6), 679–682.

[191] Kim, J. S.; Kang, S. S., Saponins from the aerial parts of *Aralia continentalis*. *Natural Product Sciences* 1998, 4, (1), 45–50.

[192] Guo, Z.; Zou, K.; Dan, F.; Wang, J.; Zhu, S.; Komatsu, K., Panajaponin, a new glycosphingolipid from *Panax japonicus*. *Natural Product Research* 2010, 24, (1), 86–91.

[193] Hosono-Nishiyama, K.; Matsumoto, T.; Kiyohara, H.; Nishizawa, A.; Atsumi, T.; Yamada, H., Suppression of fas-mediated apoptosis of keratinocyte cells by chikusetsusaponins isolated from the roots of *Panax japonicus*. *Planta Medica* 2006, 72, (3), 193–198.

[194] Liang, C.; Ding, Y.; Nguyen, H. T.; Kim, J. A.; Boo, H. J.; Kang, H. K.; Nguyen, M. C.; Kim, Y. H., Oleanane-type triterpenoids from *Panax stipuleanatus* and their anticancer activities. *Bioorganic & Medicinal Chemistry Letters* 2010, 20, (23), 7110–7115.

[195] Chan, H. H.; Hwang, T. L.; Reddy, M. V.; Li, D. T.; Qian, K.; Bastow, K. F.; Lee, K. H.; Wu, T. S., Bioactive constituents from the roots of *Panax japonicus* var. *major* and development of a LC-MS/MS method for distinguishing between natural and artifactual compounds. *Journal of Natural Products* 2011, 74, (4), 796–802.

[196] Tanaka, O.; Morita, T.; Kasai, R.; Kinouchi, J.; Sanada, S.; Ida, Y.; Shoji, J., Study on saponins of rhizomes of *Panax pseudo-ginseng* subsp. *himalaicus* collected at Tzatogang and Pari-la, Bhutan-Himalaya. *Chemical & Pharmaceutical Bulletin* 1985, 33, (6), 2323–2330.

[197] Yoo, H. H.; Kwon, S. W.; Park, J. H., The cytotoxic saponin from heat-processed *Achyranthes fauriei* roots. *Biological & Pharmaceutical Bulletin* 2006, 29, (5), 1053–1055.

[198] Nishimoto, N.; Shiobara, Y.; Fujino, M.; Inoue, S. S.; Takemoto, T.; de Oliveira, F.; Akisue, G.; Akisue, M. K.; Hashimoto, G.; Tanaka, O.; Kasai, R.; Matsuura, H., Ecdysteroids from *Pfaffia iresinoides* and reassignment of some ^{13}CNMR chemical shifts. *Phytochemistry* 1987, 26, (9), 2505–2507.

[199] Amimoto, K.; Yoshikawa, K.; Arihara, S., Triterpenoid saponins of aquifoliaceous plants. VIII. [1)] ilexosides XXIX–XXXII from the leaves of *Ilex rotunda* Thunb. [2)] *Chemical & Pharmaceutical Bulletin* 1992, 40, (12), 3138–3141.

[200] Murakami, T.; Hirano, K.; Yoshikawa, M., Medicinal foodstuffs. XXIII.[1)] structures of new oleanane-type triterpene oligoglycosides, basellasaponins A, B, C, and D, from the fresh aerial parts of *Basella rubra* L. *Chemical & Pharmaceutical Bulletin* 2001, 49, (6), 776–779.

[201] Espada, A.; Rodríguez, J.; Villaverde, M. C.; Riguera, R., Boussingoside D_1, a new triterpenoid saponin from *Boussingaultia baselloides*. *Liebigs Annalen der Chemie* 1991, 1991, (3), 291–293.

[202] Nie, R. L.; Morita, T.; Kasai, R.; Zhou, J.; Wu, C. Y.; Tanaka, O., Saponins from Chinese medicinal plants. (I). isolation and structures of hemslosides. *Planta Medica* 1984, 50, (4), 322–327.

[203] Wang, J. R.; Zhou, H.; Jiang, Z. H.; Liu, L., Two new triterpene saponins from the anti-inflammatory saponin fraction of *Ilex pubescens* root. *Chemistry & Biodiversity* 2008, 5, (7), 1369–1376.

[204] Yoshikawa, M.; Murakami, T.; Komatsu, H.; Matsuda, H., Medicinal foodstuffs. XII. [1)] Saponin constituents with adjuvant activity from hyacinth bean, the seeds of *Dolichos lablab* L. (1): Structures of lablabosides A, B, and C. *Chemical & Pharmaceutical Bulletin* 1998, 46, (5), 812–816.

[205] Kinjo, J.; Suyama, K.; Nohara, T., Triterpenoidal saponins from *Dumasia truncata*. *Phytochemistry* 1995, 40, (6), 1765–1767.

[206] Borel, C.; Gupta, M. P.; Hostettmann, K., Molluscicidal saponins from *Swartzia simplex*. *Phytochemistry* 1987, 26, 2685–2689.

[207] Lavaud, C.; Beauvière, S.; Massiot, G.; Le Men-Olivier, L.; Bourdy, G., Saponins from *Pisonia umbellifera*. *Phytochemistry* 1996, 43, (1), 189–194.

[208] Saniewska, A.; Jarecka, A.; Biały, Z.; Jurzysta, M., Antifungal activity of saponins originated from *Medicago hybrida* against some ornamental plant pathogens. *Acta Agrobotanica* 2006, 59, (2), 51–58.

[209] Bedir, E.; Kirmizipekmez, H.; Sticher, O.; Çaliş, I., Triterpene saponins from the fruits of *Hedera helix*. *Phytochemistry* 2000, 53, (8), 905–909.

[210] Kizu, H.; Kitayama, S.; Nakatani, F.; Tomimori, T.; Namba, T., Studies on nepalese crude drugs. III. on the saponins of *Hedera nepalensis* K. Koch. *Chemical & Pharmaceutical Bulletin* 1985, 33, (8), 3324–3329.

[211] Takemoto, T.; Arihara, S.; Yoshikawa, K.; Tanaka, R.; Hayashi, T., Studies on the constituents of Cucurbitaceae plants. XIII. on the saponin constituents of *Luffa cylindrica* Roem. (2). *Yakugaku Zasshi* 1985, 105, (9), 834–839.

[212] Luo, L.; Li, Z.; Zhang, Y.; Huang, R., Triterpenes and steroidal compounds from *Momordica dioica. Yao xue xue bao = Acta pharmaceutica Sinica* 1998, 33, (11), 839–842.

[213] Marston, A.; Gafner, F.; Dosssaji, S. F.; Hostettmann, K., Fungicidal and molluscicidal saponins from *Dolichos kilimandscharicus. Phytochemistry* 1988, 27, (5), 1325–1326.

[214] Domon, B.; Hostettmann, K., Saponins with molluscicidal properties from *Lonicera nigra* L. *Helvetica Chimica Acta* 1983, 66, (2), 422–428.

[215] Matsuda, H.; Li, Y.; Murakami, T.; Matsumura, N.; Yamahara, J.; Yoshikawa, M., Antidiabetic principles of natural medicines. III. structure-related inhibitory activity and action mode of oleanolic acid glycosides on hypoglycemic activity. *Chemical & Pharmaceutical Bulletin* 1998, 46, (9), 1399–1403.

[216] Matsuda, H.; Li, Y.; Murakami, T.; Yamahara, J.; Yoshikawa, M., Protective effects of oleanolic acid oligoglycosides on ethanol- or indomethacin-induced gastric mucosal lesions in rats. *Life sciences* 1998, 63, (17), PL245–PL250.

[217] Kinjo, J.; Okawa, M.; Udayama, M.; Sohno, Y.; Hirakawa, T.; Shii, Y.; Nohara, T., Hepatoprotective and hepatotoxic actions of oleanolic acid-type triterpenoidal glucuronides on rat primary hepatocyte cultures. *Chemical & Pharmaceutical Bulletin* 1999, 47, (2), 290–292.

[218] Dai, Y.; Ye, W. C.; Wang, Z. T.; Matsuda, H.; Kubo, M.; But, P. P., Antipruritic and antinociceptive effects of *Chenopodium album* L. in mice. *Journal of Ethnopharmacology* 2002, 81, (2), 245–250.

[219] Olajide, O. A.; Awe, S. O.; Makinde, J. M., Pharmacological screening of the methanolic extract of *Chenopodium ambrosioide. Fitoterapia* 1997, 68, (6), 529–532.

[220] Lall, N.; Meyer, J. J., In vitro inhibition of drug-resistant and drug-sensitive strains of *Mycobacterium tuberculosis* by ethnobotanically selected South African plants. *Journal of Ethnopharmacology* 1999, 66, (3), 347–354.

[221] Tschesche, R., *Advances in the chemstry of antibiotic substances from higher plants.* Springer: Berlin, 1971.

[222] Gadano, A.; Gurni, A.; López , M. N.; López , P.; Gratti, A.; van Baren, C.; Ferraro, G.; Carballo, M., Cytogenetic effects of aqueous extracts of the medicinal plant paico (*Chenopodium multifidum* L.). *Pharmaceutical Biology* 2000, 38, (1), 7–12.

[223] Kliks, M. M., Studies on the traditional herbal anthelmintic *Chenopodium ambrosioides* L.: Ethnopharmacological evaluation and clinical field trials. *Social Science & Medicine* 1985, 21, (8), 879–886.

[224] Gadano, A.; Gurni, A.; López, P.; Ferraro, G.; Carballo, M., In vitro genotoxic evaluation of the medicinal plant *Chenopodium ambrosioides* L. *Journal of Ethnopharmacology* 2002, 81, (1), 11–16.

INDEX

A

acarbose, 113
accessions, 193
acetic acid, 9, 20, 88, 89, 166
acetone, 108, 137
acetonitrile, 83, 87, 89, 90
acetylation, 108
acetylcholine, 14, 24
acetylcholinesterase, 114, 118
acid, vii, 1, 3, 4, 8, 9, 10, 12, 14, 15, 18, 20, 22, 24, 26, 27, 35, 39, 40, 45, 47, 48, 49, 55, 84, 88, 89, 97, 98, 99, 101, 102, 106, 108, 109, 110, 113, 114, 125, 135, 144, 147, 149, 150, 151, 152, 153, 162, 163, 165, 166, 168, 169, 170, 171, 172, 173, 174, 175, 176, 177, 178, 179, 180, 181, 182, 183, 184, 185, 187, 188, 189, 190, 191, 195, 197, 199, 200, 203
acidic, 10, 109, 134, 165
acidity, ix, 155
acne, 28
ACTH, 114
active compound, 9, 91, 113, 163, 196
active oxygen, 156, 159
active transport, 112
adaptation, 25
additives, 27, 28, 87, 88, 134, 135
adenocarcinoma, 42
adenosine, 24, 125, 129
adhesion, 23, 25, 136
adhesives, 136
adipocyte, 125, 130, 144, 152
adiponectin, viii, 121, 126, 131, 144, 152
adipose tissue, 125, 130
adiposity, 130
ADP, 146
adsorption, 81, 83, 93, 108, 140
aerospace, 139
aflatoxin, 19
Africa, 97, 168
age, 165, 191
aggregation, 9, 10, 18, 23, 39
aging process, 28
aglycones, vii, viii, ix, 1, 4, 7, 9, 10, 18, 22, 24, 26, 97, 107, 108, 109, 110, 114, 118, 155, 156, 157, 158, 161, 165, 166, 177, 178, 179, 188, 189
agriculture, 135, 193
air quality, 136
albumin, 10, 20, 36
alcoholism, 26
alcohols, 9, 165
aldehydes, 3, 144
alfalfa, 2, 10, 48, 168, 191, 193
alkaline hydrolysis, 165, 178, 179
alkaloids, 167, 193
allergy, 113
amino acids, 163
ammonia, 48
ammonium, 84, 88, 89, 140
amnesia, 127
analgesic, 31, 183, 199, 200
androgen, 16
aneuploidy, 34
angiogenesis, 112
annuals, 167
antagonism, 114
antibiotic, 28, 203
antibody, 16, 17, 33, 84, 185, 199
anti-cancer, 19, 36, 123
anticancer activity, 18
anticancer drug, 18, 26, 35
anticonvulsant, vii, 1
antidepressant, 127
antigen, 17, 45, 46, 185
antigen-presenting cell, 17
antioxidant, 19, 23, 30, 38, 124, 128, 151, 163, 183, 186, 189, 200

antitumor, 112, 183
antitumor agent, 112
apoptosis, ix, 18, 19, 24, 25, 32, 34, 37, 39, 41, 44, 48, 111, 112, 123, 126, 127, 149, 150, 152, 153, 155, 157, 198, 201
aqueous solutions, 2, 9
Argentina, 167
aromatic hydrocarbons, 141
arrest, 18, 150
arteriosclerosis, 123
artery, 23, 39, 126
arthritis, 144
ascorbic acid, 114
Asia, 31, 52, 97, 121, 129, 167, 168
asparagus, 2
assessment, 123
asthma, 33
astrocytoma, 146, 149
atherogenesis, 23
atherosclerosis, 47, 48, 123
atmospheric pressure, 88
atoms, 8, 110, 134
attachment, 4, 109, 122, 161, 177
Austria, 167

B

Bacillus subtilis, 21
bacteria, viii, 2, 10, 18, 21, 42, 133, 183
Bahrain, 200
base, 27, 47, 141, 165, 178, 182
baths, 27
beet molasses, 169, 170
beetles, 42
beneficial effect, 28, 52
benefits, vii, viii, 2, 25, 26, 27, 47, 91, 123, 133, 189, 190
benzene, 9, 166
beverages, 25, 27, 135
Bhutan, 201
bile, ix, 15, 19, 36, 42, 110, 112, 116, 119, 155
bile acids, ix, 15, 19, 36, 42, 155
biodegradability, 21
biodiversity, 163, 191
biological activities, viii, ix, 10, 11, 39, 49, 52, 114, 121, 135, 156, 158, 159, 163, 183, 184, 189, 190
biological activity, viii, ix, 10, 11, 26, 28, 40, 97, 98, 135, 155, 156, 158
biological systems, 24, 29
biomarkers, 128, 132
biosurfactant, 141
biosynthesis, 7
biosynthetic pathways, 7
blends, 27, 30
blood, 2, 18, 23, 24, 35, 40, 42, 44, 123, 125, 131, 184, 185, 198, 200
blood pressure, 24, 44, 184, 198
blood vessels, 23
BMI, 125
body weight, 125, 131, 188
Bolivia, 167
bonds, 4, 7, 9, 13, 136, 145
bone, 18, 144
bone marrow, 18
bone resorption, 144
bones, 114
brain, 23, 32, 50
breakdown, 12, 19
breast cancer, 18, 146, 147, 149, 150, 158, 159
breeding, 36, 168
bronchitis, viii, 97, 98
Bulgaria, 97
Burma, 168

C

Ca^{2+}, 13, 14, 23, 32, 49
CAD, 90
calcium, 49, 97
calorimetry, 137
cancer, viii, ix, 18, 19, 26, 28, 35, 36, 39, 44, 48, 49, 51, 52, 111, 112, 119, 123, 126, 127, 140, 146, 147, 149, 150, 151, 153, 155, 156, 157, 158, 159
cancer cells, 18, 28, 35, 36, 44, 112, 146, 147, 149, 150, 151, 153, 156, 157, 158, 159
candidates, 136, 139, 189
capillary, 20, 90
carbohydrate, ix, 2, 44, 113, 161, 163, 164, 165, 166, 178, 179, 180, 181, 182, 183, 189
carbon, 3, 7, 8, 42, 109, 134, 156, 157, 178, 179, 181, 182, 197
carbon atoms, 134
carbon tetrachloride, 42
carboxyl, 9, 10
carboxylic acid, 166, 186, 189
carcinogen, viii, 97, 111
carcinogenesis, 18, 34
carcinoma, 18, 26, 111, 115, 118, 146, 147, 149, 150, 153, 157
cardiac glycoside, 47
cardiovascular disease, 40, 49, 123
cardiovascular system, viii, 51, 52
cartilage, 114
Caryophyllaceae,, viii, 97, 107, 167
casein, 10, 119
caspases, 19

cataract, 26
C-C, 138
cell culture, 144, 192
cell cycle, 18, 126
cell death, ix, 143, 146, 147, 148, 149, 150, 151, 157
cell invasion, 153
cell lines, ix, 18, 19, 35, 39, 111, 126, 146, 147, 148, 149, 151, 152, 153, 155, 156, 157
cell membranes, 11, 13, 16, 21, 22, 27, 30, 33, 34, 40
cell surface, 2, 18, 111, 140
cellulose, 136, 137, 138, 139, 140, 141
Central Asia, 51
central nervous system, viii, 3, 14, 40, 51, 52
cerebrovascular disease, 26, 91
challenges, 177
cheese, 27, 36
chemical, vii, viii, ix, 3, 9, 12, 16, 20, 26, 29, 34, 49, 52, 81, 83, 85, 87, 88, 91, 108, 109, 110, 112, 113, 119, 121, 122, 134, 135, 136, 137, 155, 157, 158, 159, 161, 163, 168, 178, 179, 180, 186, 192, 193, 202
chemical degradation, 108, 179
chemical reactions, 109, 169, 178
chemical structures, vii, ix, 16, 29, 49, 83, 155, 157, 158, 159, 168
chemoprevention, ix, 126, 143
chemotherapy, 36, 112
Chile, 167
China, 51, 94, 167, 168, 193
Chinese medicine, ix, 38, 52, 143, 167, 187
chitosan, 140
Chitosan, 136
chloroform, 9, 84, 107, 166
cholera, 185
cholesterol, ix, 2, 9, 10, 12, 13, 14, 15, 16, 17, 25, 27, 28, 30, 31, 33, 34, 35, 39, 40, 41, 42, 43, 44, 46, 112, 114, 118, 119, 125, 130, 135, 155, 183, 184
chromatography, 3, 35, 81, 82, 83, 84, 89, 90, 107, 108, 118, 119, 144, 168
classes, ix, 8, 98, 134, 143, 163, 165, 199
classical methods, 3
classification, ix, 7, 48, 139, 156, 190
cleavage, 7, 9, 165, 178
climates, 51
clinical trials, 26, 123, 127
clothing, 136
CNS, 3, 187
coatings, 136, 139
coding, 16, 49
cognitive function, 23
collagen, 151
Colombia, 167
colon, 19, 34, 42, 44, 111, 112, 118, 147, 150, 153, 156, 198
colon cancer, 19, 44, 147, 150, 153, 156
combination therapy, 128
commercial, 15, 23, 25, 27, 28, 83, 84, 168
communication, 23, 199
complexity, 4, 9, 19, 26, 29, 107, 108, 125, 177, 189
complications, 123, 185
composition, vii, 1, 3, 9, 12, 31, 35, 49, 83, 88, 159, 165, 178, 183, 190, 191
compounds, vii, viii, ix, 1, 2, 4, 7, 9, 10, 11, 15, 16, 28, 38, 39, 44, 47, 81, 82, 84, 85, 88, 91, 108, 111, 113, 127, 133, 139, 140, 143, 161, 166, 177, 179, 181, 183, 186, 189, 193, 198, 201, 203
conductivity, 13
configuration, 81, 109, 110, 178, 179, 183, 197
conflict, 124
conformational analysis, 197
congruence, 125
connectivity, 109
consensus, 132
constituents, 29, 30, 41, 98, 113, 123, 126, 159, 168, 183, 193, 195, 196, 197, 198, 200, 201, 202
consumption, 25, 48, 85, 90
control group, 112
controversies, 127
COOH, 7, 55, 99, 102, 113, 165
cooking, 37
coronary artery disease, 126
coronary heart disease, 26
correlation, 14, 46, 109, 110, 114
correlations, 110, 180, 181, 182
cortex, 14, 37, 119
cortisol, 24, 29, 186
cosmetic, vii, 2, 3, 9, 28, 31, 166, 189
cosmetics, 25, 28, 31, 134, 135, 136
cost, 81, 85, 90, 123, 136
cotton, 140, 186
cough, 168
coupling constants, 109, 182
covering, 2, 163
CPC, 84, 108
CRF, 139
crops, 167, 192, 193
cultural practices, 122
culture, 33, 111, 118, 144
cycles, 29
cyclins, 146, 149
cysteine, 17
cytochrome, 18, 39, 147, 150
cytokines, 17, 25, 127, 144
cytomegalovirus, 188
cytometry, 43

cytotoxic agents, 43
cytotoxicity, viii, ix, 18, 32, 33, 35, 36, 97, 98, 110, 111, 116, 119, 149, 155, 156, 157, 158, 163, 193, 198

D

DCI, 39
deacetylation, 138
deaths, 123
defence, 25
degradation, 7, 108, 111
degradation process, 111
dementia, 26, 39
dendritic cell, 145
derivatives, 8, 16, 22, 24, 26, 27, 28, 35, 49, 112, 115, 144, 149, 158, 160, 163, 165, 177, 189, 197
desorption, 81, 82, 88
detectable, 26
detection, 83, 85, 87, 88, 189
detection techniques, 87
detergents, 27, 28, 166
detoxification, 45
diabetes, viii, 48, 51, 52, 91, 123, 124, 125, 126, 128, 129, 131, 164, 167
diabetic patients, 123, 129
dialysis, 82, 108
diet, 15, 16, 28, 34, 46, 47, 112, 114, 118, 124, 125, 131, 151, 184, 198, 199
dietary fat, 15
differential scanning, 137
differential scanning calorimetry, 137
digestion, 23, 36, 125
dimethylformamide, 137
diseases, 20, 23, 26, 28, 33, 51, 91, 123, 126, 144, 187
disorder, 123
disseminated intravascular coagulation, 200
dissociation, 89
distilled water, 81
distribution, 46, 141, 193, 198
diuretic, viii, 97, 98, 186
diversity, vii, ix, 1, 2, 7, 25, 29, 49, 91, 161, 164, 165, 167, 168, 192
DMF, 137
DNA, 17, 23, 24, 34, 45, 147, 150, 151, 157, 193
dopamine, 24, 45
dopaminergic, 16, 24
dosage, 201
double bonds, 7, 145
down-regulation, 144, 149, 150, 152
drug delivery, 44, 136, 141
drug discovery, 189
drugs, 25, 26, 28, 43, 47, 87, 115, 120, 159, 202
DSC, 137
duodenal ulcer, 26
durability, 136
dyeing, 168
dyslipidemia, 123

E

effluent, 88
egg, 16, 33, 44, 48
Egypt, 168, 194
electric field, 85, 90
electron, 11, 13, 29, 137, 180
electron microscopy, 11, 13, 137
electrophoresis, 90
electrospinning, 136, 137
ELISA, 90
elucidation, viii, 3, 38, 40, 45, 97, 98, 108, 109, 114, 115, 178, 189, 197
emulsifying agents, 163, 166, 183
emulsions, 10
endocrine, 43
energy, 82, 85, 121, 125, 130, 132
energy consumption, 85
energy expenditure, 125
engineering, 136, 141
environment, viii, 13, 14, 133, 136
environmental conditions, viii, 133
environments, 21
enzyme, ix, 10, 14, 19, 24, 113, 125, 151, 155
epidemic, 123, 129
epidemiology, 129
epithelium, 50, 113
equipment, 90, 139
erythrocytes, vii, 1, 2, 11, 18, 30
ESI, 84, 88, 90, 109, 110, 179
esophageal cancer, 157, 159
ester, 4, 17, 55, 99, 103, 104, 105, 106, 107, 109, 110, 134, 162, 165, 169, 170, 171, 172, 173, 174, 175, 176, 177, 178, 179, 183, 186, 187
ester bonds, 165
ethanol, 3, 9, 19, 81, 82, 83, 85, 146, 149, 166, 184, 187, 192, 193, 203
ethyl acetate, 9, 83, 84, 166
ethylene, 84
eukaryotic, 21
Europe, 33, 97, 167, 168
European Commission, 33
European Union, 27
evaporation, 3
evidence, 15, 17, 24, 25, 28, 41, 46, 112, 121, 126, 151, 156, 157, 169

evolution, 191
excretion, 15
exercise, 32
exocytosis, 111
expectorant, vii, viii, 1, 3, 97, 98
exposure, 113
extraction, 3, 9, 13, 25, 43, 44, 81, 85, 87, 89, 107, 159, 166, 168, 183
extracts, ix, x, 11, 15, 20, 25, 26, 28, 30, 33, 38, 81, 83, 84, 91, 107, 126, 131, 143, 146, 149, 152, 153, 155, 157, 158, 159, 161, 183, 185, 203

F

fabrication, 136
FAS, 125, 144
fasting, 123, 125, 199
fat, 10, 15, 27, 34, 36, 108, 124, 125, 129, 130, 131, 151
fat soluble, 108
fatty acids, 130
FDA, 27
feces, 85
feed additives, 28
feedstuffs, 163, 183, 191
female rat, 15
femur, 112
fermentation, 48, 153
fiber, 137, 140
fibers, 136, 139
fibrinolytic, 200
field trials, 203
fillers, 98
film formation, 136
films, 134, 136, 139, 141
filtration, 107, 135, 136
fish, 11, 25, 29, 33, 135, 177, 183
flavonoids, 164, 167, 192, 196
flexibility, 189
flight, 88, 89
flocculation, 27
flour, 23, 184
flowers, 49, 98, 116, 122, 165, 184, 187, 188, 201
fluid, 82
fluorescence, 87, 90
foams, 2, 10, 166
follicle, 15
food, vii, x, 1, 3, 9, 14, 22, 23, 25, 27, 28, 34, 41, 42, 46, 47, 48, 113, 124, 134, 135, 139, 140, 159, 161, 163, 166, 167, 183, 184, 189, 190, 191, 198, 199
food additive, 27, 47, 134
food additives, 27, 134, 183
Food and Drug Administration (FDA), 27
food industry, 34
food intake, 124, 184
food products, 27, 48
force, 13, 82
formation, 2, 5, 9, 10, 11, 12, 13, 19, 23, 27, 31, 40, 44, 48, 50, 114, 124, 135, 136, 137, 140, 150, 163, 165
formula, 179, 180
fragments, 157, 179, 193
free radicals, 22, 23
fructose, vii, 1, 4, 128
fruits, 21, 53, 122, 163, 165, 167, 175, 187, 188, 192, 193, 196, 202
FTICR, 88
FTIR, 137, 138
functional food, 27
fungi, viii, 22, 37, 133, 134, 138, 183
fungus, 22
fusion, 145

G

gastric mucosa, 19, 187, 203
gastric ulcer, 26
gastritis, viii, 26, 97, 98
gel, 3, 82, 83, 107, 108, 144, 169
gene expression, 24, 42, 130, 144, 152
genes, 15, 17, 19, 25, 124, 129, 144
genus, vii, viii, ix, 3, 37, 51, 52, 81, 85, 97, 98, 99, 103, 121, 143, 162, 163, 167, 168, 177, 187, 188, 191, 193
Germany, 161, 167
germination, 135, 160
ginseng, v, vii, viii, 3, 14, 15, 17, 18, 19, 20, 24, 26, 27, 32, 36, 37, 38, 39, 42, 43, 44, 45, 46, 47, 48, 49, 51, 52, 53, 54, 55, 56, 57, 58, 59, 60, 61, 63, 64, 65, 66, 67, 68, 71, 72, 75, 76, 77, 78, 79, 80, 81, 83, 84, 85, 87, 88, 89, 90, 91, 121, 122, 123, 124, 125, 126, 127, 128, 129, 130, 131, 184, 186, 199, 200, 201
ginsenosides, viii, 13, 18, 19, 23, 31, 36, 52, 53, 81, 83, 84, 85, 86, 87, 88, 89, 90, 121, 122, 123, 124, 125, 126, 128, 129, 186, 199, 200
glioma, 48
glucocorticoid, 24, 32, 33, 39, 42, 49, 125, 130
glucocorticoid receptor, 24, 32, 33, 39, 42, 49, 125, 130
glucocorticoids, 24, 29
glucose, vii, 1, 4, 14, 40, 106, 114, 123, 124, 125, 128, 129, 130, 131, 152, 165, 179, 181, 182, 183, 184, 185, 187, 197, 198
glucose tolerance, 123, 128, 185

glucose tolerance test, 185
glucoside, 55, 197, 199
GLUT4, 124, 131
glutathione, 19
glycerol, 144
glycogen, 37, 113, 117
glycones, vii, 1, 2
glycoproteins, 14, 23, 183
glycoside, 21, 38, 115, 117, 165, 180, 188, 192, 196, 197, 198, 200
glycosidic compounds, vii, 1
glycosylation, 156, 157, 185
GRAS, 26, 27
grass, 193
group B soyasaponins, ix, 23, 35, 155, 157, 158
growth, ix, 3, 15, 18, 21, 24, 28, 29, 33, 35, 45, 49, 98, 111, 112, 115, 118, 124, 133, 135, 136, 137, 140, 146, 149, 150, 155, 157, 158, 163, 184, 187
growth arrest, 150
growth factor, 18, 111, 115, 124, 140, 146, 149
Gypsophila, v, vii, viii, 3, 97, 98, 99, 107, 108, 109, 110, 111, 112, 113, 114, 115, 116, 117, 118, 119, 120, 169, 194

H

habitats, 167
hair, 27, 31, 135
harmful effects, 23
harvesting, 116
hazards, 28
healing, 51, 134, 140
health, vii, viii, ix, 2, 3, 25, 26, 27, 28, 47, 123, 125, 133, 155, 189, 190
health effects, ix, 26, 155
heart disease, 26, 123
heart failure, 127
hematopoietic system, 35
hepatic stellate cells, 146, 149, 153
hepatitis, viii, 46, 97, 98, 151, 160, 167, 186
hepatitis a, 186
hepatocytes, viii, 97, 112, 113, 114, 115, 119
hepatoma, 24, 112, 153
hepatotoxicity, 42
herbal medicine, 25
hexane, 84, 108
high fat, 34, 131, 184, 199
histamine, 19
histidine, 111
histochemistry, 193
history, ix, 33, 143
HIV, 17, 22, 26, 33, 40
HIV-1, 17, 22
homeostasis, 123, 132
hormone, 15, 29, 33, 114, 120
hormones, viii, 2, 3, 16, 24, 25, 28
HPLC-UV, 87, 88
human, 14, 15, 18, 19, 23, 25, 26, 29, 30, 31, 35, 36, 37, 38, 39, 40, 42, 44, 45, 46, 91, 111, 114, 115, 126, 128, 129, 130, 136, 146, 147, 149, 150, 152, 153, 157, 159, 188
human body, 38
human immunodeficiency virus, 45
human leukemia cells, 146, 149, 152
human skin, 136
human subjects, 14, 126
hydrogen bonds, 13, 136
hydrolysis, 9, 10, 17, 46, 98, 108, 109, 110, 165, 178, 179, 181
hydroperoxides, 23, 47, 48
hydrophilic sugar moiety, vii, 1, 2
hydrophobic sapogenin, vii, 1, 2
hydrophobicity, ix, 27, 155
hydroxide, 88
hydroxyl, 8, 22, 72, 73, 109, 138, 156, 158, 161, 179
hydroxyl groups, 138, 161
hygiene, 136
hypercholesterolemia, 39, 164
hyperglycemia, 113, 123, 184, 199
hyperinsulinemia, 131
hyperlipidemia, 184, 199
hypersensitivity, 113
hypertension, 26, 123, 126
hypertrophy, 127

I

immersion, 85
immune reaction, 17
immune response, 16, 17, 45, 46, 185, 199
immune system, viii, 16, 28, 51, 52
immunity, 17, 199
immunization, 185
immunodeficiency, 45
immunomodulatory, vii, 1, 3, 91, 98, 110, 140
immunostimulant, 17
immunostimulatory, 16
implants, 136
in vitro, 11, 15, 16, 18, 19, 23, 31, 32, 35, 36, 37, 38, 39, 41, 98, 111, 112, 116, 117, 152, 153, 159, 187, 193, 200
in vivo, 10, 16, 17, 20, 22, 30, 37, 41, 127, 141, 152, 198
induction, ix, 19, 24, 32, 33, 112, 126, 129, 149, 150, 155, 163, 198, 199
industries, vii, 2, 28, 139, 189

industry, viii, 2, 3, 26, 34
infection, 26, 33
inflammation, 17, 19, 20, 26, 32, 33, 40, 186
influenza vaccine, 32
influenza virus, 188
infrared spectroscopy, 3, 137
ingredients, 9, 23, 24, 27, 28, 33, 39, 166
inhibition, 14, 15, 19, 21, 23, 35, 112, 113, 127, 129, 140, 150, 153, 186, 187, 203
inhibitor, 24, 43, 114, 118, 130, 150
injections, 90
injury, 32, 49, 127, 160
insecticide, 167
insects, 11
insertion, 135
insulin, viii, 14, 121, 123, 124, 125, 126, 128, 129, 130, 131, 152
insulin resistance, viii, 121, 123, 124, 129, 131
insulin sensitivity, 123, 128, 152
insulin signaling, 130
integrity, 11, 113, 116, 135
interface, 136
interference, 11, 15, 85
interferons, 17
interleukin-8, 153
intermediaries, 17
intervention, 128
intestine, 14, 15, 18, 19, 23, 24, 113, 116
invertebrates, 38, 47
ion channels, 14
ion transport, 14
ionization, 41, 84, 87, 88, 109, 139, 180
ions, 12, 89
Iran, 168
iron, 9, 10, 118
ischemia, 127
isoflavone, 44
isolation, vii, viii, 3, 11, 40, 51, 52, 81, 83, 84, 98, 114, 119, 191, 202
isomers, 45, 108
Italy, 192

J

Japan, 27, 32, 51, 198

K

K^+, 13, 31
keratinocyte, 201
kidney, 2, 23, 41, 124
Korea, 49, 51, 200

L

LC-MS, 41, 89
LC-MS/MS, 41, 89
LDL, 14
lead, 7, 12, 13, 23
leakage, 46
learning, 23, 50, 127
lecithin, 44
leptin, 125, 129
lesions, 19, 45, 151, 187, 198, 203
leukemia, 126, 146, 149, 152
liberation, 33, 178
life cycle, 20
ligand, 24, 39, 49
light, 83, 87, 123
light scattering, 83, 87
lipid metabolism, 34, 129, 152, 198
lipid peroxidation, 22
lipids, 13, 22, 44, 46, 166
lipodystrophy, 126
lipolysis, 129
liposomes, 49
liquid chromatography, 3, 35, 83, 89, 108, 118, 119, 169
liver, 15, 41, 123, 158, 160, 184
liver cancer, 158
liver disease, 123
localization, 34
longevity, ix, 143
lovastatin, 125
LSD, 83, 87
lumen, 15
lung cancer, 35, 112, 119
lung secretions, 185
Luo, 93, 94, 95, 113, 115, 117, 118, 119, 120, 127, 128, 194, 203
luteinizing hormone, 15, 33
Luxemburg, 33
lymphoma, 146, 149
lyse erythrocytes, vii, 1, 2
lysis, 11, 45, 113, 141

M

machinery, 25
macromolecules, 12
macrophages, 18, 144
magnetic resonance, 34, 84, 90
magnetic resonance spectroscopy, 84
magnitude, 112, 125
malaria, 141
MALDI, 48

mammalian cells, 32
mammals, 24, 183
management, 129
MAPK/ERK, 153
marker genes, 16
marrow, 18
MAS, 116
mass, 84, 87, 88, 89, 90, 108, 139, 169, 179, 180, 195
mass spectrometry, 84, 87, 89, 108, 139, 169, 180
materials, vii, viii, 2, 3, 25, 28, 82, 84, 88, 90, 91, 112, 118, 133, 134, 135, 136, 137, 139, 141, 198
matrix, 83, 108, 150
matrix metalloproteinase, 150
measles, 188
measurements, 10, 46, 109, 180
meat, 10, 47, 135
media, 136
medical, viii, 97, 138, 139
medicine, ix, 3, 15, 26, 29, 38, 52, 84, 98, 143, 167, 187, 189, 194
Mediterranean, 168
melanoma, 146, 149
mellitus, 123, 125, 167
melting, 137
melting temperature, 137
membrane permeability, 12, 13, 17, 85, 111
membranes, 11, 12, 13, 14, 16, 17, 21, 22, 23, 27, 29, 30, 33, 34, 36, 40, 42, 46, 119, 137, 139, 140, 141
memory, 123, 127
memory function, 127
memory loss, 123
metabolic pathways, 123
metabolic syndrome, viii, 121, 123, 127, 130, 131, 132
metabolism, 15, 24, 33, 34, 35, 124, 130, 152
metabolites, 2, 19, 28, 35, 47, 49, 98, 133, 158, 164, 177, 182, 183, 192
metabolized, 19
metalloproteinase, 150
metastasis, 112, 149, 150
metformin, 124, 125, 128
methanol, 3, 9, 81, 83, 84, 85, 149, 152, 165, 198
methyl cellulose, 136
methyl group, 109, 134, 179, 182
methyl groups, 109, 134, 179, 182
methylation, 9, 108
methylcellulose, 141
methylene chloride, 84
Mexico, 167
Mg^{2+}, 13
mice, 15, 33, 34, 35, 37, 39, 40, 42, 112, 119, 123, 124, 125, 128, 130, 131, 151, 184, 186, 199, 203
microemulsion, 90
microorganism, 21, 135
microorganisms, viii, 21, 48, 133, 177
microscopy, 11, 13, 46
Middle East, 186, 187
mineralocorticoid, 24
mitochondria, 19, 147, 149, 150, 153
mitogen, 150, 153
MMP, 147, 148, 150
MMP-2, 147, 150
MMP-9, 147, 148, 150
models, ix, 12, 14, 18, 28, 125, 144, 155, 157, 186
modifications, 7, 10
molecular dynamics, 13, 39
molecular mass, 90, 108
molecular weight, 10, 81, 89, 134, 135
molecules, ix, 16, 23, 25, 39, 48, 81, 109, 134, 135, 136, 143, 155, 164, 177
monoclonal antibody, 84
monolayer, 13, 112
monosaccharide, 22, 134, 166, 178, 179, 180, 181, 182
Moon, 39, 91, 131
morphine, 19, 37
morphology, 111, 136
mortality, 123
MR, 92, 141
mRNA, 124, 125
mucosa, 17, 116, 185
multivariate, 139
mumps, 188
muscles, 33
mutation, 19
mutations, 34
Myanmar, 201
mycelium, 187
myocardial ischemia, 127

N

Na^+, 13, 23, 24, 31
Namibia, 187
nanocomposites, 136, 139
nanofibers, 136, 137, 139
nanofibrous membranes, 137, 139, 140
natural compound, 139
nebulizer, 88
necrosis, 129, 144, 146, 149
negative effects, 15, 25
Nepal, 51
nephropathy, 123
nerve, 24
nervous system, viii, 3, 14, 40, 51, 52

neurobiology, 24
neuroblastoma, 19
neurons, 49
neuropathy, 123
neuropeptides, 125
neutral, 36, 90
New Zealand, 116
NH2, 86, 124, 129
nicotine, 45
Nigeria, 1
Nile, 16, 33
NIR, 90
nitrates, 167
nitric oxide, 19, 37, 47, 126, 151
nitric oxide synthase, 19
nitrogen, 10, 161
NMDA receptors, 49
NMR, 3, 45, 84, 90, 108, 109, 110, 115, 116, 169, 178, 179, 180, 181, 182, 190, 194, 197, 200
non-polar, 81, 122, 164
North America, 51
Norway, 113
nuclear magnetic resonance, 34, 84, 90, 169, 197
Nuclear Magnetic Resonance, 108
nucleus, ix, 5, 16, 161
nutrient, 112, 117
nutrition, 31, 191

O

obesity, 28, 34, 123, 125, 126, 129, 130, 131
obstruction, 168
occlusion, 23, 39
ODS, 83, 107, 108
oedema, 20, 186
oil, 10, 20, 27, 32, 34, 90, 168
oleanane triterpenoids, ix, 155, 156
oligosaccharide, 3, 4, 108, 135, 162
olive oil, 27
one dimension, 109
organ, 49
organic solvents, 166, 168
organism, viii, 133
organs, 23, 29, 168, 193
ornithine, 156
osmotic pressure, 113
osteoclastogenesis, ix, 143, 144, 152
osteoporosis, 144
ovarian cancer, 151
overweight adults, 125
oxidation, 17, 23, 24
oxidative stress, 123, 124, 128, 153
oxygen, 19, 22, 48, 49, 156, 159

P

p53, 146, 147, 149, 150
Pacific, 97
pain, 168
paints, 139
Pakistan, 115, 192
parallel, 20, 83
parasite, 136
partition, 3, 83, 84, 108
pathogenesis, 23, 140
pathogens, 28, 141, 163, 164, 188, 198, 202
pathophysiology, 129
pathways, 7, 17, 24, 123, 124, 125, 129, 130, 149, 151
Pentacyclic triterpenoid saponins, vii, 1
permeability, 12, 14, 17, 20, 49, 85, 111, 112, 116, 117, 183, 185
peroxidation, 22
peroxide, 153
Peru, 167
petroleum, 107
pH, 9, 23, 41, 44, 112, 165
phagocytosis, 111, 119
pharmaceutical, viii, 2, 3, 9, 15, 25, 26, 28, 30, 31, 35, 166, 168, 189
pharmacology, 30, 126, 190, 191
phenotype, 125, 129
phosphate, 87, 118, 125, 144
phosphatidylcholine, 42
phospholipids, 12, 14, 17
phosphorylation, 124, 149, 151
photosynthesis, 191
physical properties, 137, 139, 163, 166
physicochemical properties, 10
phytomedicine, 159
phytosterols, 10, 47
phytotherapy, 192
PI3K, 124
placebo, 123, 128
plant growth, 135
plants, viii, ix, 2, 3, 10, 11, 14, 18, 25, 26, 28, 29, 33, 42, 44, 49, 51, 52, 53, 81, 85, 90, 91, 97, 114, 122, 125, 133, 136, 143, 153, 159, 163, 164, 165, 167, 168, 177, 182, 183, 185, 186, 188, 189, 191, 192, 194, 199, 200, 202, 203
plaque, 13
plasma membrane, 14, 113, 149
plasminogen, 130, 150
plasticizer, 136
platelet aggregation, 23, 39
platelets, 23
poison, 25

polar, 12, 14, 81, 85, 107, 122, 136, 185, 189
polar groups, 12, 136
polarity, ix, 81, 107, 155, 157
pollen, 168
polyamine, 156
polycyclic aromatic hydrocarbon, 141
polycystic ovarian syndrome, 123
polymer, 136
polymerase, 146
polymerization, viii, 133
polymers, 140
polyphenols, 23, 26, 39
polysaccharides, 151
polyunsaturated fat, 163
polyunsaturated fatty acids, 163
population, 19
precipitation, 27, 36, 108
pregnancy, 15
preparation, 31, 35, 46, 83, 85, 136, 137, 139, 140, 192
prevention, 19, 26, 36, 49, 150
priming, 127
principles, 49, 84, 128, 184, 185, 191, 203
progesterone, 16, 25, 40
pro-inflammatory, 25, 123
proliferation, viii, 15, 16, 17, 41, 42, 97, 111, 112, 126, 129, 137, 153, 157
propagation, 116
prostate cancer, 39
prostate carcinoma, 18
protease inhibitors, 195
protection, 139, 183
protein hydrolysates, 199
protein kinase C, 24
protein kinases, 19
protein synthesis, 25, 48
proteins, 10, 12, 14, 16, 19, 22, 23, 31, 40, 47, 49, 111, 123, 140, 144, 185, 199
protons, 109, 180, 182
psychostimulants, 24
purification, viii, 3, 11, 41, 43, 81, 83, 84, 97, 98, 107, 108, 178, 183, 189
purity, 3, 83, 84, 108

Q

quality control, 81, 84, 88, 91
quantification, 163
quaternary ammonium, 140

R

radicals, 22, 23
Raman spectroscopy, 90
raw materials, vii, 2, 3, 25, 28, 84, 88, 91
reactions, 7, 17, 23, 29, 109
reactive oxygen, 19, 48
reactivity, 136
reagents, 3
receptors, 14, 16, 18, 24, 32, 49
reconditioning, 167
recovery, 35, 41, 84, 108
red blood cells, 2, 42
refractive index, 87
regenerated cellulose, 137, 138, 140
regeneration, 81
regions of the world, 97
reinforcement, 136
remediation, 28
replication, 22, 200
reproduction, 15
reproductive organs, 29
residues, 7, 9, 12, 17, 109, 135, 165, 166, 178, 179, 180, 182, 183
resins, 81
resistance, viii, 10, 41, 121, 123, 124, 129, 131, 136, 140
resolution, 87, 89, 189
response, 16, 17, 24, 45, 46, 88, 151, 177
retinopathy, 123
rheumatoid arthritis, 144, 167, 193
rhizome, 88
ribose, 146
ribosome, 111, 119
rings, 110
risk, viii, 40, 113, 121, 123, 129, 140, 194
risk factors, viii, 121, 123, 129
risks, viii, 121, 123
room temperature, 9, 85
root, 10, 38, 48, 51, 83, 88, 119, 125, 128, 160, 169, 170, 171, 176, 183, 185, 195, 197, 199, 202
roots, 14, 29, 39, 47, 49, 53, 82, 87, 98, 107, 108, 110, 111, 112, 113, 114, 115, 116, 117, 118, 119, 120, 122, 128, 165, 183, 184, 185, 186, 187, 188, 191, 194, 195, 197, 199, 200, 201, 202

S

salt concentration, 9
salts, 112, 116
Saudi Arabia, 168, 194, 200
scanning calorimetry, 137
scanning electron microscopy, 137
scattering, 83, 87
schistosomiasis, 20, 189

secretion, 114, 120, 124, 129, 130, 144, 147, 150, 153
seed, 10, 19, 27, 28, 43, 45, 49, 88, 135, 159, 160, 171, 172, 173, 174, 187, 188, 193, 198, 199, 200
selectivity, 88, 188
senescence, 149, 150, 153
sensitivity, 10, 85, 88, 89, 90, 123, 128, 151, 152
sensitization, 113
serotonin, 19
serum, 10, 14, 15, 28, 36, 39, 46, 85, 90, 125, 183, 184, 185
serum albumin, 10, 36
sexual behavior, 30
sheep, 17
shoot, 116, 118
shrubs, 167, 168
Siberia, 51
side chain, 3, 4, 7, 11, 12, 165, 177, 183
signal transduction, 153
signaling pathway, 124, 129, 130
signalling, 19, 24
signals, 17, 109, 110, 125, 179, 182, 197
silica, 3, 82, 83, 108, 144, 169
simulations, 13, 39, 140
Singapore, 121, 129, 143, 155
skeleton, vii, 1, 4, 7, 8, 37, 53, 107, 110, 163, 177, 179
skin, 18, 20, 28, 31, 34, 49, 136, 167, 168, 185, 187, 199
skin diseases, 167
small intestine, 14, 15, 113, 116, 187
sodium, 49
solid phase, 87, 168
solubility, 9, 10, 83, 134, 137, 165, 200
solution, 41, 42, 82, 137, 141, 166
solvents, 9, 85, 87, 107, 137
sorption, 141
South Africa, 167, 187, 203
South America, 97, 167, 168
soy bean, ix, 155, 157, 158
soybeans, 2, 9, 25, 28, 37
species, vii, viii, 2, 19, 20, 22, 26, 48, 51, 52, 53, 83, 84, 85, 88, 89, 90, 91, 97, 98, 107, 112, 114, 116, 120, 121, 122, 125, 135, 136, 153, 159, 162, 163, 165, 167, 168, 169, 177, 182, 184, 186, 187, 188, 189, 192, 193, 194
spectroscopy, 3, 84, 90, 109, 137, 179, 190, 197, 200
sperm, 15, 31, 114
spin, 29, 182, 197
spore, 138
squamous cell, 111, 115
squamous cell carcinoma, 111, 115
Sri Lanka, 42
stability, 10, 36, 136
starch, 139
state, 23, 85, 123, 125, 186
states, ix, 143
statistics, 52
steroids, 5, 7, 24, 119, 167, 177
sterols, 10, 12, 13, 16, 22, 34, 36, 45, 107, 118, 134, 135, 193
stimulation, 14, 18, 111, 119
stomach, 14
storage, 3, 9, 10, 135, 165
stress, 17, 19, 23, 123, 124, 128, 153
striatum, 45
stroke, 123
structural changes, 42
structure, vii, viii, ix, 1, 3, 4, 9, 10, 11, 12, 17, 18, 19, 20, 22, 23, 24, 29, 30, 33, 34, 35, 40, 45, 52, 53, 81, 87, 88, 97, 98, 106, 107, 108, 109, 110, 113, 114, 115, 117, 118, 121, 122, 126, 134, 135, 138, 139, 145, 150, 151, 155, 156, 157, 159, 166, 169, 177, 178, 179, 183, 186, 189, 196, 197, 198, 201, 203
substrate, 124, 136
sucrose, 10
sugar beet, 114, 163, 195
sulfate, 99, 109, 110, 113
sulfuric acid, 3
Sun, 3, 47, 92, 118, 127, 128, 134, 141, 198
supplementation, 123, 128, 184
suppression, 14, 15, 19, 124, 144, 149, 153
surface properties, 10, 31
surfactant, 44, 133, 136, 139, 141
surfactants, 27, 28, 90, 133, 134, 136, 139, 140, 141
sweeteners, vii, 2, 3, 34
symptoms, 26
syndrome, viii, 121, 123, 127, 130, 131, 132
synergistic effect, 32, 124
synthesis, 15, 25, 29, 33, 48, 136, 141, 147, 150, 158

T

T cell, 111, 144, 185
tannins, 195
target, 12, 23, 81, 82, 83, 84, 124, 125, 144, 156
target organs, 23
taxa, 87
techniques, 3, 11, 41, 84, 85, 87, 90, 108, 109, 110, 115, 169, 178
technologies, 25, 81
technology, 82, 136
temperature, 9, 41, 44, 85, 88, 137, 165
tension, 10
terminals, 24

testing, 93, 114, 157, 158, 188
testosterone, 16
tetrahydrofuran, 89
textiles, 139, 140
TGF, 124
Thailand, 161
therapeutic agents, 183, 189
therapeutic use, 33
therapeutics, 144
therapy, 111, 119, 128
thermal stability, 136
Tibet, 167
tissue, 25, 36, 116, 125, 130, 136, 141, 156
tissue engineering, 136, 141
TNF-alpha (TNF-α), 125, 129, 144
tofu, 23
tonic, 135
toxic effect, 11, 20, 118, 136
toxicity, 11, 17, 18, 22, 26, 44, 111, 119, 136, 183
toxicology, 26
toxin, 50, 111, 115, 185
TPA, 20
trace elements, 163
traditions, ix, 161
transcription, 16, 17, 19, 24, 125, 144, 150
transcription factors, 25, 150
transduction, 153
transformations, 9
transforming growth factor, 140
translocation, 24
transmission, 16
transport, 13, 14, 24, 111, 112, 117, 124, 129
treatment, 11, 22, 26, 31, 33, 39, 42, 82, 109, 119, 124, 128, 130, 137, 149, 150, 156, 158, 165, 167, 168, 187
trifluoroacetic acid, 108
triglycerides, 125
trypsin, 10
tuberculosis, 188, 203
tumor, 35, 36, 38, 41, 48, 111, 112, 116, 119, 129, 144, 147, 149, 150, 151, 153, 190
tumor cells, 36, 48, 111, 116, 147, 149, 150, 190
tumor growth, 35
tumor metastasis, 150
tumor necrosis factor, 129, 144
tumors, 150
type 2 diabetes, 123, 128, 131
tyrosine, 23, 24

U

ulcer, 26
ultrasound, 85
United Kingdom (UK), 48, 117, 167, 168, 194
urinary tract, 187
urine, 35, 85
urokinase, 150
USA, 34
UV, 83, 87, 88

V

vaccine, 26, 29, 37, 39, 45
valve, 83
variations, 177
varieties, 193
vegetable oil, 168
vegetables, 27, 135, 163, 167, 168
versatility, 87
vessels, 23
virus replication, 22
viruses, 22, 183
viscosity, 9
vitamin D, 114
vitamin E, 46, 192
vitamins, 36, 163

W

water, 3, 9, 10, 21, 24, 27, 32, 82, 83, 84, 85, 87, 90, 107, 113, 122, 136, 137, 139, 141, 151, 163, 165, 166, 186, 200
water hydration, 10
water sorption, 141
weakness, ix, 143
weight gain, 125
western blot, 126
wetting, 9, 135
wool, 140, 168
World Health Organization (WHO), 27, 123, 125, 127
wound healing, 134, 140

Y

yeast, 22, 27, 140
yield, 26, 85

Z

zinc, 10, 118